Handbook of Neuroendovascular Surgery

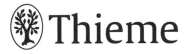

Handbook of Neuroendovascular Surgery

Eric M. Deshaies, MD
Director
SUNY Upstate Neurovascular Center
Assistant Professor of Neurosurgery
Department of Neurosurgery
SUNY Upstate Medical University
Syracuse, New York

Christopher S. Eddleman, MD, PhD
Neurosurgeon
Department of Neurological Surgery
and Radiology
University of Texas Southwestern
Medical Center
Dallas, Texas

Alan S. Boulos, MD, FACS
Herman and Sunny Stall Chair of
Neuroendovascular Surgery
Chairman
Department of Neurosurgery
Co-Director
The Neurosciences Institute
Albany Medical College
Albany, New York

Thieme
New York · Stuttgart

Thieme Medical Publishers, Inc.
333 Seventh Ave.
New York, NY 10001

Executive Editor: Kay Conerly
Editorial Assistants: Tess Timoshin and Judith Tomat
Editorial Director, Clinical Reference: Michael Wachinger
Production Editor: Kenneth L. Chumbley
International Production Director: Andreas Schabert
Senior Vice President, International Marketing and Sales: Cornelia Schulze
Vice President, Finance and Accounts: Sarah Vanderbilt
President: Brian D. Scanlan
Compositor: Prairie Papers Inc.
Printer: Sheridan Books, Inc.

Library of Congress Cataloging-in-Publication Data: Available from the publisher upon request.

Important note: Medical knowledge is ever-changing. As new research and clinical experience broaden our knowledge, changes in treatment and drug therapy may be required. The authors and editors of the material herein have consulted sources believed to be reliable in their efforts to provide information that is complete and in accord with the standards accepted at the time of publication. However, in view of the possibility of human error by the authors, editors, or publisher of the work herein or changes in medical knowledge, neither the authors, editors, nor publisher, nor any other party who has been involved in the preparation of this work, warrants that the information contained herein is in every respect accurate or complete, and they are not responsible for any errors or omissions or for the results obtained from use of such information. Readers are encouraged to confirm the information contained herein with other sources. For example, readers are advised to check the product information sheet included in the package of each drug they plan to administer to be certain that the information contained in this publication is accurate and that changes have not been made in the recommended dose or in the contraindications for administration. This recommendation is of particular importance in connection with new or infrequently used drugs.

Some of the product names, patents, and registered designs referred to in this book are in fact registered trademarks or proprietary names even though specific reference to this fact is not always made in the text. Therefore, the appearance of a name without designation as proprietary is not to be construed as a representation by the publisher that it is in the public domain.

Printed in the United States of America

5 4 3 2 1

ISBN 978-1-60406-300-4

Contents

III Treatment of Specific Disease Entities

Appendix A

Appendix B

Foreword

The evolution of vascular neurosurgery has continued and now provides a new set of tools to treat hemorrhagic and ischemic disease. Clearly, this evolution is becoming mainstream in neurosurgical training and adds to the body of knowledge that currently exists within traditional neurosurgical education. This text is an excellent reference for neurosurgical residents and fellows and, though not comprehensive, is certainly ideal for quick reference and for triggering the evaluation of further information. The topics covered in this text span the field of neuroendovascular surgery and are an absolute must for medical students, residents, and fellows who are caring for these patients.

This work is divided into sections based on introductory chapters that are appropriate in terms of discussing craniovascular anatomy of the brain and spinal cord, as well as the coagulation cascade and clotting pathways essential to understanding the various pharmacologic agents used in anticoagulation during these procedures. It is also appropriate in the introductory chapters that endovascular techniques are discussed in relation to anesthesia and medication interactions. The sections on equipment and techniques are outstanding in that they discuss radiation physics and safety, something not traditionally covered in neurosurgical circles. The discussion of vascular access and the basic discussion of endovascular tools are comprehensive for a work of this magnitude. The section on the treatment of specific disease entities is quite extensive for a work which is labeled as a handbook. The extensive nature of the disease is covered quite thoroughly and the references are appropriate for other sources.

Finally, the appendices are extremely useful and user friendly, including conversion charts, equipment and catheter sizes, shapes, vascular anatomy, and certain medications specific to endovascular interventions, as well as the neurologic scales used to assess the patients pre and posttreatment. Appendix B is also extremely useful, with pictures demonstrating vascular access, basic catheterization, coil embolization, stent placement, liquid and particle embolization, and balloon angioplasty.

Handbook of Neuroendovascular Surgery is a work that will be extremely useful to residents, medical students, and fellows who are actively participating on a neuroendovascular service. I congratulate the authors on the first extensive handbook of this type.

Robert H. Rosenwasser, MD, FACS, FAHA
The Jewell L. Osterholm, MD, Professor and Chairman
Department of Neurological Surgery
Jefferson Medical College
Thomas Jefferson University
Philadelphia, Pennsylvania

Preface

Neuroendovascular surgery is one of the most rapidly evolving disciplines in medicine. Exceedingly dependent upon advancements in material science, computer engineering, and software development, the breadth of neurovascular disease treatable by endovascular techniques appears nearly infinite. Many vascular neurosurgical diseases, treated in the past with high risk in the operating theatre, can now be safely treated in the angiography suite. This rapidly expanding specialty parallels the increasing number of neuroendovascular fellowship programs and neurosurgery, neurology, and radiology residency programs training physicians in this field.

There are many excellent textbooks dedicated to exploring the details, nuances, and idiosyncracies of neuroendovascular surgery, and their authors are applauded for their tremendous work and dedication in creating these very important works. However, these texts were not intended as, and are impractical for, daily case-by-case referencing for those being introduced to the specialty or in need of quick facts and clinical pearls while preparing for a case. Each editor of this handbook, trained in both cerebrovascular neurosurgery and neuroendovascular surgery, desperately searched for a handbook during fellowship training that would serve as a guide and quick-reference book, but found none. Out of necessity came our concept of the *Handbook of Neuroendovascular Surgery*. This handbook was written with the intent that it could be carried in labcoat pockets and easily used to review important concepts and technical information prior to a procedure. This handbook was developed and written with the newly graduated attending physician, fellow, resident, medical student, nurse, nurse practitioner, and physician assistant in mind.

In order to deliver our concept to the reader, we intentionally selected chapter authors who had recently graduated within the past five years to contribute to this handbook. Fellows and residents with neuroendovascular experience were also encouraged to coauthor many of these chapters to maintain the tenor of the handbook, which is to deliver necessary information succinctly. For us, it was imperative that the contributors have backgrounds in neurosurgery, radiology, and neurology in order to successfully impart the book with a broad range of training, viewpoints, and background.

Handbook of Neuroendovascular Surgery was organized to parallel the learning process of the reader. It was arranged to flow from the basic scientific concepts of the specialty (e.g., vascular anatomy), progress to equipment and technical aspects needed to perform the procedures, and finally describe the treatment of specific neurovascular diseases. This was accomplished by dividing the handbook into three sections: Introduction, Equipment and Techniques, and Treatment of Specific Disease Entities.

We would like to highlight two other unique features of this book that we believe will be particularly helpful to the reader when preparing for a procedure: Periprocedural Patient Care and Equipment and Technique. These chapters make this handbook particularly useful when preparing for procedures, by summarizing critical information for the reader. The reader is urged to be mindful that these chapters are meant to provide direction on how to proceed with patient care and treatment options when many individual management options and preferences may exist.

Finally, a particularly strong point of this book is the use of numerous tables and graphics throughout the text that summarize large amounts of information that the chapter authors believe are important for quick referencing. Routinely used information (e.g., anatomy, medications, and equipment) and teaching illustrations (e.g., coiling and stent procedures) has been placed in an appendices for quick and easy referencing and can also be used for patient education. Purchasers of this book will also have online access to these figures and illustrations from Thieme Medical Publishers, which can be downloaded to personal computer devices. We find this feature especially helpful as a visual teaching guide for patients when explaining procedures and obtaining their informed consent.

Handbook of Neuroendovascular Surgery is precisely what each editor was searching for during neuroendovascular training, but was unable to find. We are very excited to share this book with the neuroendovascular community! It is our sincere hope and expectation that it will become an invaluable tool for every beginner neuroendovascular surgeon's educational armamentarium and find its way to every trainee's labcoat pocket.

Contributors

Celso Agner, MD, MS, MSc
Chief of Neuroendovascular Surgery
Staff Neurologist
Michigan Neurology Associates
Mount Clemens Regional Medical
    Center
Mount Clemens, Michigan

Mohammad Ali Aziz-Sultan, MD
Associate Professor and Chief of
    Endovascular
Department of Neurological Surgery
Miller School of Medicine
University of Miami
Miami, Florida

Alan S. Boulos, MD, FACS
Herman and Sunny Stall Chair of
    Neuroendovascular Surgery
Chairman
Department of Neurosurgery
Co-Director
The Neurosciences Institute
Albany Medical College
Albany, New York

Blair Calancie, PhD
Professor
Department of Neurosurgery
SUNY Upstate Medical University
Syracuse, New York

M. Imran Chaudry, MD
Assistant Professor
Department of Radiology
Medical University of South Carolina
Charleston, South Carolina

Jesse J. Corry, MD
Senior Staff, Neurocritical Care
Departments of Neurology and
    Neurosurgery
Henry Ford Hospital
Assistant Professor of Neurology
Wayne State University
Detroit, Michigan

John C. Dalfino, MD
Assistant Professor
Department of Neurosurgery
Albany Medical Center
Albany, New York

Eric M. Deshaies, MD
Director
SUNY Upstate Neurovascular Center
Assistant Professor of Neurosurgery
Department of Neurosurgery
SUNY Upstate Medical University
Syracuse, New York

Christopher S. Eddleman, MD, PhD
Neurosurgeon
Department of Neurological Surgery
    and Radiology
University of Texas Southwestern
    Medical Center
Dallas, Texas

Randall C. Edgell, MD
Director of Interventional Neurology
Saint Louis University Hospital
Assistant Professor
Saint Louis University
St. Louis, Missouri

Mohamed Samy Elhammady, MD
Instructor
Department of Neurological Surgery
Miller School of Medicine
University of Miami
Miami, Florida

Jason A. Felton, MD
Department of Neurosurgery
Saint Louis University
St. Louis, Missouri

Ravi H. Gandhi, MD
Chief Resident
Division of Neurosurgery
Albany Medical Center
Albany, New York

Walter Jacobsen, DO
Department of Neurosurgery
Albany Medical Center
Albany, New York

Abu Yahia Lodi, MD
Professor
Department of Neurology
SUNY Upstate Medical University
Syracuse, New York

Roham Moftakhar, MD
Staff Neurosurgeon
Department of Neurosurgery
Rebound Neurosurgery
Southwest Washington Medical Center
Vancouver, Washington

David Padalino, MD
Resident
Department of Neurosurgery
SUNY Upstate Medical University
Syracuse, New York

Michael Park, MD
Resident
Department of Neurological Surgery
    and Brain Repair
University of South Florida
Tampa, Florida

Amit Singla, MD
Resident
Department of Neurosurgery
SUNY Upstate Medical University
Syracuse, New York

Fotis G. Souslian, MD
Department of Neurosurgery
University of Minnesota
Minneapolis, Minnesota

Justin Sweeney, MD
Cerebrovascular and Skull Base Fellow
Department of Neurosurgery
University of South Florida
Tampa, Florida

Ramachandra P. Tummala, MD
Assistant Professor
Department of Neurosurgery
University of Minnesota
Minneapolis, Minnesota

Aquilla S. Turk, DO
Director
Neurointerventional Surgery
Medical University of South Carolina
Charleston, South Carolina

Raymond D. Turner IV, MD
Assistant Professor of Neurosciences
Director
Cerebrovascular Neurosurgery
Co-Director
Comprehensive Stroke and
    Cerebrovascular Service Line
Department of Neurosciences
Medical University of South Carolina
Charleston, South Carolina

Madhu B. Vijayappa, MD
Interventional Neurologist
Texas Stroke Institute
Dallas, Texas

**Stacey Quintero Wolfe, MD, LCDR,
    MC, United States Navy**
Chief of Cerebrovascular Surgery
Chairman
Department of Neurosurgery
Tripler Army Medical Center
Honolulu, Hawaii

Dileep R. Yavagal, MD
Assistant Professor of Clinical
    Neurology and Neurosurgery
Faculty
Interdisciplinary Stem Cell Institute
Miller School of Medicine
Jackson Memorial Hospital
University of Miami
Miami, Florida

Junichi Yamamoto, MD, PhD
Surgeon
Albany Medical Center Neurosurgery
    Group
Albany, New York

I
Introduction

1

Cranial Vascular Anatomy

Walter Jacobsen, Eric M. Deshaies, and Jesse J. Corry

Neuroendovascular techniques not only have become an accepted modality for the treatment of neurovascular disease but also continue to evolve at an accelerated pace with progressive advancements in technology and material science. However, neuroendovascular therapies could never have developed without knowledge of the fundamentals, namely neurovascular anatomy. Thus it is appropriate that the first two chapters of this book be designed to familiarize you with basic concepts of vascular embryology and ultimately cranial and spinal neurovascular anatomy.

As with most specialties, jargon and vernacular are important to establish at the beginning so that the reader understands the concepts. Neurovascular anatomy is no different, and the language of description must first be defined so the reader may develop an internal understanding of the text that follows.

Although the neurovascular system has specific components that make it unique, it has the same fundamental building blocks as the other vascular systems in the body. More specifically, the neurovascular network is made up of arteries, capillaries, and veins, all with various sizes and functions. Each vessel has both functional and physical properties that make it unique.

The vascular tree is a continuous network made up of a multitude of varying-sized vessels (**Table 1.1**) that are continuous with one another. Arteries characteristically share the features of a well-defined lumen maintained by a muscular vessel wall, while veins are more commonly thin-walled but with large amounts of elastin fibers without large amounts of smooth muscle cells.[1] Large arteries have disproportionately thin walls for the size of their lumen, great elasticity, a thick tunica media (**Table 1.2**), and an adventitia with a high concentration of collagen and elastin. Medium-sized arteries, which constitute the majority of the named arteries of the body, have a greater proportion of smooth muscle fibers to elastic fibers in the tunica media, a thinner tunica intima than large arteries, and a prominent internal elastic membrane with a basement membrane. The adventitia of medium-sized arteries is relatively thick, with a high concentration of collagen fibers. Arterioles, which are much smaller in diameter, have a thin tunica media composed of an incomplete layer of smooth muscle. The adventitia is also thinner than that of large arteries, and the external elastic membrane is poorly defined or even absent. Capillaries, on the other hand, have very thin walls composed of an endothelium and delicate basement membrane and are classified as either fenestrated or non-fenestrated (**Table 1.3**). Blood flow through capillaries is slow, which allows diffusion to occur bi-directionally with the surrounding interstitial fluid

After an exchange of nutrients and wastes through the capillary walls, the blood flow continues through the veins (**Table 1.1**). The main function of the veins is to receive blood from tissues via the capillary system and return it to the lungs, where the blood can once again become oxygenated, and to the other filtration

Table 1.1   The Neurovasculature Is Classified According to Size

Vessel	Size	Function
Large or elastic arteries	0.4 cm – 2.5 cm	Move volumes of blood throughout the body.
Medium or muscular arteries	40 mm – 0.5 mm	Distribute blood to body and organs.
Small arteries or arterioles	0.008 mm – 0.5 mm	Deliver blood at the tissue level.
Capillaries	<0.008 mm	Exchange between blood and interstitial fluid.
Venules	~0.030 mm, variable	Smallest veins, thin-walled with no tunica media. Collect blood from the capillary beds.
Medium-sized veins	0.030 mm – 5 mm	Thin tunica media with few smooth muscle fibers. One-way valves allowing blood to travel only in one direction, toward the heart. Peripheral skeletal muscle supplies the force to squeeze peripheral veins and push blood toward the heart. External elastic layer is composed of elastic and collagen fibers.
Large veins	>5 mm	Thick layer of elastic and collagenous fibers forming the tunica externa. Thin tunica media; intrathoracic pressure delivers blood to the heart.

Table 1.2   Tunica Media

Composition	Function
Few smooth muscle fibers High density of elastic tissue	Imparts resilience to large arteries to tolerate pressure changes with cardiac contraction.

Table 1.3   Capillaries

Fenestrated	Allow select sized molecules to diffuse through the fenestrations.
Non-fenestrated	Allow solutes to pass through the vessel wall by passive and active diffusion.

systems in the body, namely the liver. A description of the exchange processes is beyond the scope of this text. Veins are generally smaller in outer diameter than the corresponding arteries but generally have larger inner diameters and can accommodate a much larger volume of blood.

The first venous structures after the capillaries are the venules, which are the smallest of the venous structures. The venules are thin walled, with no tunica media. Medium-sized veins continue, which also have a thin tunica media; however, small amounts of smooth muscle cells are present in these veins. They also have an external elastic layer that is composed of elastic and collagen fibers. Unique to veins are one-way valves, which allow blood to travel only in one direction, toward the heart. Peripheral skeletal muscle supplies the force that squeezes peripheral veins and pushes blood toward the heart. Once the force is released, the valves, which have a configuration like a trapdoor, prevent the backflow of blood. The largest veins, which also have a thin tunica media, have a thick outer layer of elastic and collagen fibers called the tunica externa. This layer continuously provides some amount of recoil in the venous system. Over time these fibers can be broken down, leading to stasis and overwhelming of the upstream venous system. Like the pressure from peripheral muscles, the intrathoracic pressure provides the force to send blood to the heart continuously.

Embryology: Aortic Arch and Head and Neck Vasculature

The development of the adult vasculature requires an infinite number of steps in both the embryonic and postnatal phases.[2,3] Variants in anatomical structure are common and typically a result of either the failure of regression of some embryonic components or overly aggressive formation of others. Rarely will the knowledge of the intimate details of embryologic development of the vasculature be necessary, so the descriptions below serve only to give one the basics of how these processes are initiated and the basic results. Any further detail should be gleaned from texts written specifically on this topic.

Vasculogenesis begins day 18 post conception in the splanchnic mesoderm of the embryonic disc, forming small capillaries. Small capillaries then coalesce into larger cords running throughout the fetus. During the fourth week of gestation, the great vessels begin to develop. The aorta develops as a series of aortic arches, as in the jawless fish that gave rise to land-based higher mammals (**Fig. 1.1**). Arches develop as a series of evolutions and regressions that result in the development of the great vessels and the vessels to the head and neck. There are five pairs of pharyngeal arches: 1, 2, 3, 4, and 6; the fifth arch either never develops or regresses quickly, so it does not contribute to the development of the vascular tree (**Fig. 1.2A**). These pairs of aortic arches fuse below as a single dorsal vessel.

Aortic Arch and Extracranial Circulation

The development of the aortic arch (**Table 1.4**) in the embryonic stages can be divided into two distinct stages, the branchial and the postbranchial.[3,4] The branchial stage, which is often seen to cease in lower vertebrates, involves a series of overlapping steps in which the six pairs of aortic arches, with the pharyngeal arches, begin to form the more-defined cephalic vessels (**Fig. 1.2B**). Anomalies at this stage

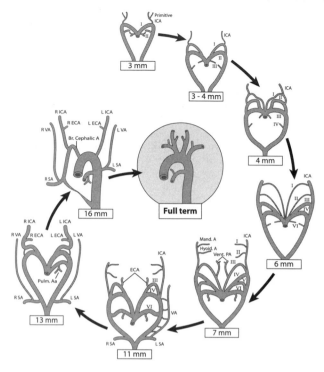

Fig. 1.1 Progressive development and organization of the aorta and its branches is depicted here, beginning with the 3 mm fetal stage to full term.

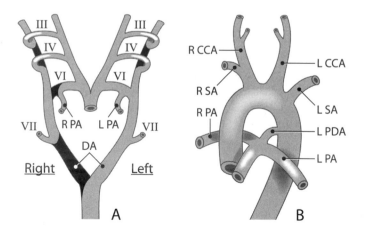

Fig. 1.2 Progressive development of the cephalic arteries (carotid, subclavian, and pulmonary arteries) from the aortic and pharyngeal arches (III to VII) is illustrated here from fetal to final adult form.

Table 1.4   Normal Development of the Aortic Arch and Great Vessels

Embryonic origin	Primitive artery	Final artery
Bulbus cordis	Truncus arteriosus	
Aortic sac	Ventral aorta	
Dorsal aortae	Carotid arteries (distal segments)	
Cervical plexuses	Cervical intersegmental arteries	
Dorsal plexuses	Longitudinal neural arteries	
Aortic arches		
I	Maxillary arteries	Portions of distal ECA (maxillofacial division, mandibular and infraorbital branches).
II	Stapedial arteries	Stapedial arteries.
III	Carotid arteries (proximal)	CCA: proximal ICA and ECA.
IV	Right and left primitive aortic arches	Right: brachiocephalic and proximal SCA. Left: aortic arch, proximal descending aorta, left subclavian artery.
VI	Ductus arteriosus	Left and right pulmonary arteries.*

*New research suggests the pulmonary arteries may develop separately in the splanchnic mesoderm and connect to the sixth aortic arch rather than originating from the arch itself.
Abbreviations: CCA, common carotid artery; ECA, external carotid artery; ICA, internal carotid artery; SCA, superior cerebral artery.

include the failure of regression of the primitive maxillary or hypoglossal arteries. The postbranchial stage involves the evolution of the adult arterial pattern (**Table 1.5**) from branchial remnants, which persist after successive interruption by the pharyngeal structures and subsequent forming and regressing of the remaining aortic arches. The most common anomaly during these stages is a failure of the regression of the primitive trigeminal artery. For a more detailed timeline of the steps of embryonic arterial vasculature development, please refer to **Table 1.6**.

Variations and Anomalies

As many in neuroendovascular surgery will attest, there is a great variety in the anatomical construction of the aortic arch, and overlooking this fact can provide numerous challenges during catheterization. As such, some variants of the aortic arch need to be known by the neuroendovascular surgeon (**Table 1.7**). The most common aortic arch configurations are the following: (1) the "bovine" arch, where there are essential two emanating trunks from the superior surface of the arch, one consisting of a common origin of the left common carotid artery and the brachiocephalic trunk and the other being the left subclavian artery; (2) the origin of the left vertebral artery directly from the aortic arch; and (3) the origin of the right subclavian artery off the ascending aorta (**Fig. 1.3**).[5]

Table 1.5 Aorta

Segments	Description	Branches
Ascending	Begins at the semilunar valve of the left ventricle and extends to the transverse curve.	Right and left coronary arteries originate from left anterior and posterior sinuses just above the aortic valve.
Transverse	Extends from the transverse curve to the left subclavian artery.	Brachiocephalic trunk Left CCA Left SCA
Isthmus	Fetal aorta narrows distal to L SCA and continues to the descending aorta.	
Descending	Starts left of the fourth thoracic vertebra and descends toward diaphragm.	

Abbreviations: CCA, common carotid artery; SCA, superior cerebral artery.

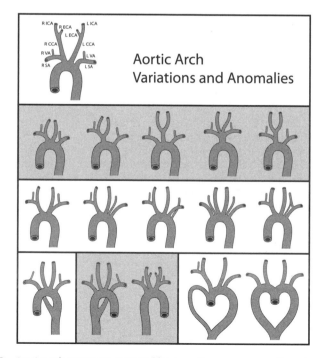

Fig. 1.3 Aortic arch variations. Depicted here are the numerous aortic arch variations and anomalies. CCA, common carotid artery; SA, subclavian artery; ICA, internal carotid artery; VA, vertebral artery.

Table 1.6   Timeline of Arterial Development

Time	Event
Day 22	Maxillomandibular arches (first pharyngeal arch) develop.
Day 26	Second aortic arch appears as first pair regresses.
Day 28	Third and fourth arches appear.
Day 29	Sixth arch appears. Second arch begins to regress. Stapedial artery develops from proximal end of second arch and contributes to the ECA.
Days 21–28 Day 35	Primitive carotid arteries deliver intracranial blood flow. They arise from the ventral aorta and third arch. Distally, the primitive carotid artery distal segment divides into cranial (future ACA) and caudal (future PCOM) segments. Dorsal segments connecting the third and fourth aortic arches regress, so that the entire blood supply of the third arch is delivered to the head.
Week 5	Third, fourth, and sixth arches are well developed, and the ICA is supplied entirely by the ventral aorta and third arch. The vascular plexuses dorsal to the third and fourth arches fuse to become the basilar artery. Transient anastomoses between the ICA and CCA and plexiform longitudinal neural arteries are trigeminal, otic, hypoglossal, and proatlantal arteries. ECA origin is unclear, but likely related to the first and second arch remnant and the ventral end of the third arch.
Week 6	Regression of longitudinal neural-ICA anastomoses. The seven cervical intersegmental arteries coalesce to form the VA. The first six proximal connections and dorsal aorta regress. The seventh segment becomes the subclavian artery. The pulmonary artery initially sprouts from the fourth arch and reconnects to the sixth arch.
Week 7	The left fourth aortic arch and dorsal aorta result in the definitive aortic arch and cranial segments of the descending aorta. The brachiocephalic artery is a remnant of the third and fourth arches. BA finishes coalescing and anastomoses inferiorly with the VA.
Week 8	Near-final configuration of aortic arch and great vessels. Ductus arteriosus remains patent, providing communication between the pulmonary trunks to the proximal descending aorta.

Abbreviations: ACA, anterior cerebral artery; ECA, external carotid artery; ICA, internal carotid artery; PCOM, posterior communicating artery; VA, vertebral artery.

Table 1.7 Aortic Anomalies

Shared brachiocephalic trunk/ Left CCA origin	Most common: the "bovine" configuration seen in an estimated 27% of patients. For 7% of patients, the left CCA originates from the proximal brachiocephalic trunk.
L SCA/CCA from a common origin and form a left brachioce-phalic trunk	Found on 1% to 2% of patients who have angiograms.
Right aortic arch	Aberrant left SCA producing mirror image branch-ing. Associated with congenital cyanotic heart disease.
Double aortic arch	Secondary to incomplete regression of paired fetal structures.
Aortic spindle	A narrow segment from the left SCA and descend-ing aorta persists into adulthood. This junction between the isthmus and spindle is marked by an inferior indentation.
Ductus diverticulum	Seen in 9% of adults. Incomplete closure of the ductus arteriosus. Identified as a bulge at the anteromedial aspect of aortic isthmus.

Abbreviations: CCA, common carotid artery; SCA, superior cerebral artery.

Intracranial Circulation

The cerebral vasculature is formed when angioblasts coalesce in areas around the cranium and form plexuses. These plexuses ultimately connect with one another, forming a single plexus covering the entire neural tube. By a series of resorptions of some components of the plexus and expansions of other components, the adult arterial configuration is developed. The internal carotid artery ascends from the aortic arches in the neck and joins the cerebral plexus. The carotid also develops branches of its own, the most important of which include the primitive trigeminal artery to supply the hindbrain through the longitudinal artery, as well as a bud that will become the ophthalmic artery in the adult. By day 30, a second communi-cation between the internal carotid artery (ICA) and the rostral longitudinal artery develops that will later become the posterior communicating artery (PCOM). By day 33 the longitudinal arteries have joined, forming the basilar artery, and the vertebral arteries have formed by the anastomoses of the cervical segmental arter-ies. By day 35 the anterior cerebral arteries, middle cerebral arteries, and internal carotid artery branches are forming. By day 44 the intracranial arteries are in the final position, and a complete circle of Willis has formed. By 70 days the arterial system is in a mature form, with arterial size and caliber still fluctuating, but with little change in organization.[3]

Circle of Willis Development

The circle of Willis develops to provide a collateral circuit to connect the anterior and posterior, and the right and left intracranial circulations (**Table 1.8**). When a complete circle develops (described later), a single patent carotid artery or vertebral artery can maintain the brain's blood supply.

Venous Development

The development of the venous system is the more complex embryological tale and has been noted throughout history to involve significantly more numerous and complex stages.[2,5] The development of the venous system lags behind arterial evolution in all embryonic stages and continues into the postnatal period. Angiographic evidence of embryonic venous structures can be seen in those who are imaged in the infant stage. As such, vascular malformations present at birth may be the result of failed regression of embryonic structures, and the venous pattern observed might not be one the physician recognizes.

The precursors of the venous system begin to take form in the third and fourth weeks. The intracranial venous system begins with a capillary plexus as well as an anterior, middle, and posterior dural plexus draining the neural tube into a lateral sinus known as the head sinus. This sinus drains into the anterior cardinal vein, a member of the primitive venous system. By day 40 post-gestation, a longitudinal sinus connects the anterior, middle, and posterior sinuses and drains into the internal jugular vein. A section of the anterior venous plexus will eventually become the superior sagittal sinus. The anterior and middle plexuses will join to form the transverse sinus, and the middle and posterior will join to form the sigmoid sinus. Over time this plexus will coalesce into the superior sagittal and transverse sinuses. The venous system lags behind arterial development considerably, and it continues to develop throughout gestation and even after birth.

The primitive extracranial venous system is composed of the cardinal veins, in which the anterior division is responsible for the drainage of the head and neck, while the posterior division drains the body. In the areas where the anterior and posterior cardinal veins converge, common cardinal veins are seen, which are the precursors of the internal jugular veins. The subclavian veins develop as bilateral vein buds in the upper extremities and ultimately anastomose with the anterior cardinal veins to form the brachiocephalic veins.

Table 1.8   Circle of Willis Developmental Segments

Cranial division	Initiates as primitive olfactory artery and gives rise to definitive ACA and MCA. ACOM forms from a plexiform vascular network.
Caudal division	Anastomoses with dorsal longitudinal neural arteries and regresses to form the PCOM. Supplies precommunicating segment of PCA BA from pair of dorsal longitudinal arteries.

Abbreviations: ACA, anterior cerebral artery; ACOM, anterior communicating artery; MCA, middle carotid artery; PCOM, posterior communicating artery.

The intracranial venous drainage develops from a series of plexiform dural channels that will ultimately form several important venous structures in the adult. The superior sagittal sinus is formed from a plexiform channel of veins covering the telencephalon and diencephalon. As the telencephalon grows posteriorly, the venous channels are stretched in a sagittal plane leading to the cortical draining veins observed in the adult. The cavernous sinus and its associated venous structures are derived from embryonic structures independent of intracranial drainage. The formation of the deep venous circulation occurs late in the embryonic stages. For a more in-depth discussion of the exact steps of embryonic venous vasculature development, please refer to **Table 1.9**.

Adult Arterial Vasculature: Extracranial Circulation

The extracranial circulation normally consists of a series of arteries that pass through the neck on the way to the cranium or arteries that supply extracranial structures in the head and neck.[3,4,6] The extracranial circulation consists of the bilateral common carotid arteries, cervical carotid arteries, external carotid arteries, and the vertebral arteries. The carotid arteries begin as a common trunk called the common carotid artery. They then split into the internal carotid artery that supplies the intracranial structures and the external carotid artery (ECA) that supplies the head and neck (**Fig. 1.4**). The left common carotid artery originates directly from the aortic arch, while the right common carotid artery is a branch of the brachiocephalic trunk behind the right sternoclavicular junction. The common carotid ascends in the neck for some distance before dividing. The most common location of the carotid bifurcation is at the C3–4 vertebral body level; however, it can occur from C2 to T3. It is always important to know where the carotid bifurcation is located, because much pathology can be localized to this area, for example, atherosclerotic disease leading to carotid stenoses. Endovascular surgeons may also encounter a non-bifurcating carotid artery, in which the ECA originates directly off the aorta as a carotid trunk. The vertebral and internal carotid arteries do not typically have any branches outside of the skull, while the external carotid supplies structures in superficial and deep head and neck.

Table 1.9 Venous Development

Adult vein	Embryonic vein
	Anterior cardinal veins drain the head and neck in the third and fourth weeks.
	Posterior cardinal veins drain the body.
Internal jugular vein	Common cardinal veins formed by the anterior and posterior cardinal veins.
External jugular vein	Formed from a capillary plexus.
Brachiocephalic vein	Subclavian veins develop as bilateral vein buds in the upper extremities and anastomose with the anterior cardinal veins to form the brachiocephalic vein.
Superior vena cava	Formed by the left and right brachiocephalic veins.

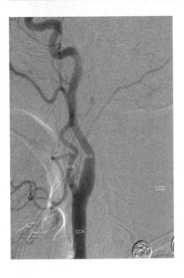

Fig. 1.4 Cervical carotid artery: left common carotid artery angiography (lateral view). The common carotid artery (CCA) bifurcates into the internal (ICA) and external (ECA) carotid arteries.

The internal carotid artery runs in the carotid sheath after bifurcating from the common carotid. In the carotid sheath, the internal carotid artery lies anteromedially to the internal jugular vein, carrying with it cranial nerves IX, X, XI, XII and postganglionic sympathetic fibers. The cervical carotid artery is congenitally absent in 0.1% of the population; most of the cases are unilateral, but some rare cases can be bilateral. The cervical internal carotid artery can be injured from anterior and lateral neck tumors, infections, or trauma, resulting in pseudoaneurysms, dissections, and fistulae. Atherosclerotic disease is the most common disease of these vessels, most often found in the aged population and treatable with carotid endarterectomy or endovascular stent placement. All of these acute and chronic vessel diseases place the patient at risk of ischemic or thromboembolic stroke in the anterior cerebral circulation, making early diagnosis and treatment critical.

At the carotid bifurcation, the external carotid artery is initially located anteromedially to ICA and then courses in a posterolateral direction. The internal jugular vein (IJV) runs posterior and lateral to these structures on its descent to meet the subclavian. The ECA is covered superficially by the sternocleidomastoid muscle and is crossed by the hypoglossal nerve in the upper cervical region. The ECA is responsible for the blood supply to the majority of the face, scalp, external and skull base auditory structures and the dura. The ECA divides into several terminal branches emanating from its main trunk, coursing both superficially, as well as deeply (**Fig. 1.5**). These arteries supply many important structures in the head and neck, as well as form collaterals with intracranial circulation (**Table 1.10**).

The vertebral arteries are paired vessels originating off the brachiocephalic trunk on the right and the left subclavian artery. In rare cases the vertebral artery may originate from the aortic arch, common carotid artery, or internal carotid artery. After their origin, the vertebral arteries normally enter the bilateral spinal foramina transversaria at C6. The artery remains contained within the foramina until the C2 body and is surrounded by a complex venous plexus. At the level of C2, the paired vertebral arteries leave the foramina and course laterally and posteri-

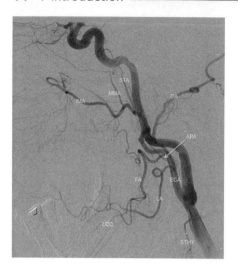

Fig. 1.5 Selective external carotid artery (ECA) injection with reflux in the internal carotid artery. The ECA and its branches are depicted: superior thyroid (STHY), facial (FA), lingual (LA), ascending pharyngeal (APA), occipital (OA), superficial temporal (STA), middle meningeal (MMA), and internal maxillary (IMA) arteries.

orly, then ascend cephalad, through the foramen transversarium of C1. The artery then courses posteromedially over the arch of C1, before turning anteromedially to pierce the atlanto-occipital membrane, becoming intracranial. Often the vertebral arteries are unequal in caliber. Fifty percent of patients are left-side dominant (having a larger left vertebral artery), twenty-five percent are right-side dominant, and twenty-five percent are co-dominant. The cervical vertebral arteries are divided into four segments (**Table 1.11** and **Fig. 1.6**).

Cervical vertebral artery injury occurs most commonly via catheter manipulations, head and neck trauma and tumors, and surgical spine fusion. As with the carotid arteries, acute injury can result in pseudoaneurysms and dissections, but atherosclerotic disease is also common and results in posterior circulation ischemic strokes and symptoms of vertebrobasilar insufficiency. Surgical treatment of vertebral artery disease is not very common now that endovascular options are available. The vertebral arteries are more difficult to access surgically than the carotid arteries because of the bony canal of the vertebrae (foramen transversarium) in which they travel along their course to the brain.

Extracranial Venous Drainage

Drainage of the head and neck occurs through the jugular venous system. The extracranial head and neck are drained primarily through the external jugular vein. The external jugular vein (EJV) begins high up in the neck, with the coalescence of the posterior auricular vein and the retromandibular vein. The occipital, posterior external, transverse cervical, transverse scapular, and anterior jugular veins later join the EJV to drain the face and head. Not all drainage of the face and scalp is superficial. Some veins drain deeply into the internal jugular vein rather than the external, and these include the occipital, facial, lingual, pharyngeal, and superior and

Table 1.10 External Carotid Artery Branches

Superior thyroid artery (STA)	First branch of the ECA; anteroinferior, courses toward thyroid gland. Supplies the larynx and upper thyroid. 20% arise above bifurcation, 10% from CC, 2% from lingual artery.
Ascending pharyngeal artery (APA)	Smallest and first posterior branch. Originates within 2 cm of the ICA/ECA bifurcation. Courses behind ICA, anterior and medial to IJV. Supplies the nasopharynx, oropharynx, middle ear, cranial nerves IX, X, XI, and meninges. Anastomoses with the vertebral artery at C3.
Lingual artery (LA)	Superior and medial course toward pharyngeal musculature. Major blood supply to tongue and floor of the oral cavity. In 15% of patients, LA and FA share a common trunk.
Facial artery (FA)	Course initially ascends, with later inferior and lateral course toward submandibular gland and crosses mandible. Supplies the face, palate, and lips. Angular branch anastomoses with the orbital branch of the ophthalmic artery.
Occipital artery (OA)	Originates from posterior ECA and runs posterior and superior between C1 vertebra and occipital bone. Supplies posterior scalp, upper cervical musculature, posterior fossa meninges. Anastomoses with the vertebral artery at C1–C2.
Posterior auricular artery	Supplies the pinna, external auditory canal, and scalp.
Superficial temporal artery (STA)	Supplies the scalp and anterior ear.
Internal maxillary artery (IMA)	A terminal branch courses within the parotid gland, behind the mandible, terminating in the pterygopalatine fossa. Supplies the deep face. Middle meningeal artery branches from here. Anastomoses with the ophthalmic artery through ethmoidal branches.

Table 1.11 Vertebral Artery Segments

Segment	Course
First	Extends from the subclavian artery to the foramen transversarium of C6.
Second	Runs through the foramen transversarium of C1–C6.
Third	Exits the foramen transverarium of C1 and courses on groove on the upper portion of C1 arch, then passes beneath the posterior atlanto-occipital membrane to enter the vertebral canal.
Fourth	Pierces the dura and passes between the hypoglossal nerve and first cervical nerve root to the anterior surface of the medulla and ends as the basilar artery at the pontomedullary junction.

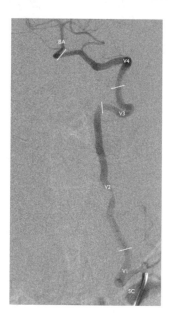

Fig. 1.6 Cervical angiography demonstrating the four anatomical divisions (V1–V4) of the vertebral artery as it courses from the subclavian to the basilar arteries. V1=extraosseous segment traveling from its origin at the subclavian artery (SC) up to its entry point into the foramen transversarium, V2=foraminal segment that travels within the transverse foramen, V3=extraspinal segment consisting of the arterial segment between C1 vertebra and the intracranial dura at the foramen magnum, V4=intradural segment often identified as a narrowing of the arterial diameter as it enters the dura and travels to the basilar artery (BA).

middle thyroid veins (**Fig. 1.7**). The external jugular vein itself also communicates with the internal jugular vein through a plexus in and around the parotid gland. The external and internal jugular veins themselves communicate with a connection through the parotid gland. The EJV ultimately crosses the sternocleidomastoid muscle superficially before piercing the deep fascia to join with the subclavian vein.

Injury and hypercoagulability disorders can cause thrombosis of the jugular veins, ultimately inhibiting adequate venous drainage of the cerebral circulation; this can result in cerebral edema and venous infarctions. In acute cases, where the patient becomes symptomatic from cerebral congestion, endovascular recanalization may be required to revascularize the vein and reestablish venous drainage of the brain.

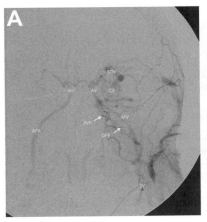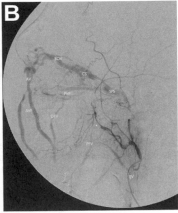

Fig. 1.7 Angiographic depiction of the extracranial veins of the face and neck on **(A)** AP and **(B)** lateral views. The angular vein (AV) begins at the medial palpebral angle and drains into the anterior facial vein (AFV). The pterygoid venous plexus (PVP) drains into the deep facial vein (DFV), which ultimately joins the superficial facial vein (SFV) before draining into the external jugular vein (EJV). The superior ophthalmic vein (SOV) and inferior ophthalmic vein (IOV) drain intracranially into the cavernous sinuses (CS), and into the superior (SPS) and inferior (IPS) petrosal sinuses to the internal jugular vein (IJV). The posterior facial vein (PFV) is also identified draining the posterior aspect of the face.

Craniofacial Circulation

The craniofacial circulation refers to the communication between the terminal branches of the external carotid and intracranial arteries (**Table 1.12**).[3,4,6] This communication can be either physiologic, in the case of the internal maxillary artery communicating intracranially through the middle meningeal artery, or it may be secondary to surgical manipulation. An example of the latter is the superior thyroid artery to middle cerebral artery bypass, or STA-to-MCA bypass (also termed ECA-ICA bypass), which is used in patients with MCA territory hypoperfusion. Hypoperfusion of the MCA territory results most commonly from Moya-Moya disease (in children), where the artery is placed on the pial surface of the brain, and from chronic MCA occlusive disease, where endovascular treatment cannot be performed. Terminal branches from the external carotid artery supplying the face and deep structures are listed in **Table 1.12** and seen in **Fig. 1.5**.

Intracranial Circulation

The intracranial circulation is composed of a combination of blood vessels through the bilateral internal cranial (ICA) and vertebral (VA) arteries.[3,4,6] The anterior circulation is formed by the ICAs, which begin in the neck and terminate intracranially. Each ICA is composed of seven segments, defined in **Table 1.13** and seen in **Fig. 1.8**. They enter the skull at the petrous part of the temporal bone and course through the cavernous sinus before becoming intradural at the distal dural ring.

Table 1.12 Facial Circulation

Artery	Description	Branches
Facial	Branches off the ECA and is the main arterial supply to the face. Wraps around the mandible anterior to the masseter. Ends with branches to the lips and nose.	Sends terminal branches to the tonsils, palate, and submandibular gland. Angular artery to the eyelids.
Internal maxillary artery (IMA)	Terminal branch of the ECA. Divides into the proximal, middle, and terminal segments.	Proximal segments (mandibular): courses anteriorly, following the bottom side of the lateral pterygoid muscle and producing the middle meningeal artery (MMA). MMA: largest IMA branch; enters skull at foramen spinosum. Largest dural artery. Accessory meningeal artery: enters skull through foramen ovale. Inferior alveolar artery: supplies mandible and lower teeth. Middle segments (pterygoid): infratemporal fossa to pterygopalatine fossa, giving rise to anterior and posterior temporal arteries and masseteric and buccal arteries. Terminal segments (pterygopalatine): distal IMA enters the pterygopalatine fossa, supplying deep face and nose. Posterior superior alveolar artery: origin rests proximal to pterygopalatine fossa, supplying teeth. Infraorbital artery: enters orbit via inferior orbital fissure, coursing anteriorly to supply cheek, lower eyelid, and upper eyelid.
Superficial temporal artery (STA)	Terminal branch of the ECA. Runs deep to the parotid gland, then posterior to the neck of the mandible and over the zygomatic process to enter the temporal fossa.	Transverse facial artery: crosses the masseter muscle to supply the parotid gland, masseter, and skin. Terminates in frontal and parietal branches to the scalp.

Abbreviation: ECA, external carotid artery.

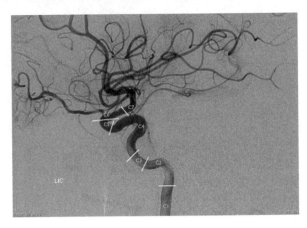

Fig. 1.8 Internal carotid artery (ICA). Understanding the anatomy of the ICA is better done by artificially segmenting (C1–C7) it based on its anatomical relations to other structures as it courses from the neck into the brain. Different systems have been created to segment the artery, but the following is the most commonly used: cervical (C1), petrous (C2), lacerum (C3), cavernous (C4), clinoidal (C5), ophthalmic (C6), communicating (C7).

The ICAs ultimately terminate as the anterior and middle cerebral arteries at the ICA bifurcation. Intracranially, the anterior circulation communicates bilaterally via the anterior communicating artery. This communication allows contralateral flow to pass between the ACAs (anterior cerebral arteries) and occasionally MCAs via retrograde flow into the M1 segment. This communication allows for a single ICA to supply both sides of the cerebrum with oxygen and nutrients.

The anterior circulation may also communicate with the posterior circulation through the posterior communicating arteries. The posterior communicating arteries branch from the final segment of the ICA prior to its bifurcation into the ACA and MCA. The PCOM courses posteriorly to anastamose with the posterior cerebral artery above cranial nerve III. There are many important perforators supplying the thalamus, hypothalamus, subthalamus, and posterior limb of the internal capsule that originate from the PCOM as it passes these structures along its course. Up to 20% of the population have a fetal PCA anomaly; the anomaly occurs bilaterally in 8%. A fetal posterior cerebral artery (PCA) is characterized by a PCOM having the same, or nearly the same, caliber as the PCA it joins (**Fig. 1.9**). In this case, some or all of the blood supply to that PCA may originate from the anterior circulation. Therefore, ICA stenosis can cause occipital strokes in some cases.

The posterior intracranial circulation is formed by the vertebrobasilar system. This system begins as the vertebral arteries pierce the atlanto-occipital membrane and enter the dura. The vertebral arteries give off the anterior and posterior spinal arteries and the posterior inferior cerebellar artery before joining the contralateral VA to form the basilar artery. The basilar artery supplies many important perforators to the brain stem as well as the anterior inferior cerebellar artery, labyrinthine artery and superior cerebellar artery before terminating as the posterior cerebral arteries (PCA) supplying the occipital lobe. The PCOM arteries anastomose with the proximal PCAs (P1-P2 junction).

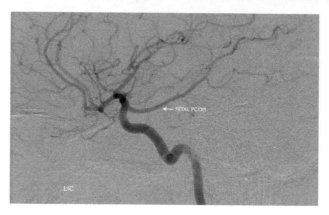

Fig. 1.9 Fetal PCOM, left ICA injection demonstrating a fetal PCOM. This artery provides blood to the posterior cerebral artery; the P1 segment is typically hypoplastic when a fetal PCOM is present.

Intracranial ICA (Table 1.13)

Various classification schemes have been described that subdivide the ICA into anatomical "segments" as it relates to its surrounding anatomical structures, during its course from the neck to the brain. Here we present the most commonly used classification system and that which the authors feel is most relevant anatomically and angiographically (**Fig. 1.8**).

The intracranial ICA begins as the artery enters the petrous bone (C2). This segment of the ICA has only two branches that are variably present, the vidian and corticotympanic arteries. These branches supply the inner ear. Persistent stapedial and otic branches are rare anomalies.

The ICA continues over (not through, a common misconception) the foramen lacerum (C3) and then enters the cavernous sinus to become the cavernous segment (C4). Here, the medial, posterior, and lateral arterial trunks branch to supply the pituitary gland, cranial nerves III-VI, and meninges. The tentorial artery of Bernasconi and Cassinari (also known as the tentorial artery or the "Italian artery") also arises from the posterior trunk of this segment to supply the tentorium. This artery is particularly important in patients with tentorial meningiomas, where preoperative embolization of this artery can significantly reduce the blood supply to the tumor.

After exiting the cavernous sinus, the ICA travels a short distance extradurally between the proximal and distal dural rings prior to entering the subarachnoid space at the level of the anterior clinoid; this is the clinoidal segment (C5). In rare cases, the ophthalmic artery can originate here, giving it an extradural origin. In up to 0.5% of the population, the ophthalmic artery may originate off the middle meningeal artery (MMA), in which case it reaches the orbit through the superior orbital fissure or a foramen in the greater wing of the sphenoid. This is important to look for when considering embolization of the MMA, because occlusion could result in monocular blindness from unintended embolization of the ophthalmic artery (OA).

Table 1.13   Internal Carotid Artery Segments

Segment	Description	Branches
C1: Cervical segment	C1 made of two parts, bulb and ascending cervical segment. Carotid bulb: Focal dilation at bifurcation from CCA. From the bulb, C1 courses within the carotid sheath. Enters at petrous temporal bone in carotid canal, and C1 ends.	No branches in this segment.
C2: Petrous segment	Vertical and horizontal segments are surrounded by a venous plexus extending from the cavernous sinus. Travels through the petrous portion of the temporal bone and exits the apex, traveling over the foramen lacerum.	Vidian artery of pterygoid canal: travels anteroinferiorly through the foramen lacerum to anastomose with the ECA. Corticotympanic artery: supplies the middle and inner ear.
C3: Lacerum segment	Smallest segment of ICA. Begins at proximal dural ring above anterior ICA genu and ends at the distal dural ring, where the ICA enters the subarachnoid space. Extradural.	Rarely, the ophthalmic artery originates here.
C4: Cavernous segment	Begins lateral to the posterior clinoid and turns forward. Terminates along the medial side of the anterior clinoid. Covered by Meckel's cave and TG ganglion. CN VI inferiorly and lateral freely through the cavernous sinus. CN III, IV, V, V2 run in the lateral wall of the sinus. Rarely, cavernous origin of ophthalmic artery (8% of autopsies).	Meningohypophyseal trunk: gives the inferior hypophyseal, tentorial, and dorsal meningeal arteries. Inferior hypophyseal artery: supplies the inferior pituitary gland. Tentorial artery of Bernasconi and Cassinari ("the Italian artery"): supplies the tentorium. Dorsal meningeal artery: supplies CN VI and clivus McConnell's capsular artery: supplies the pituitary gland capsule. Inferolateral trunk: supplies CN III, IV, VI and TG ganglion and cavernous sinus dura.
C5: Clinoidal segment	Shortest segment of ICA is extradural. Exits the cavernous sinus through the proximal dural ring and becomes intradural again as it passes through the distal dural ring at the clinoid process. Optic nerve lies superomedial; the sphenoid sinus is located anterior and inferior.	Occasionally the ophthalmic artery can be located here (extradurally).

(Continued on page 22)

Table 1.13 *(Continued)*   Internal Carotid Artery Segments

Segment	Description	Branches
C6: Ophthalmic segment	Extends from the distal dural ring to the posterior communicating artery (PCOM).	Superior hypophyseal artery: supplies anterior pituitary gland, pituitary stalk, and optic nerve chiasm. Ophthalmic artery: for course and branches, see **Table 1.11**.
C7: Communi-cating segment	Begins at posterior communicating artery (PCOM) and ends at the MCA/ACA bifurcation. Lateral to CN II; below the anterior perforated substance.	Posterior communicating artery (PCOM), anterior choroidal (ACho), anterior cerebral artery (ACA), and middle cerebral artery (MCA) further described below.

Abbreviations: ACA, anterior cerebral artery; ACho, anterior choroidal artery; ECA, external carotid artery; ICA, internal carotid artery; PCOM, posterior communicating artery; MCA, middle cerebral artery.

The ICA continues its course superiorly, medial to the anterior clinoid process, with the optic nerve being located superiorly and medially and the sphenoid sinus laterally. Before the ICA terminates as the ACA/MCA vessels, the OA originates from the ICA at the ophthalmic segment (C6). Here, the OA travels anteriorly to supply the orbital contents and retina (**Table 1.14**).

The final segment (C7) of the ICA is the communicating segment from which the posterior communicating artery (PCOM) originates. The PCOM sends multiple perforating branches to the thalamus and internal capsule. The largest branch from the PCOM is the anterior thalamoperforating artery that passes through the anterior perforating substance to supply the medial thalamus and third ventricular wall. The PCOM is the normal physiological communication between the anterior and posterior intracranial circulation, but some patients may continue to have persistent fetal connections. This persistent circulatory pattern forms a direct communication with the carotid and either the vertebral or basilar arteries. These arterial communications may be either silent anatomical variations, or pathological connections allowing thrombotic emboli to reach the circulation in a paradoxical manner (that is, carotid stenosis leading to brainstem strokes though embolic phenomena) (**Table 1.15**). A wide triangular base, or infundibulum, of the PCOM origin is sometimes seen on angiography and can be mistaken for a PCOM aneurysm. The main difference between a PCOM infundibulum and an aneurysm is that the PCOM vessel is seen coming from the apex of an infundibulum, whereas it comes from the base of an aneurysm. Sometimes the PCOM is very tiny and challenging to see on angiography, making it difficult to determine whether the bulge is an infundibulum or aneurysm.

The anterior choroidal (ACho) artery originates from the posterior wall of the ICA distal to the PCOM origin, but in rare cases it may branch proximally. It courses inferior and lateral to the optic tract, bending around the uncus and through the crural and ambient cistern before entering the choroidal fissure. The ACho supplies

Table 1.14 Ophthalmic Artery

Description	Branches
Begins anterosuperior and courses with optic nerve. The origin is intradural in 90% of patients. Lies medial to CN III and IV; inferolateral to CN II. Extensive ECA anastomoses with ethmoidal and facial braches. The anterior falx artery originates from the anterior ethmoidal artery.	Central retinal artery: runs through the optic nerve and further branches into the ciliary artery; supplies retina and choroid. Lacrimal artery: supplies lacrimal gland and conjunctiva. Superior, anterior, posterior ethmoidal arteries. Dorsal nasal artery. Palpebral artery. Medial frontal artery. Supratrochlear artery.

Abbreviation: ECA, external carotid artery.

the optic chiasm, optic tract, globus pallidus, genu of the internal capsule, posterior limb of the internal capsule, middle third of the cerebral peduncle, substantia nigra, red nucleus, ventral anterior and ventral lateral thalamic nuclei, geniculate body, optic radiations, and finally the choroid plexus. The ACho artery is not always easily identified on angiography due to its small size, but it is most easily identified on an AP or an oblique anterior view. The artery is identified as it passes posteriorly and enters the plexal point as it passes into the choroidal fissure. 2.3% of patients can have a hyperplastic ACho, which supplies the PCA distribution, and 3% can have a hypoplastic artery not identified on the angiography.

The internal carotid then bifurcates into two terminal arteries to supply the cerebrum: the anterior and middle cerebral arteries.

Table 1.15 Persistent Carotid-Vertebral Anastomoses

Primitive trigeminal artery	Most common persistent fetal circulation. 0.2–0.6% of angiograms. Associated with increased prevalence of other vascular abnormalities, such as aneurysms (14%). Connects the cavernous ICA to BA.
Primitive hypoglossal artery	Second most common persistent fetal circulation. 0.1% of cases. Connects the high cervical (C1–C2) ICA to the BA through the hypoglossal canal.
Persistent otic artery	Connects the petrous ICA to BA via the internal auditory meatus. Very rare.
Proatlantal intersegmental artery	Connects the cervical ICA (C2–C3 level) or the ECA to VA between the occiput and the arch of C1. Very rare.

Abbreviations: BA, basilar artery; ECA, external carotid artery; ICA, internal carotid artery; VA, vertebral artery.

Anterior Cerebral Artery (ACA)

The anterior cerebral artery, one of the two terminal branches of the ICA, is typically divided into three (A3) to four (A4) segments, with some authors and anatomists subdiving the ACA into as many as five (A5) segments (**Fig. 1.10**). In any case, the A3 branches typically imply the larger cortical vessels that supply the medial surface of the cerebral hemispheres, and the A4 and A5 segments typically refer to the terminal branches of the A3 segments that travel within the sulci to supply the cortical surfaces (**Table 1.16A**).

The ACA supplies the medial surface of the cerebral hemispheres. The first segment (A1) of the ACA is the pre-communicating segment that extends from the ICA origin to the anterior communicating artery (ACOM). The communicating segment has no large named branches, but it does supply perforating vessels to the optic nerve, optic chiasm, hypothalamus, septum pellucidum, anterior commissure, pillars of the fornix, and the striatum by way of the medial lenticulostriates. The ACOM complex is also the most common place for the occurrence of aneurysms. Coiling of the wide-necked ACOM aneurysms can put the perforating vessels at risk of occlusion during embolization, resulting in visual changes, hormonal dysregulation from hypothalamic dysfunction, and memory disturbance from forniceal injury.

The proximal pericallosal segment is the second segment (A2) of the ACA, extending between the ACOM and the distal ACA branches. This segment contains four main branches supplying the basal ganglia and medial sub-frontal lobe. The recurrent artery of Heubner (RAH) is usually the first branch distal to ACOM. It runs in a retrograde fashion back toward the A1 segment of the ACA before diving into the anterior perforating substance to supply the head of the caudate, the anterior limb of the internal capsule, putamen, globus pallidus, and the inferior frontal lobe. The orbitofrontal artery is the second branch from the A2 and travels to the medial inferior frontal pole. It supplies the gyrus rectus, medial orbital gyri, and the olfactory bulb and tract. The frontopolar artery is the third branch, supplying the medial frontal lobe and the superior frontal gyri. The anterior internal frontal artery is the final branch, supplying the anterior and medial frontal lobe.

The terminal segment of the ACA has many branches supplying the medial surface of the cerebral hemispheres anteriorly and above the corpus callosum. The pericallosal and callosomarginal arteries are the third segments (A3) of the ACA, both easily identifiable on lateral angiography. They supply the medial parietal lobe and precuneus, and the cingulate gyrus and paracentral lobules, respectively. The terminal branches, A4 and A5, of the ACA consist of smaller arteries that supply the medial and cortical surfaces of the frontal lobe, central sulcus, and parietal lobe, including the middle internal frontal, posterior internal frontal, paracentral, and superior and inferior parietal arteries.

There are a few anomalies of the ACA vessels. A unilateral hypoplastic A1 is the most common ACA anomaly, with a contralateral A1 usually being larger and dominant. ACOM aneurysms typically will form on the side of the dominant A1 and point toward the opposite side, consistent with the direction of the blood flow from the larger A1. A second ACA anomaly is a single A2 branch shared by both cerebral hemispheres, called an azygous ACA. Other less common ACA anomalies include a fenestrated ACOM, three A2 branches from the ACOM, and an incomplete circle of Willis from an absent A1.

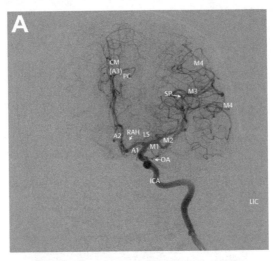

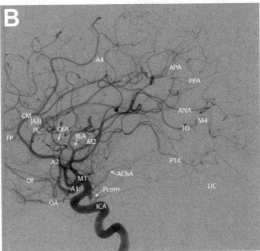

Fig. 1.10 Left internal carotid artery (ICA) injection, **(A)** AP and **(B)** lateral views. The ICA terminus (ICAt) is identified branching into the anterior (ACA) and middle (MCA) cerebral arteries. The ophthalmic (OA), posterior communicating (PCOM), and anterior choroidal (AChA) arteries are seen on the lateral views just before the ICA terminus. Branching of the ACA (segments A1–A4) into the recurrent artery of Huebner (RAH), callosomarginal (CM), pericallosal (PC), frontopolar (FP), orbitofrontal (OF), and cortical A4s is depicted here. The lenticulostriate (LS) arteries arise from the proximal MCA (M1) before bifurcating into the M2 divisions. The operculofrontal (OFA) and rolandic (RLA) arteries are seen. The sylvian point (SP), consisting of the sylvian segments (M3) of the MCA, is identified on these views. Cortical (M4) branches are also seen M4 including: posterior temporal (PTA), temporal-occipital (TO), angular (ANA), and the anterior (APA) and posterior parietal (PPA) arteries.

Table 1.16A ACA Branches

Segment	Branches	Territory supplied
A1: Pre-communicating segment	Medial lenticulostriates	A series of perforators supplying the optic nerve, chiasm, hypo-thalamus, septum pellucidum, anterior commissure, pillars of the fornix, and the striatum.
A2: Post-communicat-ing segment (aka verti-cal pericallosal part)	Recurrent artery of Heubner	Courses back toward proximal A1 and dives through the anterior perforating substance to supply the head of the caudate, anterior limb of the internal capsule, puta-men, global pallidus, and the inferior frontal lobe.
	Orbital frontal artery	Supplies the gyrus rectus, medial orbital gyri, and the olfactory bulb and tract.
	Frontopolar artery	Supplies the medial frontal lobe and the superior frontal gyri.
	Anterior internal frontal artery	Supplies the anterior and medial frontal lobe.
A3: Terminal or cortical branches	Callosomarginal artery	Supplies the cingulate gyrus and the paracentral lobule.
	Pericallosal artery	Supplies the medial parietal lobe and the precuneus.
	Middle internal frontal artery	Supplies the medial frontal lobe.
	Posterior internal frontal artery	Supplies the posteromedial frontal lobe.
	Paracentral artery	Supplies the medial frontal lobe at the central sulcus.
	Superior parietal artery	Supplies the medial and superior parietal lobe.
	Inferior parietal artery	Supplies the medial and inferior parietal lobe.

Middle Cerebral Artery

The second terminal branch of the internal carotid artery is the middle cerebral artery (MCA), which supplies the lateral surface of the cerebral hemispheres, including the frontal, temporal, parietal, and occipital lobes. The MCA is divided into four segments: M1 pre-bifurcation or horizontal segment, M2 post-bifurcation or insular segment, M3 opercular segment, and M4 cortical or terminal branches (**Fig. 1.10**).

The MCA travels through the sylvian fissure and branches out over the cortical convexities. These vessels are best viewed using an oblique view on angiography, as the vessels are overlying one another on direct AP and lateral views. M1 is the MCA segment from its origin from the ICA terminus to the bifurcation. This segment of the MCA has four important branches: (1) the uncal artery supplying the uncus and deep white matter of the medial temporal lobe, (2) the temporopolar artery coursing to the anterior-most tip of the temporal lobe to supply the temporal pole, (3) the anterior temporal artery coursing toward the anterior temporal lobe to supply the anterior temporal lobe just posterior to the temporal pole, and (4) the lateral lenticulostriate arteries consisting of a series of small perforating arteries supplying the basal ganglia and the internal capsule.

M2 extends from the MCA bifurcation into the sylvian fissure and supplies deep structures of the frontal, parietal, temporal, and occipital lobes (detailed in **Table 1.16B**). M3 completes the course of the MCA through the sylvian fissure and then exits to cover the convexities of the cerebral hemispheres, supplying blood to the cortex. M3 is identified on AP view by the sylvian point (**Fig. 1.10**), an area where the MCA abruptly turns laterally at the apex of the insula as it leaves the sylvian fissure. M4s are the named cortical branches and are described in **Table 1.16B**.

Table 1.16B MCA Branches

Orbitofrontal artery	Supplies the middle and inferior frontal gyri.
Prefrontal artery	Supplies the inferior and middle frontal gyri.
Precentral artery	Supplies the inferior and middle precentral gyri.
Central artery	Supplies the superior postcentral gyrus and anterior inferior parietal lobe.
Anterior parietal artery	Supplies the superior parietal lobe.
Posterior parietal artery	Supplies the posterior, superior, and inferior parietal lobes.
Angular artery	Supplies the posterior superior temporal gyrus and occipital gyrus.
Tempero-occipital artery	Supplies the superior, middle, and inferior temporal gyri and the occipital gyrus.
Posterotemporal artery	Supplies superior, middle, and inferior temporal gyri.
Middle temporal artery	Supplies the superior, middle, and inferior temporal gyri.

Vertebrobasilar Circulation

The vertebral arteries pierce the atlanto-occipital membrane at the foramen magnum and become intradural. Almost immediately thereafter, the anterior and posterior spinal arteries (two in number) branch to supply the lower medulla and the posterior third of the spinal cord. Injury to these vessels can result in an infarction of the posterior sensory columns of the spinal cord. The anterior spinal artery also arises from the intracranial vertebral arteries and supplies the anterior part of the lower medulla and the anterior two-thirds of the spinal cord in the cervical and upper thoracic levels. Injury to these vessels can produce an anterior spinal cord syndrome resulting in paralysis.

The posterior meningeal artery and posterior inferior cerebellar artery branch from the vertebral artery prior to joining to form the basilar artery. The posterior meningeal artery supplies the dura of the posterior fossa and falx cerebelli. The posterior inferior cerebellar artery (PICA) is divided into five segments (**Table 1.17**) supplying the medulla and inferior cerebellum (**Fig. 1.11**).

The basilar artery (BA) begins with the convergence of the vertebral arteries and ends with the bifurcation into the bilateral posterior cerebral arteries (**Fig. 1.11**). Along its course superiorly, the basilar supplies three main types of branches: (1) brainstem perforating arteries arising from the dorsal aspect of the basilar artery to supply the brainstem (pons and midbrain), (2) the anterior inferior cerebellar arteries (AICA), frequently being multiple in number (3 to 5 pairs) supplying the inferior surface of the cerebellum, and (3) the superior cerebellar arteries (SCA), supplying the superior surface of the cerebellum and arising just before the BA divides into the PCAs (**Table 1.18**).

The vertebrobasilar system is a frequent site of pathology. Basilar tip aneurysms are one of the more common types and have a higher risk of rupturing, due to their location at a bifurcation. These aneurysms are frequently wide necked, incorporating one or both PCA origins. Combined stent coiling of these aneurysms is common because of the wide-necked nature of these aneurysms. Atherosclerotic

Table 1.17 PICA segments

Anterior medullary segment	Begins at the PICA origin and extends to the most prominent portion of the olive.
Lateral medullary segment	Begins at the olive and extends to the glossopharyngeal, vagus, and accessory nerves.
Tonsillomedullary segment	Begins at glossophryngeal, vagus, and accessory nerves and extends to the mid portion of the cerebellar tonsil. Forms a caudal loop before turning superiorly, marking the caudal extent of the tonsil.
Telovelotonsillar segment	Begins midtonsillar and extends to the fissure created by the vermis, tonsil, and cerebellar hemisphere.
Cortical segment	Terminal branches supplying the vermis and hemispheres.

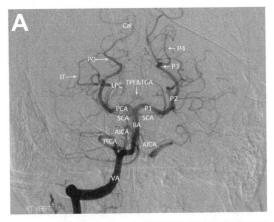

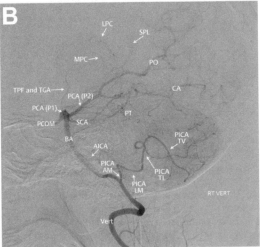

Fig. 1.11 The posterior circulation: vertebral artery angiography depicted on both **(A)** AP and **(B)** lateral views demonstrating the intracranial vertebral artery (VA) and posterior inferior cerebellar artery (PICA) identified by the hairpin loop as it travels around the cerebellar tonsils. The PICA is named according to the structures around which it courses: anterior medullary (AM), lateral medullary (LM), tonsillar (TL), telovelar (TV), and cortical segments. The anterior inferior cerebellar (AICA) and superior cerebellar (SCA) arteries are visualized coming from the basilar artery (BA), which terminates as the posterior cerebral arteries (PCA); thalamoperforators (TPF) and thalamogeniculate arteries (TGA) are seen emanating from the basilar apex and PCOM. Branches from the PCA seen here include the posterior temporal (PT), inferior temporal (IT), parietal occipital (PO), medial posterior choroidal (MPC), lateral posterior choroidal (LPC), splenial (SPL), and calcarine (CA) branches.

Table 1.18 Basilar Artery Branches

Anterior inferior cerebellar artery (AICA)	Crosses through the cerebellopontine angle cistern, inferior to CN VII and VIII. Supplies the lateral pons, middle cerebellar peduncle, and anterolateral cerebellum, as well as CN VII and VIII.
Labyrinthine artery	Supplies the labyrinth.
Superior cerebellar artery (SCA)	Travels below CN III. Supplies the vermis, deep cerebellar nuclei, and superior cerebellum.
Posterior cerebral artery (PCA)	Supplies the temporal, parietal, and occipital lobes, as well as the brainstem and choroid plexus of third and lateral ventricles. Divided into three segments.

disease is also common in the vertebral and basilar arteries. Severe stenosis of these vessels can cause hypoperfusion of the brainstem and occipital lobes, resulting in symptoms of vertigo, diplopia, syncope, and cortical blindness. Distal BA occlusion can result in "top o' the basilar syndrome," and acute thrombotic occlusion of the whole BA frequently results in coma or death.

Posterior Cerebral Arteries

The system of posterior cerebral arteries (PCA) sends arteries to the brainstem, thalamus, epithalamus, ventricular system, and temporal, parietal, and occipital lobes (**Table 1.19**). The posterior cerebral arteries are divided into several segments as they pass from the basilar apex to the PCOM segment of the PCA (P1, precommunicating or mesencephalic segment), then through the ambient (P2, ambient segment) and quadrigeminal (P3, quadrigeminal segment) cisterns, and finally through the calcarine fissure (P4, calcarine segment) to the occipital lobes (**Fig. 1.11**).

The P1 segment ends at the PCOM-to-PCA junction. Perforating vessels to the brainstem and thalamus arise from this segment. The P2 segment then travels laterally and superiorly, giving rise to the posterior choroidal and temporal arteries as it travels around the cerebral peduncles in the ambient cisterns. Here, CN III and IV are in close approximation to the PCA. The P3 segment has a very short course in the quadrigeminal cistern before dividing to form the cortical (P4) branches (**Table 1.19**). Blood flow to the PCA typically is from the vertebrobasilar circulation except when a fetal PCA is present, in which case the ICA supplies the majority of the circulation, and the ipsilateral P1 segment is hypoplastic.

Circle of Willis

The circle of Willis (COW) is a normal physiologic collateral circulation connecting the anterior and posterior cerebral circulations. The COW, which is actually a heptagon, consists of an ACOM, two A1s, two PCOMs, and two P1s. A complete circle is found in only 25% of the population at autopsy studies, with 50% of the specimens having anomalies involving one or more of its components (**Table 1.20**).

Table 1.19 PCA Segments

Segment	Description	Branches
P1 segment	Extends from the PCA origin to the PCOM	Posterior thalamoperforator arteries: supply thalamus and midbrain. Medial posterior choroidal artery: supplies choroid of third ventricle, pineal gland, thalamus, and midbrain.
P2 segment	Extends from the PCOM to the quadrigeminal plate	Lateral posterior choroidal artery: supplies the thalamus and choroid plexus of the lateral ventricle. Medial and lateral thalamogeniculate arteries: supply the medial and lateral geniculate bodies, pulvinar, superior colliculus, and crus cerebri.
P3 segment	Begins at the quadrigeminal cistern and continues distally	Posterior temporal artery: supplies the temporal and occipital lobes. Internal occipital artery: trunk with three branches. Parieto-occipital artery: supplies medial portion of the hemisphere posteriorly. Calcarine artery: supplies the occipital lobe and primary visual cortex primarily. Posterior pericallosal artery: supplies the splenium of the corpus callosum.

Abbreviations: PCA, posterior cerebral arteries; PCOM, posterior communicating artery.

Table 1.20 Circle of Willis Anomalies

Location	Anomaly
ACOM	70% are located above the optic chiasm, while 30% lie below it.
ACA	Hypoplasia or absence of one of the A1 segments.
PCOM	Hypoplasia or absence of one or both PCOM arteries.
ACA	Infra-optic origin of the A1.
ACA	Fenestrated A1—may have multiple ACA pedicles, with no ACOM.
ACA	Azygous ACA—a single unpaired vessel supplying both right and left cortex. This is associated with a high prevalence of aneurysms.
ACA	Take-off of A1 near the ophthalmic origin. Also associated with a high rate of aneurysms.

Abbreviations: ACA, anterior cerebral arteries; ACOM, anterior communicating artery; PCOM, posterior communicating artery.

It is located above the sella turcica and in the interpeduncular and suprasellar cisterns, inferior and lateral to the hypothalamus, medial and inferior to the anterior perforate substance and gyrus rectus. This communication, if complete, allows the entire cerebral vasculature to get its blood supply by only one carotid or vertebral artery if the other three vessels are occluded.

Vascular Territories and Watershed Zones

An understanding of the anatomical territories supplied by each artery is an essential tool in the neuroendovascular surgeon's armamentarium. This will be discussed briefly here. There are variations in the extent to which each arterial tree supplies a particular region and overlaps other areas supplied by different arteries; the latter is referred to as the "watershed zone."[6]

The ACA and its branches supply blood to the medial portions of the cerebral hemispheres (frontal and parietal lobes), the optic nerves, optic chiasm, hypothalamic region, corpus callosum, anterior basal ganglia, and forniceal columns (**Fig. 1.12A**). Occlusion of the ACA or its branches can lead to infarction in these areas. With regard to the motor and sensory cortex, the ACA supplies the foot, leg, and thigh segments of the homunculus.

The MCA and its branches supply the lateral convexity and sides of the cerebral hemispheres (frontal, parietal, and temporal lobes), the internal capsule, middle and posterior segments of the basal ganglia, and optic radiations (**Fig. 1.12B**). The MCA overlaps with the ACA territory over the medial convexity of the hemispheres and the anterior deep white matter and basal ganglia structures. It supplies blood to the motor and sensory cortex of the homunculus from about the hips upward.

The PCA and its branches supply the occipital lobes, inferior and posterior surfaces of the temporal lobe, medial surface of the parietal lobe, and the upper brainstem (thalamus, midbrain, and pons). The PCA blood supply overlaps that of the ACA medially, MCA laterally, and BA and its branches inferiorly. The vertebrobasilar system and its branches supply the brainstem and cerebellum.

A watershed territory describes the areas of brain that lie at the most distal regions of the arterial tree, where there is overlap in vascular territories (**Fig. 1.13**). For example, the overlap between the ACA–MCA, MCA–PCA, and ACA–PCA territories are watershed zones (**Table 1.21**). Watershed zones are nature's way of having a backup plan for vascular occlusions, so to speak. The brain tissue in these zones is susceptible to infarction during periods of systemic hypotension or reduced blood flow. Yet during normotension, the overlapping blood supply may bestow protective effects on the tissue if the unaffected vascular tree can supply enough flow to the area to prevent an ischemic stroke.

Intracranial Venous Drainage

Though often overlooked, the venous system is as important as the arterial tree, and injury to it or thrombosis can result in venous infarction, with devastating neurological consequences.[3,6] The venous drainage system of the brain can be divided into deep and superficial, and the larger, dural venous sinuses (**Fig. 1.14**). The cerebral veins and dural venous sinuses are valveless and drain as a result of a pressure gradient between arterial, intracranial, and venous pressures. The small-

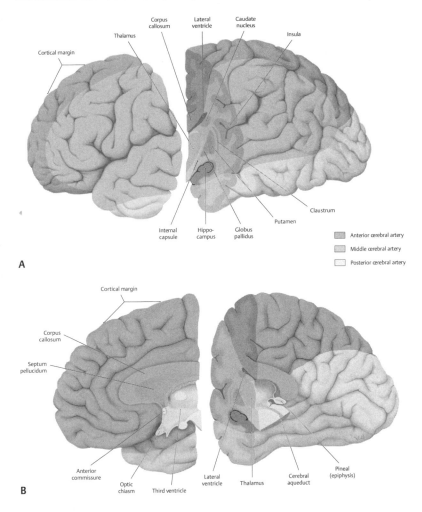

Fig. 1.12 Contributors to hemispheric blood supply. Depicted in this figure is the arterial supply to the cerebral hemispheres. (From THIEME Atlas of Anatomy, Head and Neuroanatomy, © Thieme 2007, Illustration by Markus Voll.)

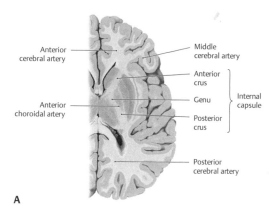

A

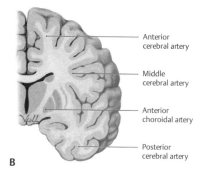

B

Fig. 1.13 Watershed territories. Artist's rendition of the watershed territories of the brain depicting overlapping anterior, middle, and posterior cerebral artery territories. (From THIEME Atlas of Anatomy, Head and Neuroanatomy, © Thieme 2007, Illustration by Markus Voll.)

Table 1.21 Watershed Territories

ACA–MCA	Cortex and deep white matter superior anteromedially.
Posterior pericallosal artery–ACA	Co-supplies the area of the splenium and medial posterior parietal cortex.
Calacrine artery–MCA	Co-supplies the posterior occipital lobe. MCA is primarily responsible for the macular representation in the cortex.
Parieto-occipital artery–ACA	Overlapping supply of the posterior third of the medial hemisphere.
Posterior temporal artery–MCA	Overlaps territories at the posterior temporal lobe.
Lenticulostriate–MCA	Co-supplies the centrum semiovale and the corona radiata.

Abbreviations: ACA, anterior cerebral arteries; MCA, middle cerebral arteries.

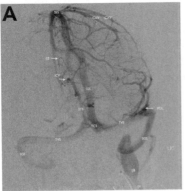 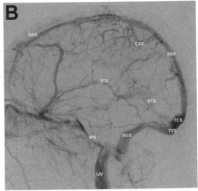

Fig. 1.14 Cerebral venous anatomy: **(A)** AP and **(B)** lateral venous phase angiography demonstrating the dural venous sinuses and the deep and superficial venous systems. (1) Dural venous sinuses: superior sagittal (SSS) and straight (STS) sinuses merge at the torcula (TCS), which then drains into the transverse sinuses (TVS) and then becomes the sigmoid sinuses (SGS) before exiting the skull and forming the internal jugular bulb (IJB) and (IJV) vein. The superior petrosal sinus (SPS) is seen draining into the TVS-SGS junction. (2) Superficial cerebral venous system. The three major superficial veins are the vein of Trolard (VOT), superficial cerebral (or sylvian fissure vein, SFV), and the vein of Labbe (VOL). Drainage from the VOT typically is into the SSS, while that from the SFV is into the SSS via the VOT or into the cavernous sinus (CVS), and the VOL drains mostly into the TVS. Many other unnamed cortical veins (CXV) are also seen. (3) Deep cerebral venous system. The deep system drains the deep structures of the brain by emptying the anterior septal (ASV), thalamostriate (TSV), choroidal (CV), anterior cerebral (ACV), and terminal (TV) veins into the larger internal cerebral vein (ICV), which then joins the basil vein of Rosenthal (BVR) to form the vein of Galen (VOG), which empties with the inferior sagittal sinus (ISS) into the straight sinus (SS).

est veins, or venules, drain the blood from the capillary beds of the cortical and deep white matter structures of the brain and coalesce to form the named veins (**Table 1.22**). The dural venous sinuses receive blood from the named veins and empty into the jugular veins of the neck (**Table 1.23**). The venous system of the brainstem is less complex but also very important, and it drains either in a transverse or longitudinal fashion (**Table 1.24**).

At the jugular foramen, the sigmoid and inferior petrosal sinuses join to form the internal jugular vein (IJV), which drains into the neck. The IJV runs in the carotid sheath with the vagus nerve and the ICA before exiting the sheath deep to the sternocleidomastoid muscle and then posterior to the clavicle. The IJV then joins the external jugular vein (EJV) to form the common jugular vein (CJV), the largest vein in the neck. The CJV ultimately receives and drains blood from the numerous veins of the head and neck, including the occipital, facial, lingual, pharyngeal, and superior and middle thyroid veins. Here the jugular vein unites with the subclavian vein to form the brachiocephalic vein.

A working knowledge of the venous anatomy from the common femoral vein (CFV) to the cerebral veins is important for navigating catheters during transve-

Table 1.22 Cerebral Veins

Location	Vein	Drainage pattern
Anterior and middle fossa	Superficial middle cerebral veins	Located in the sylvian fissure. Drain into the veins of Labbe and Trolard and into the cavernous sinus.
	Vein of Trolard	Drains the cortex superficially. Drains from the sylvian fissure to the superior sagittal sinus.
	Vein of Labbe	Drains the cortex superficially. Drains from the sylvian fissure to the transverse sinus.
	Septal vein	Runs posteriorly from the anterior horn of the lateral ventricle along the septum pellucidum, draining the deep white matter of this area.
	Anterior caudate vein	Drains deep white matter from anterior and lateral to the lateral ventricle, and the caudate. Courses on the ventricular surface of the caudate and drains into the thalamostriate vein.
	Choroidal vein	Drains the choroid plexus of the lateral ventricle. Drains into the thalamostriate vein.
	Thalamostriate vein	Runs in the groove between the thalamus and the head of the caudate, draining these structures. Drains into the internal cerebral vein. Receives blood from the anterior caudate vein.
	Atrial vein	Medial and lateral veins drain the atrium and occipital horn of the lateral ventricle into the internal cerebral veins.
	Internal cerebral veins	Paired veins located in the tela choroidea of the third ventricle travel over the thalamus and posterior to the quadrigeminal cistern. Paired veins join to contribute to the vein of Galen.
	Basal vein of Rosenthal	Drains the anterior and medial temporal lobe. Passes trough the ambient cistern. Joins with the internal cerebral veins to form the vein of Galen.
	Vein of Galen	Formed by the confluence of both internal cerebral veins, basal veins of Rosenthal, occipital veins, and an unpaired callosal vein. Joins the inferior sagittal sinus to form the straight sinus.

Location	Vein	Drainage pattern
Posterior fossa	Superior hemispheric and superior vermian veins	Plexus of veins overlying the cerebellum. Drains the tentorial surface of the cerebellum. Drains into the vein of Galen anteriorly or the straight and transverse sinuses or torcula posteriorly.
	Inferior hemispheric and inferior vermian veins	Venous plexus overlying posterior cerebellum and between the sigmoid sinuses. Drains the suboccipital surface of the cerebellum. Drains into the straight or transverse sinus or the torcula.
	Anterior hemispheric vein	Drains the pertrosal surface of the cerebellum. Unites with veins from the brainstem to drain into the superior petrosal vein.
	Vein of the cerebellomesencephalic fissure	Drains the superior half of the roof of the fourth ventricle.
	Vein of the cerebellomedullary fissure	Drains the inferior half of the roof of the fourth ventricle.
	Vein of the cerebellopontine fissure	Drains the lateral recess and lateral walls of the fourth ventricle.
	Vein of the superior cerebellar peduncle	Drains the superior cerebellar peduncle. Located in the cerebellomesencephalic fissure.
	Vein of the middle cerebellar peduncle	Drains the middle cerebellar peduncle. Located in the cerebellopontine fissure.
	Vein of the inferior cerebellar peduncle	Drains the inferior cerebellar peduncle. Located in the cerebellomedullary fissure.

nous approaches. Keep in mind that the peripheral veins, unlike the cerebral veins, do have valves that help prevent the blood from moving in a retrograde fashion away from the heart. These valves will need to be navigated by the catheter on its way into the venous circulation of the neck and brain. From the superior vena cava upward, the catheter will be going opposite the direction of the valves, but from the CFV to the inferior vena cava, it will be traveling in the same direction as the valves. This is important, because when navigating a catheter past the valves above the heart, sometimes it can be difficult to get past them and careful persistence is necessary to avoid injuring the valve.

Table 1.23 Dural Venous Sinuses

Cavernous sinus	Located on either side of the sphenoid sinus, sella turcica, and pituitary gland. Anterior border: superior orbital fissure. Posterior border: petrous apex.
Intercavernous venous connections	Named for their relation to the pituitary gland. Anterior intercavernous sinus passes anterior or anterior-inferior to pituitary gland. Posterior intercavernous sinus passes posterior or posterior-inferior to the pituitary gland. Either or both maybe absent. If both are present, called the circular sinus. May be a site of bleeding during transsphenoidal pituitary surgery.
Superior sagittal sinus	Extends from the foramen cecum anteriorly to the torcula posteriorly. Located in the midline, attached to the calvarium. Inferiorly, the dura closes to form the falx cerebri. Predominantly drains into the right transverse sinus.
Inferior sagittal sinus	Runs though the inferior edge of the falx cerebri. Drains the corpus callosum and cingulate gyrus. Joins with the vein of Galen and together they drain into the straight sinus. Predominantly drains into the left transverse sinus.
Superior petrosal sinus	Courses within the attachment of the tentorium to the petrous ridge. Drains the cerebellum and brainstem. Drains into the cavernous sinus medially and the transverse/sigmoid sinus laterally.
Inferior petrosal sinus	Located at the junction of the petrous bone with the basilar occipital bone. Begins with the posterior end of the cavernous sinus. Ends in the jugular foramen in the jugular vein.
Transverse sinus	Begins at the torcula. Courses laterally on the inner surface of the occipital bone. Ends as the sigmoid sinus at the petrous ridge.
Sigmoid sinus	Begins with the transverse sinus. Ends as the internal jugular vein in the jugular foramen.

Table 1.24 Brainstem Veins

Drainage pattern	Veins
Longitudinally draining veins	Median anterior medullary vein and median anterior pontomesencephalic vein.
	Lateral anterior medullary and pontomesencephalic vein.
	Lateral mesencephalic vein.
	Lateral medullary and retro-olivary veins.
Transversely draining veins	Peduncular vein.
	Posterior communicating vein.
	Transverse pontine vein.
	Transverse medullary veins.

Hypercoagulable states, local trauma, and temporal bone abscess all can lead to dural venous sinus thrombosis, which can cause venous infarction and hemorrhage, resulting in neurological impairment and even death. Mildly symptomatic cases or those with only partial sinus thrombosis are best managed with anticoagulation for up to six months. Severely symptomatic individuals and those with complete sinus occlusion require transvenous revascularization. Dural sinus stenosis has also been reported as a cause of pseudotumor cerebri, which, when suspected, can be tested with transvenous manometry and treated with dural sinus stent placement.

Extracranial–Intracranial Anastomoses

There are important connections between the extracranial and intracranial circulation (**Table 1.25**). This collateral flow can be advantageous and supply the brain with blood in pathological conditions such as critical aortic stenosis, Moya-Moya disease, and carotid and vertebral artery occlusions. The anastamoses may be pathological, contributing to arteriovenous malformations or dural arteriovenous fistulae, or they may be responsible for inadvertent vessel occlusions during transarterial embolization procedures. These ECA-ICA connections can also serve as a portal for infection to spread intracranially, leading to brain abscesses, meningitis, and venous sinus thrombosis. Artificial connections between the ECA and ICA circulation can be made by a neurosurgeon to revascularize vascular territories, such as the STA-MCA bypasses used to treat M1 occlusions and Moya-Moya disease.

Table 1.25 Major Arterial Anastomoses

Major artery	Branch	Anastomoses
ECA	Superior thyroid artery	Subclavian via inferior thyroid artery. Contralateral superior thyroid artery. Arteria thyroidea ima off brachiocephalic trunk.
	Ascending pharyngeal artery	ICA via C2, C2–C3, and C4 segments (caroticotympanic, vidian arteries and inferolateral trunk, respectively). ECA via occipital artery, middle meningeal, accessory meningeal, dorsal pharyngeal, and ascending palatine arteries. Hazardous during embolization of extracranial lesions. VA via musculospinal branches. Subclavian via ascending cervical artery.
	Lingual artery	ECA via facial and superior thyroid arteries.
	Facial artery	ICA via ophthalmic artery. ECA via angular, lingual, and transverse facial arteries.
	Occipital artery	ECA via ascending pharyngeal, superficial temporal, and posterior auricular arteries. VA via musculospinal branches. Subclavian artery via ascending cervical artery.
	Posterior auricular artery	ECA via occipital and superior temporal arteries.
	Superficial temporal artery	ICA via ophthalmic artery. ECA via facial, occipital, and maxillary arteries.
	Internal maxillary artery	ICA via inferolateral trunk, ophthalmic artery (deep collaterals and ethmoid), and vidian artery. ECA via infraorbital, buccal, anterior deep temporal, transverse facial, facial, and ophthalmic arteries.
ICA	ICA	BA via persistent trigeminal, proatlantal, otic, or hypoglossal arteries.
		C6: Ophthalmic segment, lingual, recurrent meningeal, middle meningeal arteries; ophthalmic, extraorbital, ethmoidal, facial arteries.
		C7: Anterior choroidal, medial posterior choriodal arteries.

Major artery	Branch	Anastomoses
Intracranial		Circle of Willis, leptomeningeal collaterals, transdural.
Extracranial	Steal syndromes	Subclavian (reverse flow in VA from a subclavian artery obstruction proximal to the VA origin). Carotid (CCA occlusion with ECA flow reversal), jaw claudication.

Abbreviations: BA, basilar artery; CCA, common carotid artery; ECA, external carotid artery; ICA, internal carotid artery; VA, vertebral artery.

References

1. Martini FH, Timmons MJ. *Human Anatomy*, 2nd ed. Prentice Hall; 1997
2. Schoenwolf GC, Bleyl SB, Brauer PR, Francis-West P. *Larsen's Human Embryology*, 4th ed. Churchill Livingstone; 2009
3. Morris P. *Practical Neuroangiography*, 2nd ed. Lippincott Williams & Wilkins; 2007
4. Osborn AG. *Diagnostic Cerebral Angiography*, 2nd ed. Lippincott Williams & Wilkins; 1999
5. Roach E, Riela A. *Pediatric Cerebrovascular Disorders*, 2nd ed. Futura Publishing; 1995
6. Schuenke M, Schulte E, Schumacher U. *Thieme Atlas of Anatomy: Head and Neuroanatomy*. Thieme Medical Publishers; 2010

Vascular Anatomy of the Spine and Spinal Cord

Raymond D. Turner IV, M. Imran Chaudry, and Aquilla S. Turk

As stated in the previous chapter, the development of the adult aortic, extracranial, and intracranial vascular networks requires an incalculable number of steps in both the embryonic and postnatal phases. The development of the vascular anatomy of the spine and spinal cord is no different. Variants in anatomical structure in the spine and spinal cord vasculature are also very common and are often unrecognized due to the redundancy of the vascular supply. As is the case with the vasculature of the head and neck, knowledge of the intimate details of the embryologic development of the spinal vasculature will rarely be necessary, so the descriptions below involve only the fundamentals of these processes. Further details should be gleaned from texts specifically written on the topic of spine and spinal cord vascular anatomy.

Early Development of Spinal Vasculature (<6 Weeks)

Until the third week of embryogenesis, 31 pairs of somites, which are segmental masses of mesoderm, develop and migrate toward the midline of the neural tube. Once reaching this phase, the somites fuse and then separate into cranial and caudal halves (**Fig. 2.1**). The caudal portion of the somite above fuses with the cranial portion of the somite below, leading to the development of the vertebral bodies. The intervertebral disc is formed from the remnant of the cranial-caudal division of the somite.

Each somite receives one pair of arteries, that is, the segmental arteries, which originate from the dorsal aorta (**Fig. 2.2**). Each segmental artery supplies blood to the corresponding ipsilateral metamer (neural crest, neural tube, and somites): skin, muscle, bone, spinal nerve, and spinal cord.[1] The segmental arteries subsequently divide into several divisions: (1) the ventral radiculo-medullary, supplying the anterior two-thirds of the spinal cord and (2) the dorsal radiculo-pial artery that supplies the epidural structures, dura mater and posterior third of the spinal cord (**Fig. 2.3**). The dorsal pial network (an anastomotic network of arteries that surround the spinal cord) eventually forms the bilateral posterolateral arteries to the spinal cord (**Fig. 2.4**).

These early stages, 3 to 6 weeks after gestation, of vascular development in and around the spinal cord are thought to be a time when vascular malformations are initiated. As the longitudinal venous channels form along both the ventral and dorsal surfaces of the spinal cord, other arterial anastomoses occur along the dorsal surface, giving an opportunity for variations in anatomical formation. Approximately 20% of those individuals harboring spinal vascular malformations have either other systemic vascular malformations or vascular malformations through-

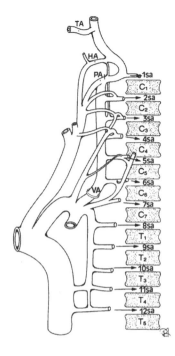

Fig. 2.1 Metameric distribution of the segmental arteries: (C) cervical, (T) thoracic, (SA) segmental artery, (TA) trigeminal artery, (HA) hypoglossal artery, (PA1) proatlantal artery, type 1, and (VA) vertebral artery. (With kind permission from Springer Science+Business Media: Lasjaunias P, Berenstein A, ter Brugge K. *Surgical Neuroangiography*, 2nd ed. Springer; 2004:73–164.)

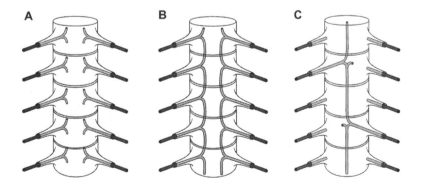

Fig. 2.2 Development of the central ventral artery. **(A)** Metameric stage, where one artery follows the spinal nerve to supply the corresponding neural tube. **(B)** Development of the longitudinal network through anastomosis of the metameric homologues. **(C)** The central ventral artery is formed through fusion and desegmentation. (With kind permission from Springer Science+Business Media: Lasjaunias P, Berenstein A, ter Brugge K. *Surgical Neuroangiography*, 2nd ed. Springer; 2004:73–164.)

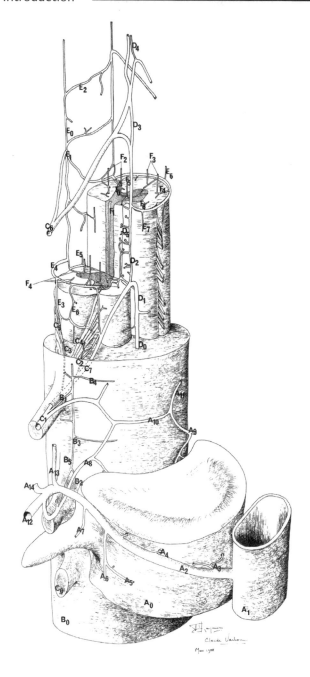

out the spinal axis. As discussed later in this handbook, spinal vascular malformations are most commonly classified into several groups, differentiated by their location, whether intradural, extradural, at the conus, or in various combinations.

Spinal Cord Blood Supply (6 Weeks to 4 Months)

Prior to the midline ventral formation of the anterior spinal artery, each longitudinal ventral neural axis provides several arterial branches, which run longitudinally and deep within the ventral sulcus and supply the anterior two-thirds of the spinal cord. These arteries provide the penetrating perforators into the spinal cord (sulcal arteries) (**Fig. 2.5**), known as the centrifugal system of Adamkiewicz.[2,3] At the cervical and lumbar enlargements, these sulcal arteries supply nearly half of the blood to the spinal cord proper, while the other half is supplied by direct ventral and pial sources (**Fig. 2.6**). In the thoracic region, the vast majority of the blood supply is derived from the ventral neural axis and pial network, not from the sulcal arteries.[4]

In conjunction with the development of the sulcal arteries, regression of the radicular arteries begins to take place as the axial organization of the spinal vasculature evolves into a longitudinal orientation. Thus, only 4–8 ventral radicular arteries and 10–20 dorsal radicular arteries remain at 4 months.[5] These remaining radicular arteries supply the entire radiculo-medullary and radiculo-pial networks. Nonfusion of the paired ventral arteries can occur during these processes, and the arteries end up as fenestrated or unfused arteries. Radiographically, they have a characteristic "diamond" shape at that segment.[6]

Within the spinal canal, longitudinal anastomotic channels form the specific vascular structures listed in **Table 2.1**.

Fig. 2.3 Detailed arterial supply of the spine and spinal cord. A0: vertebral artery, A1: aorta, A2: lumbar or intercostal artery, A3: ventral somatic branch, A4: ventromedial somatic branch, A5: ventrolateral somatic branch, A6: prevertebral anastomosis, A7: osseous branch, A8: dorsal somatic branch, A9: dorsal somatic anastomosis (ascending branch), A10: dorsal somatic anastomosis, A11: dorsal somatic anastomosis (descending branch), A12: intercostal branch, A13: paravertebral anastomosis, A14: dorsal trunk, B0: dural sheath, B1: dural artery, B2: descending dural branch, B3: ascending dural branch, B4: transverse dural branch, B5: ventrodorsal branch, C0: spinal nerve, C1: radicular artery, C2: ventral branch (radiculopial), C3: dorsal branch (radiculopial), C4: ventral root, C5: dorsal root, C6: common ventral and dorsal radiculospinal artery, C7: radiculomedullary artery, D0: ventral spinal axis, D1: descending branch, D2: ascending branch, D3: fenestrated ventral axis, D4: duplicated ventral axis, D5: perforating branch, E0: posterospinal artery, E1: bilateral posterospinal trunk, E2: dorsal medullary anastomosis, E3: lateral spinal artery, E4: coronary anastomosis, E5: dorsal funicular artery, E6: lateral funicular artery, E7: ventral funicular artery, F0: dorsal horn, F1: ependymal canal, F2: longitudinal dorsal intramedullary anastomosis, F3: longitudinal lateral intramedullary anastomosis, F4: perforating artery, F5: longitudinal medial intramedullary anastomosis, F6: longitudinal ventral intramedullary anastomosis. (With kind permission from Springer Science+Business Media: Lasjaunias P, Berenstein A, ter Brugge K. *Surgical Neuroangiography*, 2nd ed. Springer; 2004:73–164.)

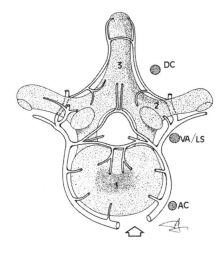

Fig. 2.4 Axial view of longitudinal spinal arterial supply: (1) vertebral body, (2) transverse process, (3) spinal process, (AC) ascending cervical artery, (VA) vertebral artery, (LS) lateral sacral artery, and (DC) deep cervical artery. (With kind permission from Springer Science+Business Media: Lasjaunias P, Berenstein A, ter Brugge K. *Surgical Neuroangiography*, 2nd ed. Springer: 2004:73–164, Fig. 2.15.)

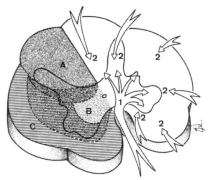

Fig. 2.5 Axial distribution of spinal cord arterial supply. The sulcocommissural (1,B) and radial (2,A,C) supply the spinal cord with multiple areas of overlap. (With kind permission from Springer Science+Business Media: Lasjaunias P, Berenstein A, ter Brugge K. *Surgical Neuroangiography*, 2nd ed. Springer; 2004:73–164, Fig. 2.76.)

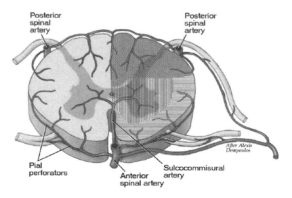

Fig. 2.6 Vascular territories of the anterior and posterior spinal arteries. (With kind permission from Elsevier: Wells-Roth D, Zonnenshayn M. Vascular anatomy of the spine. Operative Techniques in Neurosurgery Sept 2003;6(3):116–121, Fig. 5.)

Table 2.1 Developing Arteries and Their Origins

Artery of origin	Developing artery
Cervical vertebral arteries	Anterior spinal artery
Subclavian and/or supreme intercostal arteries	Upper thoracic intercostals (T2–T5)
Internal iliac arteries	Lateral sacral arteries
Caudal dorsal aorta	Middle sacral artery

Adult Spinal Arterial Anatomy

Spinal Arteries

The majority of the blood supply to the spine is credited to the segmental arterial system (**Fig. 2.7**). Other sources can and do involve the surrounding muscles of the para-axial group, such as the nuchal, interspinal, intercostal, prevertebral, scalenus, iliac, etc.; the bone; and the dura.

Two consecutive segmental arteries that normally anastomose on the posterior surface of the vertebral body bilaterally supply a given vertebral segment. Many anastomoses occur between these arteries and can supply multiple levels, often through longitudinal intersegmental extraspinal anastomoses. However, at the intercostal, lumbar, and sacral levels, direct supply from the aorta feeds each vertebral segment. Extradural anastomoses can occur in the intraspinal and extraspinal directions (**Fig. 2.8**).

Radicular Arteries

In the fully developed spinal vasculature, there are 62 segmental arteries (31 on the left, 31 on the right), one per spinal nerve root, which always travel with the spinal nerve and enter the corresponding neural foramen as they ascend with the nerve under the pedicle.[7] The segmental arteries can arise from a common trunk. The origins of the segmental arteries become more posterior the more caudal the segment examined.

The radicular artery, which travels with the spinal nerve, provides branches to both the ventral and dorsal spinal nerves. These small arteries are usually not visualized on angiography unless there is a hypervascular lesion. At the dural entry point, there is often a focal narrowing. Once intradural, the radicular arteries can be subdivided into two subtypes, the radiculo-medullary and radiculo-pial arteries.[8]

Radiculo-Medullary Arteries

Radiculo-medullary arteries are the dominant ventral supply to the spinal cord (anterior two-thirds), contributing to both the segmental system and longitudinal systems,[7] as discussed above, and often varying in number and location. The arteries are located ventral to the ventral nerve root and branch into both ascend-

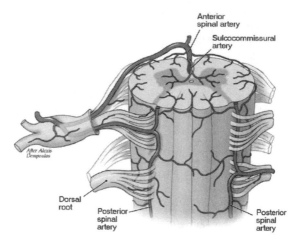

Fig. 2.7 Anterior and posterior spinal arteries. (With kind permission from Elsevier: Wells-Roth D, Zonnenshayn M. Vascular anatomy of the spine. Operative Techniques in Neurosurgery Sept 2003;6(3):116–121, Fig. 1.)

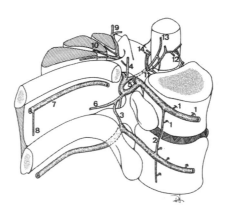

Fig. 2.8 Extradural and extraspinal branches of the intercostal system. (1) Vertebral body arteries, (2) anterolateral anastomotic artery, (3) pretransverse anastomosis, (4) pretransverse anastomosis, (5) dorsospinal artery, (6) first perforating muscular branch, (7) lateral muscular branch, (8) second perforating muscular branch and its cutaneous collateral, (9) dorsal muscular branch (medial division and longitudinal anastomosis), (10) middle and lateral muscular branches of the dorsal muscular group, (11) meningo-radicular artery, (12) retrocorporeal anastomosis, (13) dural branch, and (14) prelaminar artery or dorsal epidural branch. (With kind permission from Springer Science+Business Media: Lasjaunias P, Berenstein A, ter Brugge K. *Surgical Neuroangiography*, 2nd ed. Springer; 2004:73–164, Fig. 2.21.)

ing and descending vessels. These vessels are located in the ventral fissure of the spinal cord and are called the paired ventral neural arteries.[9] These paired arteries most often fuse in the midline to form the anterior spinal artery. The anterior spinal artery may be discontinuous focally (nonfused) and display various changes in caliber. Its normal course is from the basilar artery to the filum terminale in the subpial space within the ventral sulcus of the spinal cord, dorsal to the veins. The junction of the radiculo-medullary artery with the anterior spinal artery in the cervical region has a "Y" shape appearance, whereas in the thoracolumbar region, it has the more characteristic "hairpin" turn.

The posterolateral arteries are medullary arteries supplying the ipsilateral posterior third of the spinal cord in a centro-fugal fashion, as opposed to the pial network, which supplies the spinal cord in a centro-pedal manner.[7] The artery of lumbar enlargement, or artery of Adamkiewicz, usually arises between T9–T12 on the left side. When the artery of Adamkiewicz arises below L2 or above T8, a second ventral radiculo-medullary artery exists cranially or caudally to supply the thoraco-lumbar region[7] (**Fig. 2.9**).

Radiculo-Pial Arteries

Radiculo-pial arteries originate dorsally and travel ventrally to either the dorsal (most common) or ventral nerve root; they supply the pial network and provide branches to the nerve roots along their course. The radiculo-pial arteries do not contribute to the ventral spinal arteries and are identified angiographically by

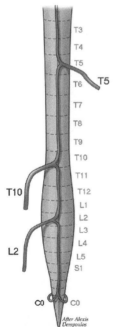

Fig. 2.9 Variations of the artery of Adamkiewicz. The most common location of the artery of Adamkiewicz is between T9–T12 (75%) followed by T5–T8 (15%) and L1–L2 (10%). (With kind permission from Elsevier: Wells-Roth D, Zonnenshayn M. Vascular anatomy of the spine. Operative Techniques in Neurosurgery Sept 2003;6(3):116–121, Fig. 4.)

hairpin turns as they join the pial network.[7] The upper cervical spinal cord derives its pial network blood supply from the vertebral arteries, posterior inferior cerebellar artery, and lateral spinal arteries.[10,11]

Pial Arterial Network

The spinal pial network can be broken down into three sections (ventral, dorsal, and lateral), all of which anastomose in the axial plane.

The ventral pial network receives its blood supply from the ventral radiculo-pial arteries, lateral pial network, and the radiculo-medullary arteries and assists the anterior spinal artery in supplying the ventral funiculus.

The dorsal network runs longitudinally (dorsolateral spinal arteries) either dorsally or ventrally to the dorsal nerve roots over the midline and supplies perforators to the dorsal funiculus.[6]

The lateral network runs longitudinally between the ventral and dorsal nerve roots, obtains blood supply from both the radiculo-pial and radiculo-medullary arteries, and provides anastomoses between the dorsal and ventral pial networks.[12] There is no true longitudinal lateral system, as it is mainly an axial plane connector between the dorsal and ventral systems. In the cervical region, the lateral spinal artery provides the blood supply of the lateral network, which, in turn, supplies the lateral funiculus.[12]

Adult Spinal Venous Anatomy

The Medullary Venous System

The spinal venous network has often been described as highly variable but with a consistent organization. Throughout the spinal cord, there is a network of capillaries that are arranged both axially and longitudinally. Their distribution throughout the spinal cord is usually symmetric; however, there is a slight ventral dominance in the thoracolumbar region and a dorsal dominance in the thoracic region.[4] Axially, there is a network of transmedullary anastomoses that connects most radial and sulcal veins (dorsal and ventral). A longitudinal anastomotic venous network is present throughout the spinal cord, but it is not responsible for direct drainage of the spinal cord (**Fig. 2.10**).

While primary pathologic malformations of the adult spinal venous network are very rare, cavernous malformations in the spinal cord will often be associated with other venous malformations. However, just as in intracranial venous anomalies, these developmental anomalies normally should not be resected, as they probably drain normal tissue of the spinal cord. Venous pathology is usually a result of fistulization and is normally not primarily venous in origin.Therefore, venous pathology normally improves once the upstream etiology is corrected.

Perimedullary Veins

The extrinsic venous network of the spinal cord consists of a pial venous network and the spinal radicular veins (**Fig. 2.11**). The pial venous network is a longitudinal system that receives drainage from the intrinsic system and is uniformly

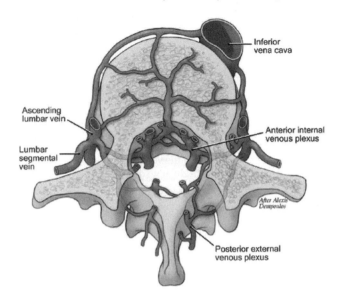

Fig. 2.10   Axial view of the venous drainage of the lumbar spine. (With kind permission from Elsevier: Wells-Roth D, Zonnenshayn M. Vascular anatomy of the spine. Operative Techniques in Neurosurgery Sept 2003;6(3):116–121, Fig. 7.)

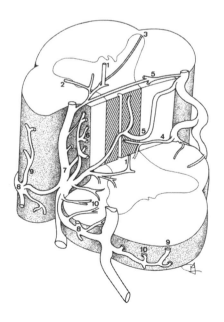

Fig. 2.11   Intrinsic and extrinsic venous network of the spinal cord. (1) Longitudinal intrinsic venous anastomosis, (2) axial anterolateral intrinsic anastomosis, (3) anteroposterior and axial anteroposterior intrinsic anastomosis, (4) deep dorsal sulcal vein, (5) transmedullary anastomosis, (6) ventral longitudinal pial anastomosis (extrinsic), (7) ventral spinal cord vein, (8) pial axial veins (extrinsic), (9) funicular vein (extrinsic), (10) radial vein. (With kind permission from Springer Science+Business Media: Lasjaunias P, Berenstein A, ter Brugge K. *Surgical Neuroangiography*, 2nd ed. Springer; 2004:73–164, Fig. 2.82.)

symmetric in its drainage pattern throughout the spinal cord. There are two main longitudinal venous systems, the ventral and dorsal.[13] However, as with the arterial anatomy, there are regional differences. For example, a single longitudinal system may exist in the cervical and lumbar regions, typically located in the midline, whereas there may be as many as three in the thoracic region, due to the increased amount of spinal cord tissue and medullary veins. This triplication of the longitudinal system in the thoracic region is also linked to the vulnerability of the thoracic vascular system to potential ischemia, given that the divergence of blood in the venous system can lend itself to stasis of flow[14] (**Fig. 2.12**).

This redundant and divergent venous system is also responsible for the congestion and stagnation of blood flow that has been associated with spinal dural arteriovenous fistulae. On the other hand, the cranial and caudal ends of the thoracic region have a more convergent venous drainage pattern into the cervical and lumbar systems and as such, have a lower incidence of vascular pathology.[15]

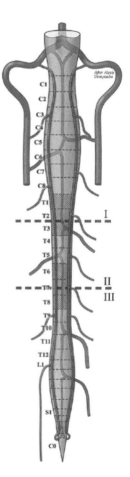

Fig. 2.12 Watershed territories of the spinal cord. The three main areas of ischemic threat are the cervicothoracic (I), midthoracic (II), and thoracolumbar (III), represented by the gray hatched lines. (With kind permission from Elsevier: Wells-Roth D, Zonnenshayn M. Vascular anatomy of the spine. Operative Techniques in Neurosurgery Sept 2003;6(3):116–121, Fig. 3.)

Radicular Veins

The medullary and perimedullary venous systems are similar to their arterial counterparts. However, the radicular veins do not adhere to the same segmentation rules as do their arterial counterparts and travel with the nerves in only 60% of the cases; the remaining ones pierce the dura between the spinal nerves.[16] Ventral and dorsal radicular veins normally occur with equal frequency. However, a known variant is the thoracolumbar venous enlargement, which is usually ventrally located.[17] The transdural portion of the radicular venous system may be as long as 1cm and have an associated narrowing, as observed with cranial dural sinuses.[13,18] It is postulated that this narrowing may represent an "anti-reflux" mechanism[18] and can lead to venous stasis and subsequent ischemia.

Epidural Venous Drainage

The epidural venous drainage system is responsible for draining the spinal cord and the adjacent bony structures. There is a clear ventral dominance of the epidural venous plexus. The epidural veins are valveless and nondistensible. In the cervical region, the vertebral veins drain into the superior vena cava via the suboccipital venous system (Batson's plexus) and the deep cervical veins[19] (**Fig. 2.13**). The upper and lower thoracic regions on the left drain into the superior and inferior hemiazygos veins, respectively. On the right side, they drain into the azygous vein. The lumbar and lumbosacral regions drain into the left renal vein, the vein of the crus of the diaphragm, and the internal iliac vein.[20]

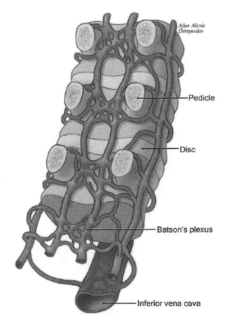

Fig. 2.13 Batson's plexus and the venous drainage of the spine. (With kind permission from Elsevier: Wells-Roth D, Zonnenshayn M. Vascular anatomy of the spine. Operative Techniques in Neurosurgery Sept 2003;6(3):116–121, Fig. 7.)

Spinal Venous Drainage

The epidural and extraspinal venous drainage is unique compared with the remainder of the circulatory system, which is heavily influenced by intrathoracic and intraabdominal pressures, which are mainly dependent on respiration. As a result, spinal venous drainage is enhanced during inspiration (negative pressure) and impeded during expiration (positive pressure).[21] This fact will often be used when performing spinal angiography to maximize opacification of spinal vessels during contrast injection.

Spinal Angiography

Spinal angiography is less common than cranial angiography. However, when there is a request for spinal angiography, it is most often to rule out a vascular malformation, generally a spinal arteriovenous malformation or dural arteriovenous fistula. To rule out spinal vascular malformations, one must be familiar with the normal spinal vascular angiographic anatomy.

The organization of the spinal vascular anatomy, as mentioned above, is in stacked transverse segments, each typically supplied by two main arteries emanating off of the aorta. Sequential catheterization of the two segmental arteries, along with the vertebrals, ascending and deep cervical, external carotids, middle sacral, and internal intercostals, makes up a complete spinal angiogram.

A typical thoracic segmental artery injection (**Fig. 2.14**) opacifies an intercostal branch (when ribs are present) and the dorsal branches to the spine and spinal cord. In segments without a specific segment supply, which often happens in the cervicothoracic region, a single segment will often supply multiple segments (**Fig. 2.15**).

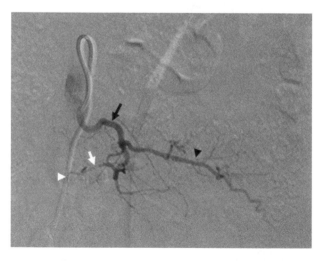

Fig. 2.14 Segmental artery injection. Injection of segmental artery (*black arrow*) off of the aorta. The ventral branch (*white arrow*) has a medial projection towards the spinal cord network (*white arrowhead*). The paravertebral artery (*black arrowhead*) fills with this injection.

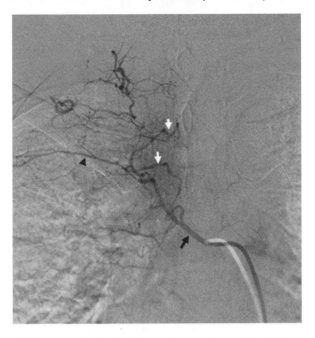

Fig. 2.15   High intercostal injection. Toward the upper thoracic levels, intercostal arteries (*black arrow*) often supply multiple levels (*white arrows*).

In the inferior segments that lack ribs, such as the lumbar segments, a typical injection often demonstrates the paravertebral anastomotic network, which may include the middle sacral artery if injecting segments for L4 or L5 (**Fig. 2.16**). Injection of a single segmental artery can often supply more than one territory (**Fig. 2.17**).

Angiographic demonstration of vascular malformations is highly varied and will be covered in Chapter 20.

Clinical Pearls

1. The midline location of the anterior spinal artery may serve as a landmark, and if there is displacement of the artery, it should be considered pathological.
2. It is critical to identify and to preserve the anterior spinal artery in cases where surgery (corpectomy) or endovascular procedures such as arteriovenous malformation (AVM) embolization put it at risk.
3. The thoracic spinal cord is a watershed zone and is at risk of infarct during prolonged hypotension and thoracic cord compression.
4. It is important to remember that the respiration of the patient may have a profound effect on the quality of spinal angiography and should be taken into account.

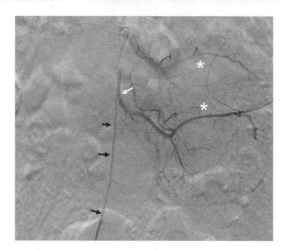

Fig. 2.16 Medial sacral artery and lumbar segmental arteries. Median sacral artery (*black arrows*) emanating off of the lumbar segmental (*white arrow*). Elaborate paravertebral artery networks (*asterisks*) can form between spinal levels.

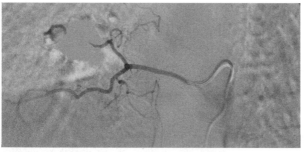

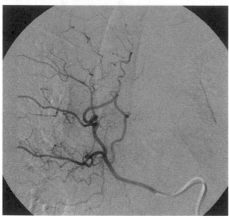

Fig. 2.17 Supply of multiple levels by one segmental artery.

References

1. Crock HV. *The Blood Supply of the Vertebral Column and Spinal Cord in Man*. Springer; 1977
2. Adamkiewicz A. Die Blutgefässe des menschlichen Rückenmarks. I. Die Gefässe der Rückenmarkssubstanze. Sitzungsber Akad Wiss Wien Math Nat Kl 1881;85:469–502
3. Margaretten I. Syndromes of the anterior spinal artery. J Nerv Ment Dis 1923;58:127–133
4. Thron AK. Vascular anatomy of the spinal cord. In: *Neuroradiology Investigations and Clinical Syndromes*. Springer; 1988
5. Tandler J. *Lehrbruch der systematischen Anatomie*, Bd. II. Leipzig; 1908
6. Gillilan LA. The arterial blood supply of the human spinal cord. J Comp Neurol 1958;110(1):75–103
7. Lasjaunias P, Berenstein A, ter Brugge K. Spinal and spinal cord arteries and veins. In: *Surgical Neuroangiography*, 2nd ed. Springer; 2001:73–164
8. Tanon L. *Les arteres de la mólle dorso-lombaire*. These, Vigot; 1908
9. Yoss RE. Vascular supply of the spinal cord: The production of vascular syndromes. Med Bull (Ann Arbor), 1950;16(11):333–345
10. Boyer P, Buchheit F, Thiebaut JB, Arrouf L, Rihaoui SA. Anatomy of intradural anastomoses between cervical nerve roots (authors' translation). Neurochirurgie 1981;27(3):191–196
11. Maillot C, Koritke JG. Origins of the posterior spinal artery trunk in man. C R Assoc Anat 1970;149:837–847
12. Lasjaunias P, Vallee B, Person H, Ter Brugge K, Chiu M. The lateral spinal artery of the upper cervical spinal cord. Anatomy, normal variations, and angiographic aspects. J Neurosurg 1985;63(2):235–241
13. Moes P, Maillot CL. Les veines superficielles de la mo'lle epiniere chez l'homme. Essai de systematisation. Arch Anat Histol Embryol Norm Exp 1981;64:5–110
14. Lazorthes G. La vascularisation arterielle du renflement lombaire. Étude des variations et des suppleances. Gouaze A, Bastide G, Soutoul JH, Zadeh O, and Santini JJ. Rev Neurol 1966;114:109–122
15. Berenstein A, Lasjaunias P, Kricheff II. Functional anatomy of the facial vasculature in pathologic conditions and its therapeutic application. AJNR Am J Neuroradiol 1983;4(2):149–153
16. Willinsky R, Lasjaunias P, Terbrugge K, Hurth M. Angiography in the investigation of spinal dural arteriovenous fistula. A protocol with application of the venous phase. Neuroradiology 1990;32(2):114–116
17. Sterzi G. Die Blutgefässe des Rückenmarks. Untersuchungen über ihre vergleichende Anatomie und Entwicklungsgeschichte. Anat H 1904;74:1–364
18. Tadié M, Hemet J, Freger P, Clavier E, Creissard P. Morphological and functional anatomy of spinal cord veins. J Neuroradiol 1985;12(1):3–20
19. Batson OV. The vertebral vein system. Caldwell lecture, 1956. Am J Roentgenol Radium Ther Nucl Med 1957;78(2):195–212
20. Gillot C, Aaron C. On the course of the branches of the left renal vein. Arch Anat Pathol 1968;16(3):A196–A202
21. Gillot C. The infrarenal inferior vena cava. Anat Clin 1981;2:301–315

Clotting Pathways and Inhibitory Medications

Celso Agner

Coagulation Cascade, Anticoagulants, and Thrombolytic Agents

The coagulation cascade is classically divided into intrinsic and extrinsic pathways, which converge to assist the conversion of prothrombin to thrombin IIa, as detailed in **Fig. 3.1**. Most often, the intrinsic is involved in vessels with damaged surfaces and requires the activation of several factors. Briefly, this contact activation pathway (intrinsic) begins with the formation of a primary complex on collagen by high-molecular-weight kininogen (HMWK), prekallikrein, and factor XII (Hageman factor). Prekallikrein and factor XII are converted to kallikrein and factor XIIa, respectively. The extrinsic pathway, which is directly activated in vessel trauma, has a more significant role in clot formation. This pathway is initiated when injured vascular endothelial cells interact with factor VII, thrombin, plasmin, factors Xa and XII, and tissue factor, which are expressed on stromal fibroblasts and leukocytes (**Fig. 3.1**).

Heparin

Heparin binds to the enzyme inhibitor factor IIa (antithrombin, AT), causing a conformational change that, in turn, inhibits factor Xa. The formation of a ternary complex between AT, thrombin, and heparin inactivates the thrombin molecule. The inhibition of the AT receptor is size dependent and, for factor Xa inhibition, it is only necessary to have a pentasaccharide binding. The development of low-molecular-weight heparin has allowed more specific binding to factor Xa that has resulted in improved coagulation blockage. One of the main complications associated with heparin is heparin-induced thrombocytopenia (or HIT syndrome). Danaparoid (Orgaran) is a combination of heparan sulfate, dermatan sulfate, and chondroitin sulfate that directly inhibits factor Xa and is often utilized for management of HIT. The absence of any heparin fragments on this drug will reduce the chances of cross-reactivity to under 10%.

Warfarin (Coumadin)

Warfarin (Coumadin) inhibits vitamin K epoxide reductase, an enzyme that recycles oxidized vitamin K to its reduced (active) form; vitamin K participates in the carboxylation of blood coagulation proteins (II, V, VII, X, and proteins C and

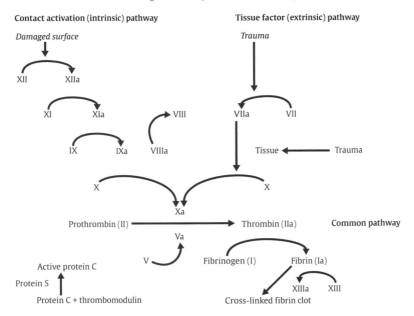

Fig. 3.1 Coagulation cascade.

S). Initially, warfarin promotes clot formation because the half-lives of proteins C and S (anticoagulants) are shorter than those of the calcium-dependent clotting factors (II, VII, IX, and X). Reduced levels of protein S reduce the activity of protein C, which in turn degrades factors Va and VIIIa, which leads to a temporary prothrombotic state. Initiation of warfarin therapy should be bridged with heparin or low-molecular-weight heparin until the INR is therapeutic. Reversal of warfarin therapy includes replacement of clotting factors with fresh frozen plasma (FFP), vitamin K, and, in emergency situations, factor VIIa or VIIIa infusions.

Thrombolytic Agents (Table 3.1)

Tissue plasminogen activator (tPA), used for stroke lysis therapy, is a serine protease located on the endothelial cell surface that catalyzes the conversion of plasminogen to plasmin. Plasmin, like trypsin, belongs to the family of serine proteases and breaks down fibrin clots. Plasminogen is made in the liver, secreted into the blood stream, and converted into plasmin by tissue plasminogen activator, urokinase plasminogen activator (uPA), and factor XIIa. Plasmin in turn, is deactivated by α_2-antiplasmin, a serine protease inhibitor. As with most enzymes, its action depends on its effective binding to a surface receptor.

Table 3.1 Function of Anticoagulation and Antiplatelet Agents

Agent	Function	Dosing
Heparin	Factor IIa binding	
Warfarin (Coumadin)	Vitamin K epoxide reductase inhibitor	
t-PA	Tissue plasminogen activator	
Aspirin	Cyclooxygenase inhibitor	
Clopidrogel (Plavix)	ADP receptor antagonist	
Ticlopidine	ADP receptor antagonist	
Prasugrel	ADP receptor antagonist	
Abciximab (Rheopro)	IIb/IIIa inhibitor	
Epitifibatide (Integrillin)	IIb/IIIa inhibitor	
Tirofiban	IIb/IIIa inhibitor	

Abbreviation: ADP, adenosine 5′-diphosphate.

Platelet Biology and Antiplatelet Agents (Table 3.1)

Activation of the thromboxane A2 (TxA2) IIb-IIIa, and ADP (adenosine 5′-disphospate) platelet surface receptors induces platelet activation and aggregation, and therefore, these receptors have been targeted by pharmacological agents to inhibit clot formation (**Fig. 3.2**).

Aspirin, a salicylate, inhibits the action of cyclooxygenase and thromboxane A2, resulting in decreasing TxA2 production and inhibiting platelet aggregation (**Fig. 3.2**).

Clopidogrel and ticlopidine, both thienopyridines, inhibit the ADP receptor, which is a platelet ATP-mediated receptor that induces calcium-dependent platelet conformational changes, resulting in platelet aggregation (**Fig. 3.2** [3]). The degree of receptor inhibition can be profound and affect the thrombogenicity of implants, such as intracranial stents and other devices. In most circumstances, inhibition of those receptors by either clopidogrel or ticlopidine can last from five to ten days. However, resistance to clopidogrel can exist in 10%–20% of cases, due to the lack of the converting enzyme. This resistance can result in the underestimation of effect and lead to thromboembolic complications. A new generation of thienopyridines (e.g., prasugrel) have been released and have a shorter time of onset, more consistent inhibition, longer half-life, and are thought to have lower rates of patient resistance.

Controversy still exists as to what test determines the appropriate measurement of platelet inhibition/aggregation; however, most modern neuroendovascular centers have the ability to determine the amount of platelet inhibition/aggregation.[1,2] The adequate amount of platelet inhibition necessary to significantly reduce thromboembolic complications is also controversial.

- Clopidogrel is a prodrug with irreversible inhibition of the P2Y12 subtype of the platelet surface ADP receptor. The ADP receptor is important in the cross-linking of platelets with fibrin. Blockage of this receptor also inhibits plate-

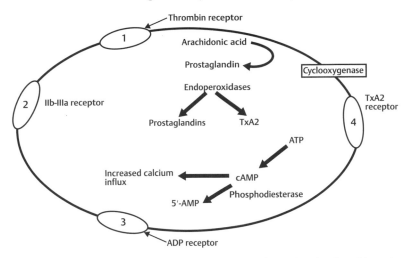

Fig. 3.2 Platelet receptors: (1) Thrombin receptor, indirect site of action of heparin and heparinoids; (2) IIb-IIIa receptor, site of action of IIb-IIIa inhibitors; (3) ADP receptor, site of action of clopidogrel and ticlopidine; (4) TxA2 receptor, indirect site of action of aspirin.

let aggregation by impeding activation of the IIb/IIIa glycoprotein pathway. The latter receptor is the final step in platelet aggregation and cross-linking of platelets with fibrin. Since this reaction is irreversible, clopidogrel's antiplatelet action may last up to 10 days. Its main uses are in the prevention of thomboembolic phenomena from platelet adhesion to implanted devices, such as stents.
- Ticlopidine is a drug with a very similar chemical structure to clopidogrel, but with a much higher incidence of hematologic side effects. It works similarly by inhibiting the ADP receptor and decreases platelet aggregation. However, the increased incidence of thrombotic thrombocytopenic purpura significantly reduced its clinical use.
- Prasugrel is a prodrug with the same irreversible inhibition of the P2Y12 subtype of the platelet surface ADP receptor.

The IIb-IIIa receptor (**Fig. 3.2** [2]) is involved in platelet-platelet aggregation and can be inhibited by IIb-IIIa antagonists, such as eptifibatide, abciximab, and tirofiban. These agents are frequently utilized in the neuroendovascular suite due to their effective antiplatelet effect with a short half-life. Abciximab is generally the preferred drug due to its fast onset of action and short elimination half-life, allowing for excellent antiplatelet effects and rapid reversal with platelet transfusion.[3,4]

- Abciximab is a fragment of a monoclonal antibody derived from human cell culture. It also affects the vitronectin receptors on platelets, endothelium, and smooth muscle cells. Since it is a fragment of an antibody, it binds to the IIb-IIIa receptor on platelets with very high affinity, leading to prolonged receptor inhibition and, therefore, prolonged thrombolytic effects in vivo.

- Epitifibatide (Integrilin) is a protein found in the venom of the southeastern pygmy rattlesnake, *Sistrurus milliarus barbouri*. It reversibily binds to the IIb/IIIa receptors on the platelet surface and prevents platelet aggregation and adhesion to the underlying cell matrix. Dissociation between eptifibatide and platelets results in a cessation of the drug effect. Since the binding has less affinity than abciximab, eptifibatide's half-life is much shorter (approximately 2.5 hours) and its action is reversed by platelet transfusion. Normal platelet function returns in less than 48 hours. Inhibition generally occurs in up to 80% of platelets and is concentration dependent.

Clinical Pearls

1. Anticoagulation with warfarin requires the simultaneous initiation of heparin or low-molecular-weight heparin (Lovenox) to avoid thrombotic events from the initial hypercoagulable state induced by the longer half-life of the vitamin-K dependent proteins C and S.
2. The effects of antiplatelet drugs can last up to ten days; no antiplatelet drug inhibitor exists, but platelet infusion can improve coagulation when emergent reversal is needed.
3. Tissue plasminogen activator (tPA) is a serine protease located on the endothelial cell surface and catalyzes the conversion of plasminogen to plasmin, a serine protease that breaks down fibrin clots.

References

1. Pongrácz E. Measurement of platelet aggregation during antiplatelet therapy in ischemic stroke. Clin Hemorheol Microcirc 2004;30(3–4):237–242
2. Zwierzina WD, Kunz F. A method of testing platelet aggregation in native whole blood. Thromb Res 1985;38(1):91–100
3. Gralla J, Rennie AT, Corkill RA, et al. Abciximab for thrombolysis during intracranial aneurysm coiling. Neuroradiology 2008;50(12):1041–1047
4. Jones RG, Davagnanam I, Colley S, West RJ, Yates DA. Abciximab for treatment of thromboembolic complications during endovascular coiling of intracranial aneurysms. AJNR Am J Neuroradiol 2008;29(10):1925–1929

Endovascular Anesthesia and Medications

Celso Agner

As neuroendovascular surgery becomes more sophisticated with regard to procedural and medication variety, careful preprocedural patient risk stratification is essential for determining potentially dangerous side effects and/or interactions secondary to medication administration. This chapter discusses the core preprocedural and periprocedural care, medications, and endovascular agents associated with neuroendovascular procedures.

Sedation

As angiography suites have advanced in terms of equipment used, such as flat-panel displays, so have the staff involved in the care of the patients: for example, angiography/neurospecific nursing, using patient monitoring capabilities, neuroanesthesia, etc. As a result, an increasing number of neuroendovascular procedures are being performed with sedation as opposed to general anesthesia. Consequently, in 2002 the American Society of Anesthesiologists (ASA) redefined sedation levels (**Table 4.1**).[1]

Table 4.1 ASA Definition of Sedation

Type of anesthesia	Definition
Minimal sedation	Patient has normal response to verbal stimulation, the airway is not compromised, and the ventilatory and cardiovascular functions remain unaffected.
Moderate sedation/analgesia (conscious sedation)	Patients have purposeful response to verbal or tactile stimulation, no airway intervention is required, there is adequate spontaneous ventilation, and usually cardiovascular function is unaffected.
Deep sedation/analgesia	Patient has purposeful response after repeated or painful stimulation. There may be a need for airway intervention, with a possibility of inadequate spontaneous ventilation and with usually intact cardiovascular function.
General anesthesia	Patients are not arousable, even with painful stimulation. Airway intervention is required, spontaneous ventilation is frequently inadequate, and cardiovascular function may be impaired.

Risk Stratification

The ASA Physical Status Classification[2] addresses risks associated with the performance of surgical procedures based on the patient's presurgical morbid state (**Table 4.2**).

The Mallampati Score[3]

The Mallampati score (**Table 4.3**), utilized to determine the ease of intubation, is based on oropharygeal anatomy (**Fig. 4.1**) and vocal cord visualization. The thyromental distance assesses ease of intubation. If the distance is less than 6 cm, intubation is likely to be difficult. When combined with neck flexibility, this score provides the practitioner a good idea of the potential risks of endotracheal intubation if deeper sedation becomes necessary.

Before determining the type of sedation, the interventionist must investigate preprocedural morbidities to avoid inadvertent complications amenable to prevention. It is important to determine such conditions as a history of arterial hypertension, diabetes mellitus, or renal insufficiency; allergies to shellfish, contrast agents, sulfa drugs, or anesthetic agents; familial hyperthermia secondary to anesthesia (malignant hyperthermia); intolerance to local anesthetics; intolerance or resistance to anticoagulant and antiplatelet agents; and hypersensitivity to heparin, protamine, aspirin, clopidrogel, and diverse antibiotics.

Table 4.2 ASA Classification

Score	Description
1	Normal, healthy patient
2	Mild systemic disease
3	Severe systemic disease
4	Severe systemic disease, at constant risk of death
5	Moribund patient, not expected to survive the operation
6	Brain-dead patient

Table 4.3 Mallampati Preintubation Scoring System

Score	Description
Class I	Soft palate, fauces, uvula, and pillars well visible
Class II	Soft palate, fauces, portions of uvula
Class III	Soft palate, bases of uvula
Class IV	Hard palate only

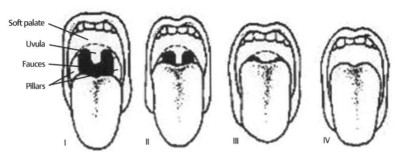

Soft palate
Uvula
Fauces
Pillars

I   II   III   IV

Fig. 4.1   Mallampati anatomical landmarks.

Sedation-Agitation Scores

Sedation-agitation scores were developed to help assess the depth of sedation in patients during procedures or in those unable to cooperate with the neurological examination. Progression from one level of sedation to another helps in determining preventive or reversal measures.[3] Evaluation of sedation and pain in children may be challenging but is rather important, in particular with the increasing number of neuroendovascular procedures performed on the pediatric population. The following are the most commonly used scales:

1. *Ramsay Sedation Scale:* Developed to assess the level of consciousness during titration of sedative medications. Easy to use and reproduce (**Table 4.4**).
2. *Sedation Agitation Score:* Developed to determine the depth of sedation in the general ICU. Easy to use, although not appropriate for non-English-speaking, hearing-impaired, or neurologically compromised patients[4] (**Table 4.5**).
3. *Richmond Sedation Scale:* Developed to assess the daily level of sedation in the general intensive care unit. Easy to administer, it values eye contact between patient and examiner as a key point on sedation assessment. Reliable and reproducible[5] (**Table 4.6**).
4. *Critical Care Pain Observational Tool (CCPOT):* Integrates different pain assessment tools into one useful scale for pain assessment in adults who are awake or intubated[3] (**Table 4.7**).
5. *University of Michigan Sedation Scale (UMSS):* Developed for rapid, reproducible, and reliable evaluation of sedation in children[6] (**Table 4.8**).
6. *The Bi-Spectral Index:* An EEG modality for interpreting cortical activity. Scores vary from 0 (no cortical activity) to 100 (fully awake). It may interfere with electromyography if patients are not adequately sedated. However, it has shown excellent correlation with other available sedation scales.[7–9]

Table 4.4 Ramsay Sedation Scale

Score	Definition
1	Anxious, agitated, restless, or all of them
2	Cooperative, oriented, and tranquil
3	Responds to simple commands only
4	Brisk response to light glabelar tap or loud auditory stimulation
5	Sluggish response to light glabelar tap or loud auditory stimulation
6	No response to light glabelar tap or loud auditory stimulus

Table 4.5 Sedation Agitation Score

Score	Definition	Description
7	Dangerous agitation	Pulling catheters, climbing over bedrail, combative
6	Very agitated	Requires restraints, does not calm down despite frequent verbal enforcement
5	Agitated	Agitated but calms down to verbal commands
4	Calm and cooperative	Calms, awakens easily, follows commands
3	Sedated	Awakens to verbal and tactile stimuli but drifts down shortly afterwards
2	Very sedated	Arouses to physical stimulation, does not communicate or follow commands. May move spontaneously.
1	Unarousable	Minimal or no response to noxious stimuli. No commands or communication.

Table 4.6 Richmond Sedation Scale

Term	Description	Score
Combative	Immediate danger to staff	4
Very agitated	Pulls or removes tubes, catheters, or is aggressive to staff	3
Agitated	Frequent non-purposeful movements or patient-ventilator dys-synchrony	2
Restless	Anxious or apprehensive but movements not aggressive or vigorous	1
Alert and calm		0
Drowsy	Sustained, greater than 10 seconds awakening, with eye contact, no voice	−1
Light sedation	Briefly (<10 seconds) awakens with eye contact to voice	−2
Moderate sedation	Any movement to voice, without eye contact	−3
Deep sedation	No response to voice but any movement to physical stimulation	−4
Unarousable	No response to voice or physical stimulation	−5

Table 4.7 Critical Care Pain Observational Tool

Indicator	Description	Score
Facial expression	No muscular tension observed	0
	Presence of frowning, brow lowering, orbit tightening, and elevator contraction	1
	All of the above facial movements plus eyelid tightly closed	2
Body movements	Does not move at all	0
	Slow, cautious movements, touching pain site	1
	Pulling tube, attempting to sit up, moving limbs/thrashing, striking at staff	2
Muscle tension	No resistance to passive movements	0
	Resistance to passive movements	1
	Strong resistance to passive movements, inability to complete them	2
Compliance with the ventilator	Alarms not activated, easy ventilation	0
	Alarms stop spontaneously	1
	Asynchrony	2
OR vocalization (extubated patients)	Normal voice tone or no sound	0
	Sighing, moaning	1
	Crying, sobbing	2

Table 4.8 University of Michigan Sedation Scale (UMSS)

Score	Description
0	Awake and alert
1	Minimally sedated: tired/sleepy, appropriate response to verbal conversation and/or sound
2	Moderate sedation: somnolent/sleeping, easily aroused with light tactile stimulation or simple commands
3	Deeply sedated: deep sleep, arousable only with significant physical stimulation
4	Unarousable

Presedation Check List

Before the beginning of any procedure, whether diagnostic or interventional, all aspects of both patient care and procedural ability should first be checked. All interventional procedures should have an outlined approach regarding the type of sheath, guide, microcatheters, and interventional equipment to be used, as well as bail-out or salvage plans and closure devices. If all equipment is known to be available before the procedure begins, it will ensure efficient use of time and an absence of scrambling if unexpected events occur. Reassessment of the patients and all of their information is also necessary before beginning any procedures. This will ensure that all people involved in the patient's care are well versed on the patient's potential for tolerance of the procedure as well as what patient access is available in case any resuscitative maneuvers are necessary. A presedation check list that can be used is offered in **Table 4.9**.

Medications in Neuroendovascular Surgery

Local Anesthetic Agents

The most common local anesthetic agents used in neuroendovascular surgery are presented in **Table 4.10**. These medications are used to decrease minor pain and discomfort due to arterial puncture, catheter manipulation, and pressure. Always determine a patient's allergy status prior to anesthetic infusion.[10] Aspiration prior to injection prevents accidental intra-arterial infusion. Test the surrounding area prior to puncture to make sure the injection was effective before beginning the procedure. Administration of an additional dose of local anesthetic prior to insertion of closure devices ensures maximum patient comfort.

Ideally, local anesthetic would have either intermediate or long action, a minimal side effect profile, and achievement of effective topical concentrations upon direct injection. Maximal doses are determined by weight and can be increased by ⅓ when epinephrine is added. Onset of action generally occurs in 2–5 minutes. Duration of action is generally between 30 and 45 minutes.

The main mechanism of the anesthetic's action is blockage of voltage-gated sodium channels and, occasionally, potassium channels. Epinephrine is generally

Table 4.9   Presedation Checklist

1. Peripheral access lines

   a. Preferably two large-bore access lines, in case rapid fluid resuscitation or drug infusion is necessary

2. Arterial lines

   a. A direct arterial line is preferred for endovascular interventions rather than transducing through an arterial sheath, due to the dampening of the blood pressure readings and the inability to transduce blood pressures once the sheath is removed at the conclusion of the procedure. Accurate blood pressure monitoring is essential in allowing rapid treatment of abrupt periprocedural blood pressure fluctuations.

3. Foley catheter

   a. Preferably in all patients where the procedure is likely to be prolonged or when the patient will receive high volumes of intravenous fluids

   b. All patients undergoing intracranial procedures, such as aneurysm coil embolization, AVM embolization, and tumor embolization

4. Mallampati score and ASA

5. Co-morbidities:

   a. Diabetes mellitus

   b. Hypertension

   c. Illicit drug use

   d. Pregnancy

   e. Baseline neurological and physical examination

   f. Baseline recent laboratory work, including glucose levels, CBC, basic metabolic profile

   g. Time of last food/liquid intake

   h. Medications: dose and last time taken

   i. Room logistics

      i. Crash cart available?

      ii. Medication check list, including availability of reversal agents and ease of drug access

      iii. Intubation material check list, including tube extension, status of gas outlets

      iv. Proximity of the anesthesia equipment

   j. Positioning of patient in relation to EVD, lines, etc.

   k. Procedure type and anesthesia considerations, time-out to determine correct patient and procedure

   l. Potential complications and backup mechanisms

   m. Pulse oximetry monitor placed on the same foot where the arterial sheath will be introduced would provide early sign of femoral artery obstruction or flow compromise

   n. Are all lines well secured?

Table 4.10 Local Anesthetics

Drug	Class	Half-life (main compound)	Metabolism	Dosage	Onset of action	Duration of action	Side effects	Contraindications
Lidocaine (Xylocaine)	Amino-amide	1.5–2 hours	Hepatic	~40 mL. In general, around 10 mL topical injection. Maximum dose 5 mg/kg without epinephrine. Maximum dose can be increased to 7–8 mg/kg once epinephrine utilized.	1–5 minutes	60–180 minutes	Hypotension, hypertension, GI disorders, nausea, vomiting, bradycardia, convulsions (rare)	Hypersensitivity to local anesthetics of the amide type or components of the solution, sodium bisulfide, and/or citric acid in solutions containing epinephrine.
Mepivacine (Carbocaine)	Amino-amide	Unknown	Hepatic	Maximum 5 mg/kg (axillary block). Maximum dose can be increased to 7–8 mg/kg once epinephrine utilized. In general, 10 mL topical injection.	10–20 minutes	60–180 minutes	Excessive doses may cause CNS or cardiac depression, leading to convulsions, hypotension, and arrhythmias. Persistent paresthesias may occur secondary to topical mepivacaine injection.	Hypersensitivity to amide-type anesthetics.
Bupivacaine (Sensorcaine, Marcaine)	Amino-amide	3.5 hours (adults), 8.1 hours (neonates)	Hepatic	Maximum 3 mg/kg	15–30 minutes	180–360 minutes	Excessive doses may cause CNS or cardiac depression, leading to convulsions, hypotension, and arrhythmias. Those are rare if drug utilized correctly. Lipid rescue useful in cardiovascular toxicity.	Hypersensitivity to amide-type anesthetics.

Abbreviation: CNS, central nervous system.

added to local anesthetics to promote vasoconstriction of small α-adrenergic capillaries. This decreases local absorption and thus concentrates the action of the local anesthetic to the area of interest. It may, however, increase the systemic exposure to local anesthetics.

Side effects are usually related to their effect on excitable tissue. Therefore, the actions of cardiac, muscular, and nerve tissues may be altered, depending on the local tissue concentration. Central nervous system (CNS) side effects are dependent on the local anesthetic concentration. They may involve restlessness, seizures, loss of consciousness, confusion, and death, if high concentrations are achieved rapidly, with subsequent generalized neuronal depression, followed by respiratory and cardiovascular arrest.

Cardiovascular side effects are more common whenever inadvertent intravascular injection occurs and when high systemic concentrations are achieved rapidly. There is a higher potential for generating cardiac arrhythmias, which are more common with certain classes of local anesthetics and depend on systemic concentrations achieved.

Hypersensitivity to local anesthetics generally manifests as topical dermatitis or a typical asthmatic attack, and it is more common with ester anesthetics.

The metabolism of ester anesthetics is generally through plasma esterases. Amides are usually degraded by the cytochrome P-450 system. Therefore, if patients have severe liver insufficiency, the interventionist should take a more careful approach when considering the use of anesthetics of the amide type. Older patients have different levels of protein binding and, therefore, more bioavailability, leading to a higher potential for toxicity. Lower peripheral binding in neonates and children may increase the chance for local anesthetic toxicity.

Sedative-Hypnotic Agents

The main sedative drugs used before and during neurendovascular procedures are summarized in **Table 4.11**. Preference is based upon ease of response and ability to reverse actions quickly when neurological evaluation is recommended. In some situations, toxicity, baseline medical conditions, and age determine the right drug choice. In the particular situation of neuroendovascular procedures, the ideal drugs have a short half-life, fast onset of action, beneficial effects on the intracranial pressure, and a low incidence of side effects like hypotension or bradycardia. In addition, drugs that can be easily titrated are preferable to drugs that accumulate in the body or have a long half-life, allowing for a slow decrease in action between loading. There is still a lack of a good randomized study in which the effects of the opioids are summated to the side effects in patients with conditions like renal insufficiency or hepatic failure.

Multiple studies have addressed the onset of awakening after use of propofol and midazolam. For acute management, there is no statistical difference between the awakening times for propofol and midazolam. However, multiple studies seem to show that the prolonged use of propofol promotes a faster awakening time than midazolam.[11–13] Additionally, it has been consistently reported that there is a synergistic effect of propofol and midazolam on sedation of patients in multiple conditions. Interactions between different classes of drugs should always be considered when choosing a sedative in the NICU. The effects on ICP, evidence of clinical seizures, or concomitance with other medical conditions will determine which agent will be the most appropriate for each case scenario.

Reversal of action of benzodiazepines is sometimes desired, once functional neurological tests and/or repeated neurological assessments are required. Fluma-

Table 4.11 Sedative Agents

Drug	Class	Half-life (main compound)	Metabolism	Dosage		Administration
Midazolam (Versed)	Benzodiazepine	3–11 hours	Liver	Preoperative sedation		IM: 0.07–0.08 mg/kg 30–60 minutes prior to procedure (generally 5 mg). Maximum dose 10 mg.
						IV: 0.02–0.04 mg/kg with repetition every 5 minutes until desired effect (maximum 0.1–0.2 mg/kg).
				Conscious sedation	Adults	IV: 0.5–2 mg slow infusion (over 2 minutes), titrate over 2–3 minutes to maximum 2.5–5 mg. Repeat every 2 minutes if needed. Doses vary according to patient's clinical condition. Dose should be reduced 30% if other sedatives/hypnotics are being used concomitantly.
					Children	IV: Doses based upon ideal body weight. Caution with IM dosing, since children may present with toxic effects earlier.
					Elderly	IV: Initial 0.5 mg slowly. No more than 1.5 mg in a 2 minute period. If further titration needed, give no more than 1 mg slowly over 2 minutes.
Diazepam (Valium)	Benzodiazepine	3–20 hours		Sedation	Adults	IV: 2–10 mg; may repeat in 3–4 hours, if necessary. Tailor for clinical effects. Reduce dose in debilitated or COPD patients.
					Children	Oral: 0.2–0.3 mg/kg (maximum dose 10 mg) 45–50 minutes prior to procedure.

Lorazepam (Ativan)	Benzodiazepine	8–15 hours	Preoperative sedation		IM 0.05 mg/kg administered 2 hours before surgery; maximum 4 mg/dose.
					IV 0.044 mg/kg; 15–20 minutes before surgery (maximum 2 mg/dose).
				Elderly	IV 0.5–4 mg/day. Initial dose not to exceed 2 mg.
Propofol	Phenol/Anesthetic	26–32 hours	Loading dose/continuous infusion		5 mcg/kg/min initial injection for the majority of patients. Increments of 5–10 mcg/kg/min over 5 to 10 minutes until desired effects appreciated. Maintenance rates of 5–50 mcg/kg/min.

Abbreviations: IM, intramuscular; IV, intravenous.

zenil is the main drug used for complete reversal of benzodiazepine action. Its properties, side effects, and precautions are summarized in **Table 4.12**.

Most sedation protocols are directly linked to analgesic protocols to attempt to decrease the overall painful sensation associated with many neuroendovascular procedures. The main characteristics of analgesics are the ability to promote pain relief with minimal sedation. Also, their half-lives should be short enough to permit frequent neurological assessment. The main analgesic drugs used in neuroendovascular surgery are summarized in **Table 4.13**.

Antiplatelet, Thrombolytic, and Anticoagulant Agents[14]

Antiplatelet agents are essential in the preprocedural, intraprocedural, and postprocedural management of patients undergoing neuroendovascular procedures, in particular during prolonged periods of parent vessel occlusion, such as during balloon-assisted coiling of intracranial aneurysms, balloon-test occlusion, or standard embolization procedures in the central nervous system. Their use is also considered whenever there is a possibility of stent implantation or during acute stroke management. The choice of agent is based upon the drug's ability to promote effective and fast effects with a short half-life and the potential for pharmacological or hematological reversal of its action. Since the mechanisms of action vary among different classes of drugs, their action is often synergistic and additive. The main antiplatelet agents used in neuroendovascular procedures are presented in **Table 4.14**.

In addition, anticoagulation is essential in prevention and treatment of the thromboembolic complications associated with many endovascular procedures, either as prohylaxis during known difficult catheterizations or as a part of the procedure in the beginning, after the introduction of the guiding catheter in elective procedures, after the first coil embolization in emergent aneurysm rupture, or after observed thromboembolic complications in diagnostic and/or therapeutic interventions. A summary of the actions, side effects, reversal, and indications of various anticoagulants is provided in **Table 4.14**.

Despite the well-documented prevention of thromboembolic events with antiplatelet agents, 20–30% of patients have been found to be resistant to antiplatelet agents. Three of the most common assays for antiplatelet effectiveness are light transmission aggregometry, thromboelastography, and impedance aggregometry.[19,20] Although the results of these assays have not been standardized, it is clear that antiplatelet ineffectiveness may be related to the patient's antiplatelet resis-

Table 4.12 Flumazenil (Benzodiazepine Reversal Agent)

Drug	Dosage	Onset of action	Duration of action	Side effects
Flumazenil (Romazicon)	0.2 mg IV initial in 15 seconds, may repeat 0.2 mg at 1 minute intervals (maximum 1 mg). If there is need for re-sedation, repeated doses can be given at 20 minute intervals to maximum of 1 mg/dose and 3 mg/hour.	1–3 minutes. Peak in 6–10 minutes	Approximately 1 hour	Vomiting, nausea, headaches, agitation, dizziness, fatigue, seizures

Table 4.13 Analgesic Drugs

Drug	Class	Half-life (main compound)	Metabolism	Dosage	
Haloperidol	Butyrophenone	18–54 hours	Liver	Initial intermittent IV dose	0.03–0.15 mg/kg every 0.5–6 hours
				Continuous dose/infusion	0.04–0.15 mg/kg/hr
Fentanyl	Opioid agonist	1.5–6 hours	Liver oxidation	Initial intermittent IV dose	0.35–1.5 mcg/kg IV q 0.5–1 hour
				Continuous dose/infusion	0.7–1.0 mcg/kg/hr
Remifentanyl	Opioid agonist	1–1.5 minutes	Plasma esterase	Initial intermittent IV dose	15–30 mg IV q 6 hours. Decrease for age >65, weight <50 Kg, or renal impairment

Table 4.14A Antiplatelet Agents

Drug	Mechanism of action	Half-life (main compound)	Metabolism	Dosage		Onset of action	Duration of action	Side effects	Contra-indications	Reversal of action	Monitoring	Interruption prior to procedures
Aspirin (Bayer Aspirin, Ecotrin)	Blocks thromboxane A2 (cyclo-oxigenase inhibitor), maximum effect with 160 mg of daily aspirin (range 50–320 mg daily), larger doses don't increase efficacy	20 minutes (plasma) Plasma peak level 30 minutes	Liver	Loading dose	325 mg PO/per rectum	20–30 minutes	4–6 hours	Gastric irritation, nausea, abdominal irritation, ringing in ears	Active gastrointestinal bleeding, hypersensitivity to aspirin, and patients younger than 13 years old.	Drug interruption and platelet transfusion	N/A	N/A
				Maintenance	325 mg PO daily							
Clopidogrel (Plavix)	Blocks platelet ADP-binding site. Inhibits ADP-mediated activation of GP IIb/IIIa complex	8 hours for the main compound. 2% of platelets are covalently bound to clopidogrel by day 11		Loading dose	300–600 mg PO/per rectum	2 hours. Steady state platelet inhibition 3–7 days after utilization	5–11 days once steady state reached (40–60% platelet function inhibition)	Bleeding, allergic reactions, ecchymoses	Acute bleeding, hypersensitivity to the drug			5–7 days
				Maintenance	75–150 mg PO daily							

| Ticlopidine (Ticlid) | Persistently inhibits ADP-mediated platelet-fibrinogen binding and subsequent platelet-platelet interactions | 2 hours to 5 days (elderly patients) | Liver | Maintenance | 250 mg PO BID | 2 hours. Steady state within 5 days | 14–21 days (platelet inhibition rises to 60–70%) | GI bleeding, diarrhea, rash, nausea, and severe neutropenia, agranulocytosis (FDA boxed warnings), leukemia, pancytopenia, and thrombocytosis | GI bleeding, liver and kidney failure | Methylprednisolone 20 mg IV (prolonged bleeding time normalized after 2 hours) | CBC prior to starting treatment and every 2 weeks for 3 months | 10–14 days |

Table 4.14B Thrombolytic Agents

Drug	Mechanism of action	Half-life (main compound)	Metabolism	Dosage			Onset of action	Duration of action	Side effects	Contra-indications	Reversal of action	Monitoring	Interruption prior to procedures
Alteplase	Binds to fibrin in a thrombus and converts entrapped plasminogen to plasmin. This will initiate fibrinolysis with limited systemic proteolysis.	Less than 5 minutes	Liver	Acute stroke (NINDS trial)	Bolus	0.1 mg/kg	5–10 minutes (80% of alteplase unbound after 10 minutes)	1 hour	Bleeding, allergic reactions, ecchymoses	Active internal bleeding, history of stroke, recent intracranial or intraspinal surgery (3 months), intracranial neoplasms, severe uncontrolled hypertension	Stop medication immediately and transfuse fresh frozen plasma + packed red cells or whole blood.	N/A	N/A
					Infusion	0.8 mg/kg over 1 hour							
				Acute stroke (IMS trial)	Bolus	0.1 mg/kg							
					Infusion	0.6 mg/kg IV, 0.3 mg/kg IA							
				Intervention		6–22 mg at clot level							

Table 4.14C   Anticoagulant Agents

Drug	Mechanism of action	Half-life (main compound)	Metabolism	Dosage		Onset of action	Duration of action	Side effects	Contra-indications	Reversal of action	Monitoring	Interruption prior to procedures
Heparin	Inactivation of factor X, inhibiting conversion of prothrombin to thrombin. After thrombosis development, larger amounts of heparin prevent conversion of fibrinogen to fibrin.	90 minutes	Liver	Intraprocedural	50–100 units/kg bolus at positioning of guide-catheter, followed by 1,000 units every hour till the end of procedure, to achieve ACTs between 200–300. Higher doses generally considered for higher-risk procedures.	Immediate after IV injection, delayed after SC injections	2–4 hours	Thrombocytopenia	Hemophilia, recent surgery, clotting disorders	Protamine sulfate 10 mg for every 1,000 units of heparin given. However, dose should be calculated based upon the time of last heparin infusion. Between 30–60 minutes of infusion, half a dose of protamine should be sufficient to reverse heparin effects.	N/A	N/A
				Maintenance	12–18 units per kilogram to achieve PTT between 70 and 90							

Table 4.14D IIb/IIIa Inhibitor Agents

Drug	Mechanism of action	Half-life (main compound)	Metabolism	Dosage		Onset of Action	Duration of action	Side effects	Contra-indications	Reversal of action	Monitoring	Interruption prior to procedures
Eptifibatide (Integrillin)	Reversibly inhibits platelet aggregation and prevents fibrinogen, von Willebrand factor, and other adhesive ligand binding to GP IIb/IIIa. Dissociation between eptifibatide and platelet results in cessation of effects.	2.5 hours	Liver	Loading dose	180 mcg/kg bolus for normal creatinine clearance. If ClCr <50 mL/min, give 180 mcg/kg prior to the procedure, followed by a second bolus of 180 mcg/kg 10 minutes after the first.	15 minutes after bolus, there is 84% of platelet inhibition utilizing the standard doses	4–6 hours (elimination half-life 2.5 hours)	Hemorrhage, allergic reactions, ecchymoses, intracranial hemorrhages	History of bleeding diathesis, hypertension, major surgery within the past 6 weeks, history of stroke within the past 30 days, patients on renal dialysis, known hypersensitivity to the product	Drug interruption and platelet transfusion	N/A	N/A
				Maintenance	2 mcg/kg/min for normal ClCr. 1 mcg/kg/min for ClCr <50 mL/min.							

Drug	Mechanism	Half-life	Metabolism	Route	Dose	Onset	Offset	Side effects	Contraindications	Reversal	
Abciximab (Reopro)	Binds to IIb/IIIa platelet receptors and inhibits platelet aggregation	Several minutes to 30 minutes	Liver	Intravenous	0.25 mg/kg bolus, followed by 0.125 mcg/kg/minute infusion	10 minutes	After IV infusion, effects decrease substantially after 10 minutes; platelet function generally recovers within 48 hours of administration, although the drug may remain in the circulation for up to 15 days.	Bleeding (10–25%), thrombocytopenia, allergic reactions, hypotension, bradycardia, anxiety, vertigo	Active internal bleeding, recent (within 6 weeks) GI or GU bleeding, bleeding diathesis, oral anticoagulants within seven days, thrombocytopenia, recent surgery or trauma, intracranial neoplasm, uncontrolled hypertension, h/o vasculitis	N/A	N/A N/A
				Intra-arterial	Range 2–30 mg intra-procedural for thromboembolic complications						
Tirofiban (Aggrastat)	Reversible inhibition of GP IIb/IIIa receptor in a dose-dependent manner. Over 90% platelet inhibition obtained in a concentration-dependent manner	2 hours	Limited, urinary excretion	Intravenous (not FDA approved for stroke management)	0.4 mcg/kg/min for 30 minutes then continued infusion to 0.1 mcg/kg/min. Renal patients should receive half the dose	Immediate	4–8 hours after drug is interrupted	Hemorrhage, which may be severe, requiring massive platelet transfusions.	Known hypersensitivity to any component of the product, active internal bleeding, intracranial hemorrhage, intracranial neoplasms, aneurysm, major surgical procedures, aortic dissection, severe hypertension, another concomitant IIb/IIIa inhibitor.	Platelet transfusion and drug interruption	N/A N/A

tance. The reasons for antiplatelet resistance are thought to be multifactorial and related to genetics, medications, environmental factors, and systemic co-morbidities, such as diabetes.[20]

Blood Pressure Modulating Agents

Blood pressure modulating drugs are very important in neuroendovascular surgery. Their desired property is an ability to manage hypo/hypertension without affecting the patient's mental status or intracranial pressure. They should also allow for quick blood-brain barrier equilibrium and a fast action in the intracranial vasculature. Multiple neuroendovascular procedures, including embolization of arteriovenous malformations and balloon occlusion testing, may require drugs that allow for the induction of controlled hypotensive episodes. In addition, rescue vasopressor medications should be readily available to induce rapid recovery of normotension if patients become symptomatic during induced hypotension. Beta-adrenergic agents and calcium channel blockers, as well as nitrates, are the main drug categories used in blood pressure modulation during neuroendovascular procedures and are summarized in **Table 4.15**.

Anti-Arrhythmic Agents

Manipulation of the extracranial internal carotid arteries often leads to bradycardia and, in rare occasions, asystole. Besides the normal agents of a well-equipped neuroangio suite, pharmacological agents need to be readily available to allow rhythm control and the patient's return to baseline neurological examination. In other instances, patients with acute strokes or ruptured intracranial aneurysms may have diverse cardiac rhythm changes that will eventually interfere with the progress of the intervention. Those agents should, therefore, be available in the room for immediate use when requested.

Contrast Agents

Multiple items should be addressed prior to the performance of neuroendovascular procedures. Among those, the following factors should be considered and determined:

1. Whether the procedure should be done and, if needed, what is the contrast agent of choice.
2. Whether there any contraindications to the use of iodine contrast agents. Was any prior reaction noticed? If so, how severe was it? What contrast agent was utilized when reaction occurred?
3. Whether there are any contrast agent/sulfa drug allergies.
4. Whether there is any active asthma treatment.
5. Whether any history of cardiac disease will limit the amount of contrast injected.
6. Whether there is any history of kidney failure.
   a. Is the patient on dialysis?
   b. If so, when is the next dialysis scheduled?
   c. If there is a history of kidney transplant, is the patient on immunosuppressive therapy?

Table 4.15 Blood Pressure Modulating Agents

Drug	Class	Half-life (main compound)	Onset of action	Duration of action	Metabolism	Dosage		Side effects	Contraindications
Labetalol	Non-selective β-blocker/α-blocker	6–8 hours (PO), 5.5 hours (IV)	Approximately 5 minutes	2–6 hours	Liver	Loading	20 mg over 2 minutes, 40–80 mg at 10 minute intervals if needed with maximum 300 mg.	Fatigue, dizziness, dyspepsia, nausea, nasal stuffiness	Bronchial asthma, obstructive airway disease, overt cardiac failure, > 1st degree heart block, cardiogenic shock, severe bradycardia, prolonged hypotension
						Maintenance	200 mg at rate of 2 mg/min. May switch to tabs later in the hospital to 200–400 mg q 6–12 hours on Day 1.		
Nicardipine	Calcium channel blocker	2–4 hours initial, 8.6 hours once it reaches steady state	Approximately 5 minutes	2–4 hours	Liver	Loading	5 mg/hr (initial blood pressure drop maximum 15 mg/hr).	Headache, hypotension, tachycardia, nausea, vomiting	Advanced aortic stenosis
						Maintenance	3 mg/hr after initial BP reduction achieved.		
Esmolol	Selective β1-blocker	3.7 hours	9 minutes	3.7 hours	Hydrolysis of ester linkage in red blood cells to methanol and free acid	Loading	Immediate blood pressure control: 80 mg bolus over 30 seconds.	Hypotension, dizziness, diaphoresis, somnolence, confusion, headache, agitation, bronchospasm, nausea, infusion site reactions	Sinus bradycardia, heart block greater than 1st degree, cardiogenic shock, and overt heart failure
						Maintenance	0.15 mg/kg/min. May titrate up to 0.3 mg/kg/min.		

(Continued on page 84)

Table 4.15 (Continued) Blood Pressure Modulating Agents

Drug	Class	Half-life (main compound)	Onset of action	Duration of action	Metabolism	Dosage		Side effects	Contraindications
Nitroprusside	Arterial and venous dilator (more prominent venous dilator)	2 minutes (metabolites; several days)	Seconds	2–3 minutes	Blood	Maintenance	0.3–0.5 mcg/kg/min. Titrate for desired blood pressure.	Hypotension and cyanide toxicity.	Aortic coarctation or arteriovenous shunting
Nitroglycerin	Venous dilator, to a lesser degree arteriolar dilator	1–4 minutes	Seconds	3–4 hours elimination half-life	Liver	Loading	5–10 mcg/min	Severe hypotension	Aortic coarctation or arteriovenous shunting
						Maintenance	5 mcg/min increments every 3–5 minutes until some response is noted.	Headaches are the most common side effects	
Hypertensive Drugs									
Neosynephrine	Alpha-1 adrenergic receptor agonist	2–3 hours	Minutes	2–3 hours	Liver	Maintenance (Shock)	100–180 mcg/min IV until BP stable.	Arrhythmias, hypotension	Hypersensitivity to similar drugs. Hypotension, severe asthma, heart shock, diabetes mellitus, caution in elderly patients
Norepinephrine	Sympathomimetic amine	1 minute	Minutes	1–2 minutes	Liver, kidney, plasma	Loading	8–12 mcg (diluted in D5W) and observe response.	Bradycardia, hypotension, injection site necrosis, visceral vasoconstriction	Mesenteric ischemia or thrombosis, cardiac autonomic irritability, ventricular tachycardia and fibrillation, hypercarbia
						Maintenance	Escalate dose up to desired BP control.		

7. Whether there is any history of diabetes.
   a. Any history of oral hypoglycemic agent usage?
8. What is the laboratory assessment?
   a. BUN, creatinine, clearance of creatinine
   b. Hemoglobin/hematocrit/platelet count prior to puncture to determine whether the patient has any bleeding disorder or coagulopathy.
9. What vessels will be catheterized?
   a. If patient is awake and external carotid artery branches will be injected, choose low ionic contrast agents or dilute contrast agents, since discomfort tends to be lower with lower ionic compounds.
10. Attempt to utilize the lowest amount of contrast, particularly for patients with history of kidney and heart failure.
11. Always choose the correct agent for the procedure, including agents that will not incur increased risks of complication or pain.

The main contrast agents utilized in the neuroangiography suite are listed in **Table 4.16**.

Major side effects, such as kidney insufficiency, severe skin reactions, hypervolemia, and pain, are experienced in patients receiving highly osmotic and ionic agents. In addition, procedures like external carotid artery injections or preparation for meningioma embolization through external carotid artery branches should be performed with the use of the least ionic compound available and/or a dilute ionic compound, to allow for better patient comfort.

More recently, agents such as gadolinium have been used for performance of cerebral angiography when kidney insufficiency is a concern. There is a still significant amount of controversy regarding the possible nephrotoxic potentials of gadolinium infusion for the performance of diagnostic angiography. According to the most re-

Table 4.16 Contrast Agents

Drug	Class	Trade name	Iodine content	Osmolality	Relative osmolality	Comfort during angiography
Sodium and/or methylglucamine diatrizoate	High osmolality - ionic	Hypaque	141	633	High osmolar	↓
			282	1415		
			370	2016		
Iopamidol	Non-ionic monomer	Isovue 370	370	796	Low osmolar	↑
Iohexol	Non-ionic	Omnipaque 350	350	884	Low osmolar	↑
Iodixanol	Non-ionic dimer	Visipaque 320	320	290	Iso-osmolar	↑ ↑

cent evidence, gadolinium does not appear to be a safer contrast agent than iodinated compounds, particularly when doses higher than 0.4 mmol/kg are used.[15,16] The current understanding is that studies should be tailored specifically to the patient's needs and that contrast agents should be used sparingly once a procedure is planned.

Unlike peripheral angiography, CO_2 is not recommended as a contrast agent for lesions above the diaphragm, since it will predispose to air embolism and further complications.

Medical Management of Cerebral Vasospasm

Angiographic cerebral vasospasm occurs in up to 70% of patients with a history of subarachnoid hemorrhage. In 20–40%, it can become clinically significant, although patients with Fisher Grade 3 and 3+4 are at a higher risk. In addition to aggressive neurointensive care management, pharmaceutical spasmolysis is frequently required for moderate to severe cerebral vasospasm. The main drugs used for spasmolysis are listed in **Table 4.17**.

Special Situations

Radial and brachial access for performance of cerebral angiography and interventions has been more commonly accepted, due to the common difficulty with peripheral arterial approaches in patients with diffuse vascular disease, atherosclerosis, and physical conditions that obstruct the normal performance of angiography. In those particular scenarios, the Allen test is performed to determine if the collateral supply to the hand by the ulnar artery is sufficient. After an oxygen saturation probe is placed at the hand to be examined, the radial artery is occluded once the wrist is flexed at 20 degrees (to avoid false-negative results), and the artery is compressed for a period of time to allow decreased oxygen saturation. Subsequently, the examiner releases the ulnar artery and measures the capillary refill time for a peripheral saturation of at least 92%. A refill time of less than 5 seconds is normal, between 5–15 seconds intermediate, and above 15 seconds abnormal. If there is a normal reperfusion, a solution of heparin (5,000 IU/mL), verapamil (2.5 mg), lidocaine (2%, 1 mL), and nitroglycerin (0.1 mg) is infused locally prior to insertion of the sheath and catheter. Depending on the size of the artery, interventions can also be performed via this route.[17]

Clinical Pearls

1. Reduce mistakes by planning ahead. Always think about the procedure to be performed, the required equipment, and any possible complications to determine the type of sedation required to complete the procedure safely.
2. Monitor depth of sedation closely throughout the procedure, using the sedation scales discussed in this chapter and continuous monitoring of vital signs; be prepared to use reversal agents when needed.
3. Assess the patient's airway and check all possible allergies, drug interactions, and underlying medical conditions of the patient before beginning the procedure.
4. Evaluate the appropriate contrast agent to be utilized, take precautionary measures, and ensure adequate hydration to avoid inadvertent kidney injury. In

Table 4.17 Spasmolytic Agents

Drug	Class	Mechanism of action	Half-life	Duration of action	Dosage	Disadvantages
Papaverine	Benzylquinolone	Inhibition of muscular cAMP and cGMP, blockage of calcium ion channels	<1 hour	Approximately 3 hours	3 mg/mL at 6–9 mL/min for a total of 300 mg per vascular territory	Short action and need for multiple treatments; mild improvement in cerebral blood flow. Potential increase in ICP.
Milrinone	Bipyridine methyl carbonitrile	Inhibition of cardiac and vascular muscular cyclic AMP phosphodiesterase III (facilitates calcium reuptake). Inotropic properties in addition	50 minutes	Unknown, higher than papaverine	0.25 mg/mL at a rate of 1 mL/minute for a total of 5–15 mg per arterial territory	Ventricular arrhythmias, ventricular fibrillation, hypotension, pain. Infusion should be slow to avoid severe associated reactions.
Verapamil	Phenylalkylamine calcium channel blocker	Suppresses the sinoatrial node. Negative inotropic properties. Increases CBF linearly in accordance to changes in blood pressure during treatment.	5–12 hours (lower for intra-arterial use)	Many hours	2.5 to 10 mg of verapamil over 5–10 minutes	Hypotension, headaches, swelling.
Nimodipine	Calcium channel antagonist	Blocks influx of extracellular calcium into L-type voltage-gated calcium channels	8–9 hours (lower for intra-arterial usage)	Many hours	2–5 mg of nimodipine per vessel over 5–10 minutes	Diaphoresis, congestive heart failure.
Nicardipine	Calcium channel antagonist	Blocks influx of extracellular calcium into L-type voltage-gated calcium channels. More selective for vascular smooth muscle cells than cardiac muscles	40 minutes	Many hours	0.075–0.15 mg/kg/hour intravenously; 10–30 mg total intra-arterial infusion (in general, 5–10 mg of nicardipine per vessel treated)	ICP elevation, hypotension, diaphoresis.

Abbreviations: AMP, adenosime monophosphate; cAMP, cyclic AMP; cGMP, cyclic GMP; ICP, intracranial pressure.

many circumstances, patients may have had other contrast examinations (e.g., CTA) before coming into the angiography suite. Be specific and targeted during the angiographic study to avoid unnecessary drug exposure to the patient.

References

1. American Society of Anesthesiologists Task Force on Sedation and Analgesia by Non-Anesthesiologists. Practice guidelines for sedation and analgesia by non-anesthesiologists. Anesthesiology 2002;96(4):1004–1017
2. Mak PH, Campbell RC, Irwin MG; American Society of Anesthesiologists. The ASA Physical Status Classification: inter-observer consistency. Anaesth Intensive Care 2002;30(5):633–640
3. Sessler CN, Grap MJ, Ramsay MA. Evaluating and monitoring analgesia and sedation in the intensive care unit. Crit Care 2008;12(Suppl 3):S2
4. Ryder-Lewis MC, Nelson KM. Reliability of the Sedation-Agitation Scale between nurses and doctors. Intensive Crit Care Nurs 2008;24(4):211–217
5. Ely EW, Truman B, Shintani A, et al. Monitoring sedation status over time in ICU patients: reliability and validity of the Richmond Agitation-Sedation Scale (RASS). JAMA 2003;289(22):2983–2991
6. Malviya S, Voepel-Lewis T, Tait AR, Merkel S, Tremper K, Naughton N. Depth of sedation in children undergoing computed tomography: validity and reliability of the University of Michigan Sedation Scale (UMSS). Br J Anaesth 2002;88(2):241–245
7. Mondello E, Siliotti R, Noto G, et al. Bispectral Index in ICU: correlation with Ramsay Score on assessment of sedation level. J Clin Monit Comput 2002;17(5):271–277
8. Riker RR, Fraser GL, Simmons LE, Wilkins ML. Validating the Sedation-Agitation Scale with the Bispectral Index and Visual Analog Scale in adult ICU patients after cardiac surgery. Intensive Care Med 2001;27(5):853–858
9. Simmons LE, Riker RR, Prato BS, Fraser GL. Assessing sedation during intensive care unit mechanical ventilation with the Bispectral Index and the Sedation-Agitation Scale. Crit Care Med 1999;27(8):1499–1504
10. Catteral WA, Mackie K. Local anesthetics. In: Brunton LL, Lazo JS, Parker KL, eds. *Goodman and Gilman's The Pharmacological Basis of Therapeutics*, 11th ed. McGraw Hill; 2006:369–386
11. Bewlay MA, Laurence AS. Sedation for neuroradiology revisited: comparison of three techniques for cerebral angiography. Eur J Anaesthesiol 2003;20(9):726–730
12. Boyd O, Mackay CJ, Rushmer F, Bennett ED, Grounds RM. Propofol or midazolam for short-term alterations in sedation. Can J Anaesth 1993;40(12):1142–1147
13. Carrasco G, Molina R, Costa J, Soler JM, Cabré L. Propofol vs midazolam in short-, medium-, and long-term sedation of critically ill patients. A cost-benefit analysis. Chest 1993;103(2):557–564
14. Majerus PW, Tollefsen DM. Blood coagulation and anticoagulant, thrombolytic, and antiplatelet drugs. In: Brunton LL, Lazo JS, Parker KL, eds. *Goodman and Gilman's The Pharmacological Basis of Therapeutics*, 11th ed. McGraw Hill; 2006:1467–1488
15. Boyden TF, Gurm HS. Does gadolinium-based angiography protect against contrast-induced nephropathy?: a systematic review of the literature. Catheter Cardiovasc Interv 2008;71(5):687–693
16. Ailawadi G, Stanley JC, Williams DM, Dimick JB, Henke PK, Upchurch GR Jr. Gadolinium as a nonnephrotoxic contrast agent for catheter-based arteriographic evaluation of renal arteries in patients with azotemia. J Vasc Surg 2003;37(2):346–352
17. Levy EI, Boulos AS, Fessler RD, et al. Transradial cerebral angiography: an alternative route. Neurosurgery 2002;51(2):335–340, discussion 340–342
18. Mallampati SR, Gatt SP, Gugino LD, et al. A clinical sign to predict difficult tracheal intubation: a prospective study. Can Anaesth Soc J 1985;32(4):429–434
19. Kasotakis G, Pipinos II, Lynch TG. Current evidence and clinical implications of aspirin resistance. J Vasc Surg 2009;50(6):1500–1510
20. Coccheri S. Antiplatelet drugs—do we need new options? With a reappraisal of direct thromboxane inhibitors. Drugs 2010;70(7):887–908

II

Equipment and Techniques

Radiation Physics and Safety

M. Imran Chaudry, Raymond D. Turner IV, and Aquilla S. Turk

Neuroendovascular surgery involves an extensive list of equipment, devices, and techniques. However, one element is ever-present but intangible, colorless, odorless, and largely unnoticed—radiation, without which no neurointerventional procedure would be done. Knowledge of radiation, from the basic physical principles that govern its behavior to safety measures that can reduce exposure to not only the patient but also the interventionalist, is paramount.

Physics of Fluoroscopy

Fluoroscopy involves imaging the body using radiation, which is defined as the transfer of energy in the form of particles or waves. In most fluoroscopy units, a tungsten target is bombarded with energized electrons, where approximately 1% of their kinetic energy is transformed into waves of photons of electromagnetic radiation, called X-rays. X-rays, which contain more energy than other forms of electromagnetic radiation (e.g., ultraviolet, infrared, microwaves, or visible light), have sufficient energy (>30 eV) to cause ionization, where an outer shell electron is displaced (**Fig. 5.1**).[1]

To generate X-rays, a cathode, consisting of a heated filament, generates high-energy electrons, which are accelerated to the tungsten target by the aid of an anode, that is, a high-voltage terminal that attracts the electrons. The energy gained by the electron is equal to the potential difference between the anode and the cathode. As the electrons interact with the tungsten nucleus, they release energy in the form of X-rays, whose production is termed braking (deceleration) or bremsstrahlung radiation.

The distribution of X-ray energy levels is continuous, given the variable degree of interactions by the accelerated electrons with the tungsten target. Most low-energy X-rays are either absorbed within the fluoroscopy unit or filtered out using various techniques, which contribute to reducing X-ray exposure levels. Some X-rays are produced with a discrete level of energy and are termed characteristic X-rays. The resulting X-ray spectrum therefore consists of characteristic and bremsstrahlung radiation.[1]

Components of the Angiography Suite

Most modern angiography suites consist of a biplane angiography unit, capable of simultaneous imaging of two image planes using two X-ray tubes (anteroposterior and lateral planes), and either two image intensifiers or flat-panel digital detec-

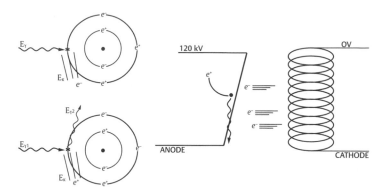

Fig. 5.1 Production of X-rays through bremsstrahlung radiation.

tors (**Fig. 5.2**), the angiographic table, and a suspended rack of monitors, which display a variety of information, including but not limited to the current angiographic views, the patient's vital signs and cardiac monitoring, and saved images for roadmapping or 3D volume-rendered images. The X-ray tube/intensifiers/detectors have the ability to rotate 360 degrees in the anteroposterior plane while the movement in the craniocaudal plane is limited due to the table. As a result, most angiographic views can be obtained.

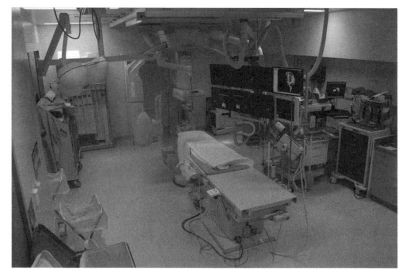

Fig. 5.2 Standard interventional suite.

Dynamic Fluoroscopy

Dynamic fluoroscopy allows angiographic images to be displayed continuously in real time. This allows for dynamic radiographic imaging, which is important for examining the dynamic flow of contrast through vascular lesions, collateral circulation, or normal cerebral circulation. Fluoroscopy is now performed at relatively low radiation doses because of better filtering and detection, which requires fewer X-rays to produce a high-quality image.[2] When image intensifiers are used, this low dose can result in high levels of image mottling (also known as quantum mottle or noise), which limits the ability to detect subtle and low-contrast lesions. However, modern fluoroscopy utilizes digital radiographic receptors, which have a much wider exposure range, thereby significantly reducing the amount of noise and increasing the ability to detect low levels of contrast. Digital fluoroscopic imaging also permits various forms of image overlay and subtraction, so that roadmapping strategies for catheterizing difficult vessels and progressive coil embolization monitoring can be performed (**Fig. 5.3**).

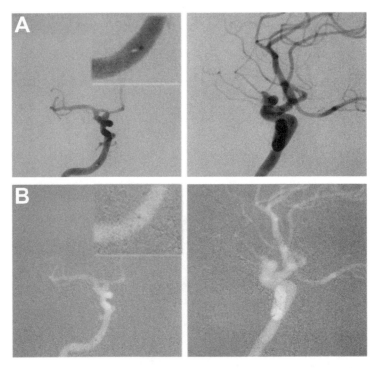

Fig. 5.3 Roadmap navigation. Images are acquired at the desired viewing angles. The microcatheter can be seen in the insert image. This image is then reversed and overlayed onto an active image, thus allowing the visualization of any radiopaque structure, such as a wire. The angio table must not be moved; otherwise, the images become offset, and either the roadmap has to be reset or the table must be placed back into the identical position.

Digital Subtraction Angiography (DSA)

In digital subtraction angiography (DSA), a digital image (or mask) of the native image (no contrast) is subtracted from subsequent images with contrast administration to show only the opacified structures (**Fig. 5.4**).[2] DSA is very sensitive to artifacts created by patient motion, which can be corrected with re-masking or "pixel-shifting." Most modern angiography systems use charge-coupled device (CCD) cameras, which record the images in digital format. If conventional TV cameras are used along with image intensifiers, the images for digital subtraction must first be digitized. An important property of DSA images is their ability to undergo post-processing, which may include changing windowing levels, filtering, or applying digital tools to measure distances and densities quantitatively. Other advantages of digital imaging include speed of acquisition, instant transfer to viewing stations, and easy archiving options.

Radiation Safety (Tables 5.1 and 5.2)

Now that we understand how X-rays are generated and what equipment is used to capture them, we must now focus on the negative effects of radiation exposure and ways to minimize both patient and operator exposure.

Several important factors must be taken account when quantifying the amount of radiation exposure; these include, but are not limited to, intensity of the source, the nature and energy of the source, and the area exposed to the source.[3] The most common unit of radiation exposure is the "effective dose" (HE), a standardized unit allowing comparisons between procedures. The calculation of total HE requires accounting for energy deposition in tissues, the responsiveness of tissue to radiation, and partial body exposure effects.

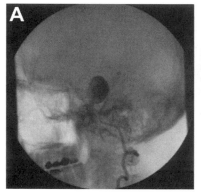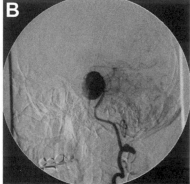

Fig. 5.4 Digital subtraction angiography **(A)** Unsubtracted image demonstrating the X-ray image of the skull as well as the injected posterior circulation. **(B)** Removing the skull image through subtraction allows the injected posterior circulation to be visualized more effectively.

Table 5.1 Stochastic and Deterministic Effects of Radiation Exposure

	Stochastic	Deterministic
Radiation Exposure	<2 Gy	>2 Gy
Damage	Genetic	Direct tissue
Results	Solid tumors	Skin erythema, alopecia, cataract induction, and sterility
Latent Period	Long term	Short term, immediate

Abbreviation: Gy (Gray), unit for measuring ionizing radiation exposure.

Radiation can affect humans in two different ways, producing genetic and somatic effects.[4] The genetic effects are generally less noticeable than the somatic effects, due to the difficulty in demonstrating generational effects of exposure. Somatic effects are clearly more obvious, because they directly affect the individual undergoing exposure. Somatic effects can be broadly classified into local effects, such as skin erythema, necrosis, or retrolenticular opacities, and carcinogenic effects. These effects can further be described as deterministic and stochastic effects.

Deterministic Effects

One deterministic effect of ionizing radiation can be a loss of function in the irradiated organ or tissue. Because most organs and tissues require a certain percentage of functional cell loss before the organ itself is disabled, a threshold dose of radiation for this deterministic effect must therefore exist. The principal unit for measuring the dose of ionizing radiation is the Gray (Gy), where 1 Gy = 1,000 mGy. Skin dose entry rates in fluoroscopy range from 10 to 100 mGy/min. The threshold dose for the induction of deterministic effects is ~2 Gy. It is important to note that below 2 Gy, deterministic effects (such as skin erythema, alopecia, cataract induction, and sterility) are very infrequent. The severity of deterministic effects increases proportionately with increased dosing. For example, skin erythema can occur at doses of 2 Gy and skin necrosis at 30 Gy.

Table 5.2 Radiation Risks

Stochastic Effects	<2 Gy
Deterministic Effects	>2 Gy
Skin Erythema	>2 Gy
Cataract Induction (Acute)	>2 Gy
Cataract Induction (Chronic)	>5 Gy
Skin Necrosis	>30 Gy

Stochastic Effects

Below the threshold dose for deterministic effects, exposure to ionizing radiation can still affect cellular function; this is more likely on the genetic level through damage to DNA. These effects involve both the somatic carcinogenic side effects as well as the potential genetic effects. These effects are termed stochastic effects. Although the probability of a stochastic effect is proportional to the dose of radiation, the severity of the effect is independent of the dose. Because radiation effects are more likely on actively dividing cells, the bone marrow, lining of the lungs, stomach and colon, and lymphoid organs are especially radiosensitive and are at risk for the induction of solid tumors. Normally, there is a latency period before the appearance of radiation-related malignancies. The latency period is usually between two and six years for leukemia and fifteen to twenty years for solid tumors.

Dosimetry

As mentioned above, radiation exposure can be expressed as the "effective dose" (HE), which involves many factors. The international unit for expressing the biologic equivalence of radiation dose is the sievert (Sv), where 1 Sv equals 1,000 mSv. The probability of a radiation-related malignancy is related to the radiation dose, but the severity of the effect is independent of that dose (**Table 5.3**).[3,4] Whole-body dose limits for radiation workers is 50 mSv per year. The effective dose is the best single parameter for quantifying the total amount of radiation a patient receives during any radiological examination. However, as stated, the effective dose involves many factors and is difficult to calculate. The dose-area product (DAP), a dose metric currently available on most modern interventional units, quantifies the amount of radiation that is incident on the patient. Knowledge of the DAP for patients allows for comparison of radiation doses for a type of examination against local and national averages, as well as between different physicians. The DAP can also be used to generate approximate values for the patient effective dose, and these in turn may be converted into a nominal quantitative risk of malignancy if the patient demographics are taken into account.

Table 5.3 Annual Dose Limits

Occupational Exposure	50 mSv/yr
Public Exposure	1 mSv/yr
Lens of the Eye	150 mSv/yr
Skin	500 mSv/yr
Extremities	500 mSv/yr

Limiting Radiation Exposure

Limiting radiation exposure should be a primary concern for all persons involved in neurointerventional procedures.[4] Physicians, nurses, and technologists involved in neurointerventional procedures tend to be exposed to the highest cumulative doses, and their radiation exposure is normally monitored via thermoluminescent dosimeter (TLD) badges, which are monitored by an institutional radiation safety officer. Since any exposure to radiation poses some undetermined health risk, radiation exposure and dosing should be kept as low as reasonably achievable.

Strategies that serve to reduce patient radiation exposure will also reduce radiation exposure and dosing to the interventionalists, anesthesia team, and procedure staff (**Table 5.4**).[4] Examples include minimizing the use of radiographic/geometric magnification, filters, high frame rates, and DSA runs, while increasing the use of collimators, lead screens, and shields, as well placing the source as close to the patient as possible, thus significantly reducing radiation scatter. Finally, it is necessary to encourage the use of complete lead coverage, including a thyroid collar.

The occupational radiation limits are 50 mSv, but the most highly exposed individuals, such as interventional fellows, are likely to receive approximately 5 mSv per year.[4] Lead shielding is required by OSHA to ensure that radiation doses to the public do not exceed 1 mSv per year. Other methods for protecting staff rely on the three (IRS) principles of radiation protection (**Table 5.5**):

1. Increased distance: The intensity of radiation decreases as the square of the distance between the source and detector increases. Although the inverse-square law applies to point sources of radiation, it may be used as a guide for scatter radiation.
2. Reduced exposure time: Radiation doses are proportional to the length of the exposure time. Reducing the overall time of the procedure or reducing fluoroscopy rates will reduce radiation exposure.
3. Shielding: The effectiveness of shielding depends on the thickness and type of barrier. Common barriers are lead shields and protective clothing (lead aprons, thyroid shields, and lead glasses). Protective clothing should be at least 0.25 mm lead (Pb) equivalent, and it is commonly 0.5 mm Pb equivalent. A 0.5 mm Pb apron attenuates approximately 95% of incident radiation, providing a substantial degree of protection.

Table 5.4   Actions to Reduce Patient Radiation Exposure

Collimation beam reduction
Exposure reduction
Small image format intensifiers

Table 5.5   Actions to Reduce Staff Radiation Exposure

Increase distance from radiation source
Reduce exposure
Shield with 0.25 to 0.5 mm lead apron

Clinical Pearls

1. X-rays, which contain more energy than other forms of electromagnetic radiation (e.g., ultraviolet, infrared, microwaves, or visible light), have sufficient energy (>30 eV) to cause ionization, in which an outer shell electron is displaced, and hence they can produce free radicals.

2. A deterministic effect is dose dependent, results in loss of cellular function, and normally occurs at radiation doses greater than 2 Gy.

3. A stochastic effect occurs below the threshold radiation dose for deterministic effects and affects cellular function on the genetic level through damage to DNA. Although the probability of a stochastic effect is proportional to the dose of radiation, the severity of the effect is independent of the dose.

4. Neurointerventionalists and staff should wear thermoluminescent dosimeter (TLD) badges that are monitored by the institutional radiation safety officer, so their radiation exposures can be determined and evaluated.

5. Radiation exposure is reduced by increasing distance from the source, reducing exposure time, and effective shielding.

References

1. Huda W, Slone R. *Review of Radiologic Physics*, 2nd ed. Wolters Kluwer; 2003
2. Bushberg JT, Seibert JA, Leidholdt EM. *The Essential Physics of Medical Imaging*, 2nd ed. Lippincott Williams & Wilkins; 2002
3. Grainger RG, Allison DJ. *Grainger and Allison's Diagnostic Radiology: A Textbook of Medical Imaging*, vol. 1, 3rd ed. London: Harcourt Publishers; 1997
4. Morris P. *Practical Neuroangiography*, 2nd ed. Lippincott Williams & Wilkins; 2007

Vascular Access and Arteriotomy Closures

Stacey Quintero Wolfe, Roham Moftakhar,
and Mohammad Ali Aziz-Sultan

Arterial Anatomy and Access

Femoral Artery

Anatomy

The common femoral artery is the distal extension of the external iliac artery. It begins after the take-off of the epigastric artery as it travels deep to the inguinal, or Poupart's, ligament. Distally, it branches into the superficial and deep femoral artery, and the deep femoral artery branches at the knee into the anterior and posterior tibial arteries. The dorsalis pedis artery is the distal extension of the anterior tibial artery. The common femoral artery is bordered medially by the femoral vein and laterally by the femoral nerve.

The optimal location for femoral artery access is over the femoral head (which provides a firm surface for manual compression), distal to the epigastric artery (which prevents retro- or intra-peritoneal hemorrhage), and proximal to the common femoral bifurcation (which prevents occlusion with large-bore vascular sheaths and allows usage of a closure device) (**Fig. 6.1**). The puncture site can be estimated to be within 1 cm to 2 cm craniocaudally of the midpoint of the inguinal ligament, which runs from the anterior superior iliac crest to the lateral edge of

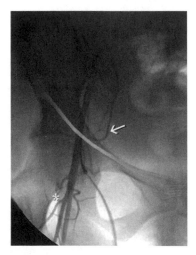

Fig. 6.1 Anatomy of the femoral artery. Common femoral artery angiogram showing the bifurcation (*asterisk*) into the profundus and superficialis branches distal to the femoral head and cannulation over the upper, inner quadrant of the femoral head to prevent vascular complications. Note the location of the inferior epigastric artery (*arrow*) just above the inguinal ligament.

the symphysis pubis. At this area, the point of maximal pulse intensity may be felt, which usually correlates with the common femoral artery. The common femoral artery overlies the femoral head in 92% of patients, and the bifurcation is above the inguinal crease 78% of the time.[1]

Equipment

Below are listed the basic pieces of equipment necessary for intra-arterial access, whether through the femoral or radial arteries or even the femoral vein.

Access Needle
Typically, a micropuncture set is used, containing a 21 gauge needle, microwire, and microsheath dilator. In some arteries that are difficult to access, an 18 gauge needle and Benston wire can be used, but their use increases the risk of arterial injury.

Guidewire
- 0.038 inch J-tip guidewire or Benston wire
- For difficult access cases (stenosis or tortuosity) when it is not possible to pass a J-wire or Benston wire, an access microwire or floppy straight-tipped glidewire may be used to gain access safely, using direct visualization with fluoroscopy.

Vascular Sheath
- Sheaths vary in length from 10 to 90 cm. Longer sheaths should be used in older patients with tortuous arteries (45 cm) and patients undergoing intervention (65–80) to decrease the redundancy and friction on the catheter and to improve stability.
- Sheaths vary in diameter from 4 to 10 French. Most diagnostic angiograms are performed through a 4 Fr or 5 Fr diagnostic sheath. Pediatric angiograms should be performed either through a 4 Fr sheath or without any sheath to prevent common femoral artery occlusion. Most adult interventions can be performed through a 6 Fr sheath, although the use of additional balloons, stents, or thrombolytic devices may require a larger bore for access.

Access Technique

Prior to performing angiography, it is essential to assess the pulses at the dorsalis pedis and the posterior tibial with palpation and Doppler for baseline comparison. After the initiation of local anesthesia (without epinephrine to avoid vasoconstriction) and intravenous conscious sedation (Chapter 4), both groins are sterilely prepped and draped.

Before arterial cannulation is performed, it is imperative that all vascular catheters and sheaths are available, properly set up, and flushed. All flush lines and Touhy-Borst adapters should be carefully checked for microbubbles, as air embolization into the distal circulation can cause occlusion. For routine diagnostic angiography, we attach the vascular sheath to a pressurized flush line of heparinized saline (1000 units/L). All wires and catheters are flushed and soaked in saline, followed by laying out all the equipment on the table in preparation. The use of a flush line connected to the diagnostic catheter is useful to prevent thrombus from forming in the catheter while setting up the diagnostic views or preparing other equipment for use. Some angiographers, however, do not attach the diagnostic catheter to a flush line and therefore must be particularly careful about preventing air and clots from either entering the catheter during wire/syringe exchange or forming inside the catheter from stagnant blood. For prevention of clots forming in the catheter, "double-flushing" the catheter by first drawing back 2 to 5 cc of blood and then using a second saline-filled syringe is recommended to flush and clean the inner lumen of the catheter. Most angiographers who do not use a flush line will advance the diagnostic catheter with a syringe connected to the catheter, intermittently "puffing" contrast to reduce the amount of stagnant blood in the catheter.

At this point, the area of arterial puncture is estimated by using palpation of the pulse with the anatomic landmarks discussed above, and a radiopaque object can be used to confirm the location of the upper, inner quadrant of the femoral head (**Fig. 6.2**). It is sometimes helpful to compress manually the area medial to the artery and trap it with slight lateral pressure prior to puncturing the artery, to prevent the artery from rolling away from the needle. If the patient is awake, local anesthesia (2% lidocaine) will be administered to the local and deep areas where the sheath will be placed. For patients with particularly tough skin, a history of several prior angiograms, or anticipated placement of a closure device, a small cutaneous nick with a scalpel can be made. The tract may be dilated to further accommodate the sheath and closure device, but dilation is not absolutely necessary. Although double-wall puncture (or through-and-through technique) is still used to ensure intra-luminal arterial access, the risk of hematoma may be unnecessarily high in patients on anticoagulation or antiplatelet medications. For this reason, many angiographers prefer a single-wall puncture technique, in which arterial entry is confirmed by brisk arterial blood flow. For patients on antiplatelet or anticoagulation therapy, pediatric patients, elderly patients with a high probability of atherosclerosis, or patients with poorly definable pulses (such as ones dealing with obesity), a micropuncture set can reduce the risk of arterial injury, pseudoaneurysm formation, and subcutaneous/retroperitoneal hematoma.

Once the micropuncture needle is in the artery and arterial backflow is confirmed by the color and pulsitility of flow, the microwire is advanced. Fluoroscopy is often used to visualize the advancement of the microwire, allowing confirmation of the left of midline position that usually ensures arterial cannulation.

Once arterial cannulation is confirmed, a Cope Mandril (Cook Medical), 0.038 J- or Benston wire is placed using the Seldinger technique through the 18 gauge needle or microsheath. During the sliding of the needle over the wire with the right hand, compression of the artery is maintained with the left hand to minimize subcutaneous hematoma formation. The wire can be stabilized with the left thumb to prevent inadvertently pulling out the wire. The wire is then wiped with a damp Telfa dressing (preferred over cotton-based gauze to prevent a microembolic shower from particulate cotton materials) to remove blood clots. If a dilator is used, it is then placed, and the Cope Mandril wire is removed. Once the cap is removed from the microdilator, the left thumb should be held over the opening to prevent the excessive escape of blood. The 0.038 J- or Benston wire is then placed through the dilator. Once again, the left hand is used to hold pressure and stabilize the wire while the right hand removes the dilator from over the wire. The wire is again wiped with a damp Telfa dressing, and the sheath is placed with gentle pressure and a slight twisting motion.

After placement, back-bleeding and flushing the sheath ensure the absence of air and clot in the access sheath. It then can be affixed to the skin with a clear adhesive covering or stitch, to prevent inadvertent removal of the sheath and to maintain direct visualization of the groin site for hematoma.

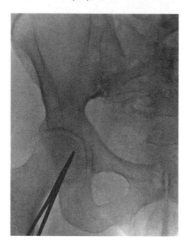

Fig. 6.2 Localization of the area of micropuncture. A scout radiograph showing the tip of a hemostat over the upper, inner quadrant of the femoral head.

Pediatric Nuances

Vascular access in pediatric patients is similar to that in adults, but the arterial caliber is smaller, and the arteries are more mobile and more prone to vasospasm. For this reason, we always perform micropuncture access with a gentle advancement of the wire without rotation. A 4 Fr short vascular sheath can be used and advanced without rotation to prevent tearing or spasm of the artery. As the sheath is short, it must be affixed to the skin with a sterile adhesive. We also may administer low doses of verapamil and heparin into the sheath to prevent clotting or vasospasm. In infants and toddlers, it is possible to use the catheter directly through the skin without a sheath to avoid arterial occlusion with the sheath. Distal occlusion, however, is a rare issue, as children often have significant collateral circulation in the lower extremities.

Radial Artery Access

Anatomy

At the elbow, the brachial artery branches into the radial and ulnar arteries. As the larger of the two branches, the radial artery runs along the radial side of the forearm to the wrist. It then winds around the lateral side of the carpus, beneath the tendons of the abductor pollicis longus and extensor pollicis longus and brevis into the palm of the hand, where it unites with the deep volar branch of the ulnar artery to form the deep volar arch (**Fig. 6.3**).

Equipment

- Micropuncture set with 4 Fr introducer sheath
- Antispasmodic cocktail **(Table 6.1)**
- Dilators ranging from 5–8 Fr, depending on the size of sheath
- Vascular sheath

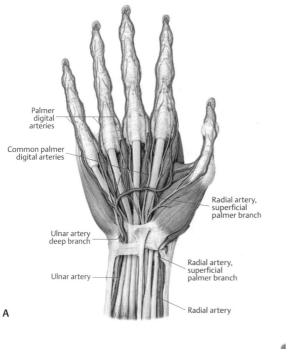

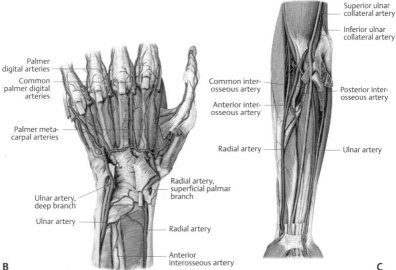

Fig. 6.3 **(A–C)** Arterial anatomy of the hand and brachium. (From THIEME Atlas of Anatomy, General Anatomy and Musculoskeletal System, © Thieme 2005, Illustration by Karl Wesker.)

Table 6.1 Radial Artery Antispasmodic Cocktail

Heparin (5000 IU/mL)
Verapamil (2.5 mg)
Lidocaine (2% without epinephrine, 1.0 mL)
Nitroglycerin (0.1 mg)

Technique

A finger pulse oximeter is placed on the same side that the sheath will be placed to monitor hand oxygenation throughout the procedure. After confirmation of adequate blood supply to the hand with the Allen's test (see below), the forearm and the hand are prepared and draped in the usual sterile fashion. Placing the patient's arm on an arm board makes it easier to gain access. Once access is obtained, the patient's arm could be placed at his or her side or left on the arm board, depending on the comfort of the angiographer. However, the patient's arm must be secured to the table in case the patient inadvertently withdraws the arm during the procedure.

After local anesthetic (without epinephrine) is administered, a micropuncture set is used to cannulate the artery and insert the sheath. At times, it is necessary to use ultrasound to locate the radial artery for cannulation. Once the artery is cannulated with the introducer sheath, the antispasmodic cocktail is administered into the artery (**Table 6.1**). Then a 0.038 inch wire is placed through the 4 Fr introducer sheath and the introducer sheath is removed. Depending on the size of the intended sheath, the artery is dilated to that size and the sheath is inserted. Vascular sheaths up to 8 Fr have been reported to be placed in the radial artery, and 6 Fr shuttles can be used here for carotid stenting.

At the conclusion of the procedure, the sheath is removed, and manual compression of the artery is performed until hemostasis is achieved. A pressure dressing is then applied. Vascular closure devices are contraindicated, due to the small size of the vessel and high risk of arterial occlusion with the devices.

Allen Test

The radial artery is accessed at the wrist, in a manner similar in location to placement of an arterial line for blood pressure monitoring. The Allen test ensures adequate collateral circulation from the ulnar artery. The examiner compresses both the radial and ulnar arteries simultaneously. The patient is instructed to flex and extend the fingers to drain the hand of residual blood. The examiner releases the ulnar artery and measures the time to achieve visual capillary refill and at least 92% oxygen saturation at the finger pads. Capillary refill time of less than 5 seconds is normal; 5 to 15 seconds is equivocal; greater than 15 seconds is abnormal. It is important for patients to maintain their wrist at 20 degrees of flexion to avoid false-positive results, which can be induced by hyperextension.

Brachial Artery Access

Anatomy

The brachial artery begins at the lower margin of the teres major as a continuation of the axillary artery (**Fig. 6.3**). It travels along the humerus, and at the distal humerus, the median nerve and the brachial artery pass through the antecubital fossa underneath the lacertus fibrosus, which takes its origin from the biceps tendon and the fascia of the flexor-pronator mass. The brachial artery then ends approximately 1 cm distal to the elbow, where it divides into the radial and ulnar arteries.

Equipment

Refer to the section on radial artery access for a list of equipment. An exception is that an antispasmodic cocktail is not typically needed, because the caliber of the brachial artery is larger than that of the radial artery.

Technique

At the elbow, the brachial artery dives into the antecubital fossa (**Fig. 6.3**). Therefore, arterial puncture 1 cm above the anticubital fossa is preferred. A strong pulse can usually be felt at this location that allows for the brachial artery to be compressed against the distal humerus at the end of the procedure. The arm is secured to the table and prepared and draped in the usual sterile fashion. The arm should be extended to palpate the pulse better. After local anesthetic is injected, a micropuncture set is used to cannulate the artery. Dilators are used to place the sheath of choice (4–8 Fr).

At the conclusion of the procedure, the sheath is removed, and manual compression of the artery is performed until hemostasis is achieved. A pressure dressing is then applied, and the patient must keep the arm straight for preferably up to 6 hours. Vascular closure devices are contraindicated, due to the small size of the vessel and high risk of arterial occlusion.

Arterial Cut-Down Procedures

Common Carotid Artery

Anatomy and Exposure

In rare instances, the arterial vasculature may be incompatible with catheter navigation into the carotid artery. In these cases, it is relatively simple for a neurosurgeon or vascular surgeon to expose the common carotid artery surgically for direct catheterization (**Fig. 6.4**).[2] A small transverse incision at the level of the thyroid cartilage will expose the common carotid artery, medial to the internal jugular vein. The external, internal, and common carotid arteries should be dissected free and demarcated with vessel loupes.

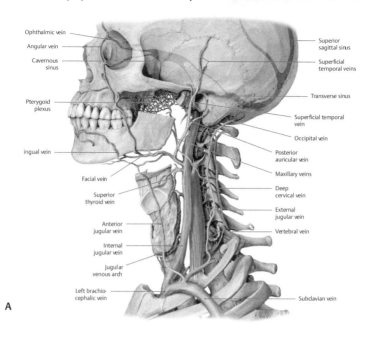

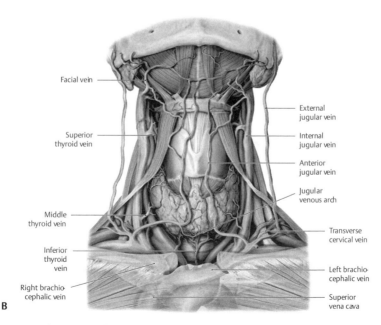

Fig. 6.4 (A,B) Internal jugular venous anatomy. (From THIEME Atlas of Anatomy, Neck and Internal Organs, © Thieme 2006, Illustration by Karl Wesker.)

Equipment

- Micropuncture kit
- 5–0 or 6–0 Prolene (Ethicon, Inc.) stitch
- 4–6 Fr short sheath

Technique

A purse-string suture should be placed around the site of the common carotid artery access before the artery is punctured. The microneedle puncture should occur in the middle of the purse-string suture. The Seldinger technique is used to advance a microwire and sheath or catheter. A vascular sheath may then be placed and secured with the purse-string, and the intervention performed. It is important to remember that the wires will not need to be advanced as far as with a groin puncture and should always be observed with fluoroscopy to avoid inadvertent advancement into and perforation of the intracranial vasculature. Following removal of the sheath, the purse-string suture should be tied securely to close the arteriotomy site.

Vertebral Artery

Anatomy and Exposure

In cases of severe vertebrobasilar tortuosity, as in direct carotid exposure, direct exposure of the vertebral artery may be necessary. This exposure is commonly performed by a neurosurgeon. The vertebral artery is located at the lateral margin of the foramen magnum, where the dural entry zone is located. The exposure involves a several centimeter vertical skin incision, placed 2 cm medial to the mastoid process. The muscular layers (3) are carefully dissected until the medial arch of C1 is localized, from which the vertebral artery can be found laterally. At this point, the vertebral artery is carefully dissected and punctured with a 21 gauge needle.

Equipment

- Micropuncture kit
- 5–0 or 6–0 Prolene stitch
- 4 Fr to 6 Fr short sheath

Technique

A micropuncture catheter is used to place a 4 Fr vascular sheath, which can be advanced approximately 2 cm and secured to the surrounding muscle before beginning the intervention. It is important to remember that the wires will not need to be advanced as far as with a groin puncture, and they should always be observed with fluoroscopy to avoid accidental advancement into and perforation of the intracranial vasculature. Following removal of the sheath, the arteriotomy can be repaired with a 6–0 suture.

Venous Anatomy and Access

Femoral Vein

Anatomy

The femoral vein is located just medial to the common femoral artery (**Fig. 6.1**). It is a continuation of the popliteal vein and ends at the inguinal ligament, where it becomes the external iliac vein. One may navigate through the external iliac vein into the inferior vena cava, past the heart and into the superior vena cava, and then to the internal jugular vein. From there the sigmoid and transverse sinuses, the inferior petrosal sinus, the basilar plexus, and facial vein can be cannulated. Like the artery, the vein should be punctured over the femoral head to allow for post-procedural compression, but the puncture should be below the inguinal ligament to prevent a retroperitoneal hematoma.

Equipment

The equipment needed is the same as in femoral artery access.

Technique

The technique used is the same as in femoral artery access.

Internal Jugular Vein

Anatomy

The internal jugular vein drains blood from the brain, the superficial parts of the face, and the neck (**Fig. 6.4**). At its origin, proximal to the sigmoid sinus, it is somewhat dilated and often referred to as the jugular bulb. A common trunk draining the anterior branch of the retromandibular vein, the facial vein, and the lingual vein joins the internal jugular as it travels laterally by the carotid artery and unites with the subclavian vein to form the brachiocephalic vein (innominate vein).

Equipment

The equipment needed is the same as in femoral artery access.

Technique

The internal jugular vein may be punctured directly in the carotid triangle and lateral to the carotid artery, with a 4 Fr micropuncture kit. This technique is useful if it is impossible to navigate from the femoral vein due to stenosis, although this is rarely necessary.

Venous Cut-Down Procedures

Superior Ophthalmic Vein

Anatomy and Exposure

The superior ophthalmic vein (SOV) may be cannulated from the internal jugular through the facial and angular veins (**Fig. 6.5**). However, direct surgical cannulation of the SOV may be an excellent alternative when catheterization from the femoral or jugular veins is not possible.

Equipment

See the list of equipment used for vertebral artery access.

Technique

A 2 cm incision is made medially in the skin crease above the upper eyelid. An operating microscope is used to incise the orbicularis oculi muscle and open the orbital septum, under which the arterialized SOV is found. Sutures are placed around each end of a 10–15 mm segment to straighten and control the vein, and a small incision is made in the vein. A 4 Fr vascular sheath is placed, and the distal suture tied to ligate the SOV. This technique is particularly useful for access to the cavernous sinus for embolization of carotid-cavernous fistulae.

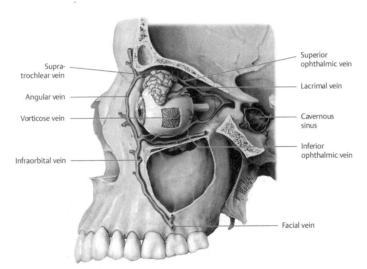

Fig. 6.5 Supraophthalmic vein exposure. (From THIEME Atlas of Anatomy, Head and Neuroanatomy, © Thieme 2007, Illustration by Karl Wesker.)

Arteriotomy Closure Techniques

Manual Compression

Manual compression has traditionally been used for closure of a percutaneous arteriotomy. The fingertips of both hands are placed just proximal to and over the arteriotomy site. Pressure is held until hemostasis is achieved; the time required depends on sheath size and anticoagulation use. The pulse should always be felt to ensure that complete arterial occlusion is not occurring, as this may cause thrombosis and occlusion in small caliber, atherosclerotic vessels. Manual pressure may be held following diagnostic procedures, but with the use of anticoagulation, it is less desirable following interventions. Once pressure has been held for an adequate time interval (**Table 6.2**), it is slowly released while the groin is observed for any hematoma formation. Distal pulses should also be periodically checked. Should a hematoma begin forming, pressure should be held for an additional 10 to 15 minutes. If oozing from the groin site is still present or if the hematoma continues to get larger, a manual compression device, such as the FemoStop (Radi Medical Systems Inc., Reading, MA) or sandbags, can be used to maintain pressure for longer periods of time. Close monitoring of the hematoma size can be done by outlining the site with a marker. Persistent increases in hematoma size should be followed up with a femoral artery ultrasound to rule out pseudoaneurysm formation. In very rare cases, the artery must be repaired surgically.[3]

Closure Devices

A variety of arterial closure devices have been developed to reduce immobilization. These devices are described in **Table 6.3** and illustrated in **Fig. 6.6**.

Potential Complications of Vascular Access and Closure

See Chapter 10 for information on potential complications.

Table 6.2 Recommended Compression Following Arterial Catheterization

Sheath	Type of procedure	Antiplatelets	Time (minutes)
4–5 Fr	Diagnostic	No	10
4–5 Fr	Diagnostic	Yes	15–20
6–8 Fr	Intervention	No	20–40
6–8 Fr	Intervention	Yes	30–60

Table 6.3 Closure Devices

Hemostatic patches	Description	Contra-indications	Arteriotomy
1. Syvek (Marine Polymer Technologies) 2. Chito-Seal (Abbott Vascular) 3. Clo-Sur P.A.D. (Scion Cardio-Vascular) 4. D-Stat Dry (Vascular Solutions) 5. Neptune Pad (TZ Medical, Inc)	Technique: Used in conjunction with compression. Mechanism: Acts on contact with blood or exposed tissue to accelerate the clotting cascade. Active ingredients: thrombin, glucosamines, or alginate	None	Any size; good for larger skin incisions

Mechanical closure devices	Description	Contra-indications	Arteriotomy
FemoStop (Radi Medical Systems, Inc)	External mechanical compression. Secure device with a strap beneath the patient and inflate bulb to 20 mmHG > SBP for 10–15 minutes. Maintain longer for anticoagulation by deflating below SBP with monitoring of distal pulses to prevent limb ischemia or arterial occlusion.	None	Any size
Angioseal (St. Jude Medical)	Mechanical seal by sandwiching the arteriotomy between a bio-absorbable anchor and collagen sponge. Dissolves within 60–90 days. Repeat puncture can be performed 1 cm above or below previous closure.	Artery <4 mm Puncture at or below CFA bifurcation	6 Fr Angioseal: 5–6 Fr 8 Fr Angioseal: 7–8 Fr
Perclose (Abbott Laboratories)	Delivers a monofilament suture via two needles deployed through the arterial wall with a pre-tied knot, which is tightened and cut outside of the arterial wall.	Artery <4 mm Puncture at or below CFA bifurcation	5–8 Fr
Starclose (Abbott Laboratories)	Extravascular closure with a nitinol clip with 360° apposition of the arterial wall. Avoids intrusion and narrowing of the vessel lumen.	Puncture at or below CFA bifurcation	5–6 Fr
Mynx (Access|Closure)	Extravascular polyethylene glycol sealant that expands in the sheath tract by blood absorbtion. A balloon protects the vessel lumen during placement. Dissolves in 30 days.	Artery <4 mm May use near bifurcation	5–7 Fr

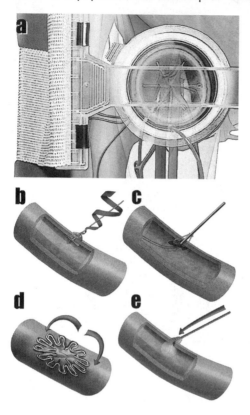

Fig. 6.6 Closure devices. A sagittal view through an artery showing the **(a)** FemoStop (Radi Medical Systems Inc.), **(b)** AngioSeal (St. Jude Medical), **(c)** Perclose (Abbott Vascular), **(d)** StarClose (Abbott Vascular), and **(e)** Mynx (Access|Closure) closure devices.

Clinical Pearls

1. Named after Dr. Sven-Ivar Seldinger (1921–1998), a Swedish radiologist, the Seldinger technique revolutionized the field of angiography in 1953 by allowing rapid and safe vascular access. Prior to the description of the Seldinger technique, sharp trocars were used to create lumens through which devices could be passed, resulting in a high rate of complications.
2. A scout flouroscopic image should be performed prior to puncture to ensure that cannulation occurs over the upper, inner quadrant of the femoral head to prevent vascular complications. Femoral angiography should be performed in all patients to assess arterial anatomy.
3. Due to the mobile nature of the femoral vessels, trapping the vessel by placing one's fingers medially and pulling the vessel lateral helps to secure it for puncture.
4. Short, rapid thrusts with the needle in a "spear-fishing" technique may be helpful in cannulating difficult arteries.

5. Using a twisting motion with wires, dilators, and catheters during cannulation allows for ease of cannulation and minimizes tissue damage. However, this technique should not be used in the pediatric population to prevent tearing the fragile arterial wall.

6. In patients where fluid management is a concern, it is not necessary to place continuous flushes on venous catheters. The rate of intraprocedural thrombosis is very low.

References

1. Garrett PD, Eckart RE, Bauch TD, Thompson CM, Stajduhar KC. Fluoroscopic localization of the femoral head as a landmark for common femoral artery cannulation. Catheter Cardiovasc Interv 2005;65(2):205–207

2. Ross IB, Luzardo GD. Direct access to the carotid circulation by cut down for endovascular neuro-interventions. Surg Neurol 2006;65(2):207–211, discussion 211

3. Sherev DA, Shaw RE, Brent BN. Angiographic predictors of femoral access site complications: implication for planned percutaneous coronary intervention. Catheter Cardiovasc Interv 2005;65(2):196–202

Introduction to Endovascular Equipment

John C. Dalfino, Ravi H. Gandhi, and Alan S. Boulos

The selection of equipment is a critical step in the planning process for any neuro-interventional procedure. As with open surgical procedures, there are few times when only one tool can do the job. Nevertheless, frustration and failure can often be avoided with the careful selection and use of the appropriate devices.

This chapter is designed to provide a detailed description of the design, function, and use of the most commonly employed neurointerventional devices. Tables describing the various permutations of each device are provided as quick reference tools to aid in the selection process. Recommendations regarding the effective use of some devices are also provided.

Preparation

Before any neurointerventional procedure can be started, several items must first be arranged and set up. Throughout the procedure, there is either behind or on the side of the interventionist an equipment table that contains not only a workspace but also space for equipment that may or may not be used later in the case (**Fig. 7.1**).

At or near the foot of the bed are the heparinized pressurized flush lines that are connected to the various catheters to prevent stagnation of blood inside them, as well as a power injector with sterile tubing that is placed on the field. These lines must be cleared of all air within them to prevent air emboli through the catheters. Some interventionists choose to use filters to reduce the incidence of air in the flush lines. The flush rate of the catheters is also highly variable, but most interventionists choose 1 drop/second. Lastly, depending on the size of the catheter that is to be flushed, the interventionist may choose to run a micro versus a macro flush line, which can limit the volume going through the catheter in patients who may be sensitive to extra volume during longer cases. The ends of the flush lines are normally connected with the catheters through a stopcock and a Y-Touhy-Borst connector. The stopcock allows a place to connect either syringes of contrast or the power injector line. The Touhy-Borst Y-valve (**Fig. 7.2**) allows a continuous flow of heparinized saline during either catheter or wire manipulation. This connector also has a rotating adjustable seal that can conform to either the wire or the catheter so that it can still be moved without backflow of saline or blood from the back of the connector.

Several important items are normally located on the equipment table (**Fig. 7.1**). The essential elements are a sharps container, dry 4×4 gauze pads, wet Telfa pads, towels, wire bowls, smaller cups for either saline or contrast, and a varying array of syringes used for injection of either saline or contrast. The gauze pads, when damp, are useful for wire manipulation. The wet Telfa pad is used for wiping wires

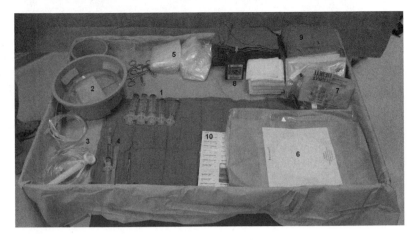

Fig. 7.1 Basic angio table setup. Common supplies on a basic angio table setup: (1) multiple syringes for injection of saline or contrast, (2) bowls used to contain wires or catheters when not in use, normally filled with heparinized saline, (3) multiple sets of tubing to connect flush lines to the catheters, (4) scalpel and local anesthetic syringe, (5) sterile covers for the radiation shield and X-ray detectors, (6) patient drape with cutouts for groin access, (7) bag to collect waste of saline and contrast, (8) sharps container, (9) gowns for the operators, and (10) stickers to label all syringes and tubing.

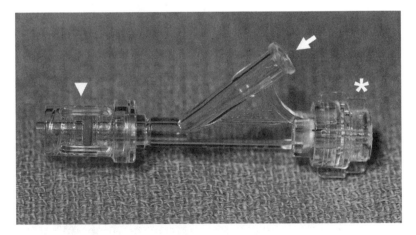

Fig. 7.2 Touhy-Borst rotating hemostatic valve. This is normally connected to the catheters, allowing them to be connected to a continuous flush (*arrow*). The connector (*arrowhead*) rotates. The valve (*asterisk*) can be opened to allow placement of other catheters or wires and turned to provide a secure seal, which does not allow outflow of the saline flush or blood from the catheter.

so that small blood clots do not form on them and become thromboemboli when a catheter is exchanged over them. Wire bowls, usually one for macrowires and catheters and another for microwires and catheters, are partially filled with saline and are used not only to wet the equipment before use but also to store equipment when it is not in use.

Various syringes are used in neurointerventional procedures, depending on the desired volume of injected material. It is very important to mark these syringes with the labels provided so that the contents of the syringes do not get mixed up. Larger (30 mL) syringes are often used only for saline. Medium-sized (10 mL) syringes are used only for contrast. Sometimes these syringes may be colored, often blue, yellow, and red. This is where labeling becomes important. There is no generally accepted convention. Smaller syringes (1–3 mL) are used for injections into microcatheters.

For vascular access equipment, for example, a micropuncture set, please see Chapter 6. Once access is obtained, the following review describes equipment that will be helpful to formulate a concise and effective neurointerventional plan.

Introducers (Sheaths)

An introducer (sheath) is a small tube that is inserted through the skin and into a vessel to provide access to the intravascular space. Introducers consist of four parts: tip, hub, shaft, and dilator (**Fig. 7.3**).
- The tip of the sheath provides an opening into the intravascular space. The tips of most introducers are tapered so that the tip of the sheath does not dig into the vessel wall (**Fig. 7.4**).
- The proximal end of a sheath is its hub. Most sheaths have a built-in hemostatic valve that prevents blood loss while devices are introduced. A side port, which

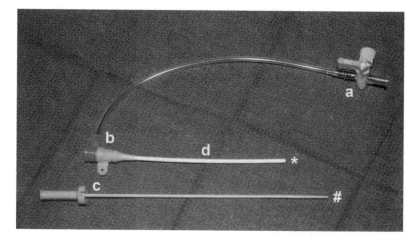

Fig. 7.3 Introducer sheath. The introducer sheath allows multiple types of catheters to be placed and held securely. Each sheath has several notable parts, namely **(a)** stopcock, **(b)** hub, **(c)** introducer stylet/dilator with a rounded tip (*pound sign*) for minimal trauma upon placement, and **(d)** sheath shaft with a tapered tip (*asterisk*).

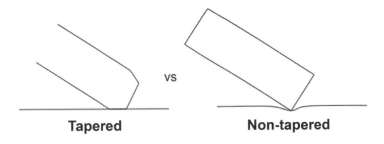

Fig. 7.4 Tapered introducers. The tips of most introducers are tapered to reduce the risk of vessel injury.

is accompanied by a stopcock and a flush line, can be used to inject contrast, draw blood for laboratories, or connect to a heparinized saline flush.

- The shaft of the sheath is the tube between the tip and the hub. A sheath is described by the diameter of its working lumen (inner diameter) and the length of its shaft. For instance, a 10 cm 6 Fr introducer has a shaft 10 cm long and will accommodate a device up to 2 mm (6 Fr) in size. The size of the arteriotomy created by the sheath will vary depending on the thickness of the walls of the sheath, but is usually 1–2 Fr larger. It is particularly important to know the outer diameter of the introducer if a closure device will be used.
- The dilator is a removable inner cannula that is coaxially inserted into the sheath while it is advanced through the skin and into the target vessel. It extends from the tip of the introducer and tapers to a soft, blunt tip. The dilator makes it easier to insert the relatively blunt sheath through the skin. It also prevents the walls of the sheath from "snow plowing" into vessel walls when the sheath is advanced (**Fig. 7.5**).

Recommendations for Selecting the Length of the Introducer

- Short (10 cm) introducers are used for most diagnostic procedures, because they are easy to insert and cause the least damage if inserted incorrectly.
- Medium-length introducers (25 cm) will help to straighten out tortuous iliac anatomy in older patients. Consider using a wider-diameter sheath for even better kink resistance.
- Long introducers (70 cm or more) will provide direct access to the supra-aortic vessels and tend to provide more proximal support than guide catheters, because they are stiffer.
- Long armored sheaths can provide additional support in tortuous anatomy but may increase the risk of vessel injury and vasospasm.
- Wet the outside of the introducer to make it easier to push.
- Avoid using a sheath that is too long. Any excess catheter outside the patient effectively lengthens the working distance from the hub to the target position of the microcatheter (**Fig. 7.6**).

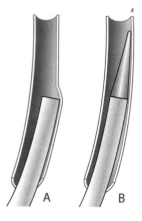

Fig. 7.5 Snow plowing. **(A)** Pushing a straight stent through a vessel can result in vessel injury as the edge of the sheath's tip "snow plows" into the vessel wall. **(B)** Adding a smooth dilator eases the transition and reduces the risk of vascular injury.

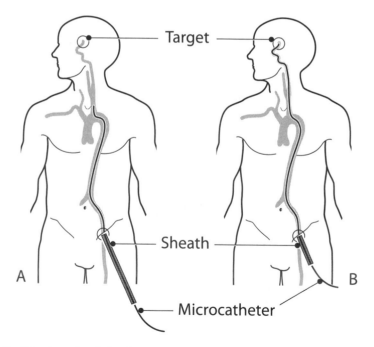

Fig. 7.6 Long sheath. **(A)** If the sheath is too long for the patient the excess length will lengthen the working distance between the hub and the target. **(B)** An appropriately sized sheath will protrude less than a few centimeters beyond the skin.

Recommendations Regarding the Diameter of the Introducer

- The sheath must be large enough to accommodate any devices that will be used during the procedure.
- Dual microcatheter techniques and stents will generally require a 6 Fr or larger introducer.
- The introducer must be small enough to fit in the parent vessel without occluding it. Consider more proximal placement of the sheath when accessing smaller vessels.

Catheters

Like introducers, catheters have a tip, a hub, and a shaft. They are inserted through a separate introducer rather than through the skin, so they do not require a dilator. Catheters are generally sized by their outer diameter. This is an important distinction from introducers. A 6 Fr catheter is 2 mm in diameter and will go through a 6 Fr introducer. The tips of catheters are typically straight, pre-shaped, or shapeable either by steam or hand, so that they can be better navigated into the lesion or vessel desired.

Diagnostic Catheters

Almost any catheter can be used for a diagnostic angiogram, but not all are equally safe. Large, stiff catheters are easy to steer and hold their position well when devices are passed through them, but they are more likely to cause a dissection or dislodge an embolus than softer catheters. For most diagnostic procedures in adults, a 4 Fr or 5 Fr diameter catheter with a soft, hydrophilic, non-braided tip is sufficient. 3.2 Fr diagnostic catheters are available for pediatric cases.

Considerations for Diagnostic Catheter Selection

Diagnostic catheters are available in a variety of preformed shapes (**Fig. 7.7**). Convenience and frugality lead most interventionalists to use a single catheter during a diagnostic procedure. Consider changing out the catheter for a different shape if difficulty is encountered in selecting a vessel.

- In younger patients with a Type I arch, nonrecursive catheter shapes (**Fig. 7.7A**), such as a multipurpose or Judkins right coronary catheter, can be used with or without a wire to select pre-cerebral vessels efficiently.
- In older patients with more tortuous anatomy (Type II or III arch) or a bovine arch, a recursive catheter shape (**Fig. 7.7B**) such as the Simmons-2, Newton, or Vitek catheter will make it easier to engage the carotid origin.
- When other catheters fail, consider using a headhunter shape to access the right subclavian and vertebral artery. This shape, combined with a shapeable 0.035 glide wire formed in a large "C" shape, will often select a difficult right subclavian or vertebral artery when other combinations fail.

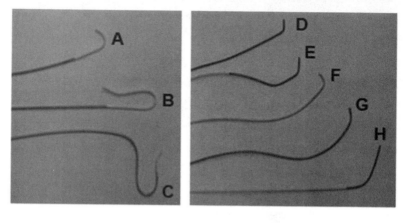

Fig. 7.7 Diagnostic catheters. Common catheter shapes used in diagnostic cerebral angiograms. (Left) Nonrecursive catheter shapes: A, internal mammary; B, Simmons 1; C, Vitek cerebral. (Right) Recursive catheter shapes: D, angled glide; E, Headhunter 1 (H1); F, Judkins right 4 (JR4); G, modified JR4; H, long vertebral.

Guide Catheters

Guide catheters are larger, stiffer catheters through which other, smaller catheters and devices can be passed. A guide catheter gets its support from a braided stainless steel core that runs along the entire length of the catheter. The added stiffness from this core helps to reduce the tendency of the catheter to herniate back into the arch when devices are passed through it.

The stiffness of the guide catheter varies along its length. Proximally, the catheter is stiff to help straighten out tortuous vessels and to provide a safe conduit for passing devices to their intended targets. Distally, a guide catheter is made more pliable to reduce the risk of vessel trauma. Like diagnostic catheters, guide catheters are available with pre-shaped tips to facilitate vessel selection off the arch. However, due to their larger sizes and stiff characteristics, they are manipulated forward only with the presence of a wire or other catheter. There are rare circumstances where guide catheters are manipulated forward without an inner device present.

Traditional and Intermediate Guide Catheters

Traditional guide catheters are generally positioned as high up in the target cervical vessel as possible for good support, but they are too stiff to safely pass intracranially. In tortuous anatomy, however, even high cervical placement of the guide catheter may not lend enough support to prevent it from herniating back into the arch while passing stiff devices through it (**Fig. 7.8**). Intermediate guide catheters, such as the Neuron (Penumbra, Inc.) or the DAC (Concentric Medical, Inc., Mountain View, CA) are soft enough to be positioned intracranially. Like traditional guide catheters, intermediate guide catheters have a braided metal core. In the

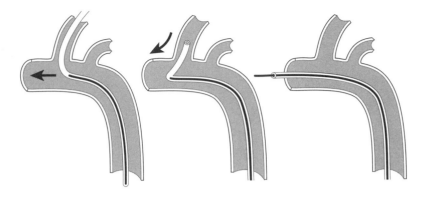

Fig. 7.8 Stiff catheters. Catheters that are too stiff or not in a stable position can be knocked out of a vessel while pushing devices through them.

DAC, the stainless steel braid is softer near the tip to make it less traumatic than a traditional guide catheter. A similar result is obtained with the Neuron guide catheter by transitioning the stiff stainless steel braid in the proximal shaft with a platinum coil at the tip (**Table 7.1**).

Balloon Guide Catheters

A balloon guide catheter is similar to a standard guide catheter except that it has an externally mounted compliant balloon at the tip. Currently, the only FDA-approved balloon guide catheter available is the Merci Balloon Guide Catheter (Concentric,

Table 7.1 Traditional and Intermediate Guide Catheters

Name	Outer diameter	Inner diameter	Length (cm)	Special features
Envoy	5.0 Fr/6.0 Fr	5.3 Fr (0.070″)	90, 100	Multiple shapes, more stiff.
DAC 038	3.9 Fr (0.050″)	2.9 Fr (0.038″)	125, 136	Smallest intermediate guide catheter.
DAC 044	4.3 Fr (0.056″)	3.3 Fr (0.044″)	115, 130, 136	Compatible with Merci microcatheters.
DAC 057	5.2 Fr (0.068″)	4.3 Fr (0.057″)	115, 125	Long working length available.
Neuron 6 F 070	6.0 Fr/6.0 Fr	(0.070″)	95, 105	Straight or angled tip available.
Neuron 6 F 053	6.0 Fr/5.0 Fr	(0.053″)	105, 115	Straight or angled tip available. Distal flexible zone choice on each catheter 6 cm or 12 cm.

Mountain View, CA). This catheter is designed to arrest flow in the internal carotid artery (ICA) during Merci clot retrieval to reduce the risk of distal embolic complications. The Merci Balloon Guide Catheter is available in several sizes and lengths to accommodate balloon occlusion of either the ICA or common carotid artery (CCA) (**Table 7.2**).

Other Uses of Balloon Guide Catheters

- A balloon guide catheter is a convenient and cost-effective method for performing a test balloon occlusion of the internal carotid artery. Unlike a stand-alone balloon, the lumen of the balloon guide catheter can be continuously flushed with heparinized saline to reduce the risk of thromboembolic complications.
- A balloon guide catheter can slow or stop antegrade flow through the carotid artery while accessing a carotid-cavernous fistula to aid in visualization during angiography.
- Consider using a balloon guide catheter during embolization of high-flow tumors or arteriovenous malformations (AVMs) to slow flow through the lesion during embolization to prevent premature occlusion of the venous drainage system.
- A balloon guide catheter can arrest and (with aspiration) reverse flow while crossing or stenting the carotid artery as a form of "proximal protection," particularly when a distal protection device is not feasible (**Fig. 7.9**).

Recommendations for Choosing a Guide Catheter

- For young adult patients with favorable anatomy, the simplest solution is to use a traditional guide catheter with an angled tip, such as the MPC Envoy (Cordis, Endovascular, Miami Lakes, FL). A guide catheter can be navigated high into the cervical vasculature without performing an exchange or using a separate selection catheter. For extra support, consider using a Simmons-shaped guide catheter. Its curves will gently press against the vessel walls to help hold it in place.
- In tortuous anatomy, consider using a guide sheath. A guide catheter can be placed inside the sheath in a coaxial arrangement for more distal access, if required. Armored sheaths can provide even greater proximal support but have a greater chance of causing vasospasm or dissection.
- Consider an intermediate guide catheter in very tortuous anatomy or in small-caliber vessels where a traditional guide catheter or sheath would be occlusive.
- Avoid using an excessively long guide catheter. If there is an excessive amount of catheter outside the patient, the micro-devices may not be long enough to reach the lesion (**Fig. 7.6**).

Table 7.2 Merci Balloon Guide Catheters

Outer diameter (proximal)	Inner diameter	Length
8 Fr (0.105″/2.7 mm)	0.078″ (5.9 Fr/1.9 mm)	80 cm
8 Fr (0.105″/2.7 mm)	0.078″ (5.9 Fr/1.9 mm)	95 cm
9 Fr (0.118″/3.0 mm)	0.085″ (6.4 Fr/2.1 mm)	80 cm
9 Fr (0.118″/3.0 mm)	0.085″ (6.4 Fr/2.1 mm)	95 cm

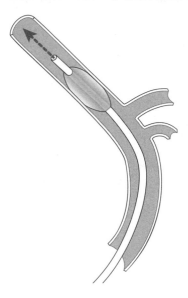

Fig. 7.9 Balloon occlusion of ICA. If a balloon guide catheter is used for ICA test occlusion, the central lumen can still be flushed with heparinized saline to prevent distal thromboembolic events.

Microcatheters

Microcatheters are small catheters (less than 3 French) designed for intracranial use. Some common characteristics of microcatheters used for neurointerventional procedures include:

- A tapered shaft with a useable length of ~150 cm.
- A hydrophilic coating to enhance trackability through small vessels.
- A shaft with a braided metal core for torqueability.
- One or two distal markers.
- A pre-shaped tip or tip shapeable with steam.

Classes of Microcatheters

Although alternative classifications exist, perhaps the most functional classification is to separate them based on their size, specifically the outer diameter (OD) of their tips.

- Small microcatheters (less than 1.5 Fr tip) are used mostly for AVM embolizations.
- Medium-sized catheters (1.5–2.0 Fr) are well suited for aneurysm coiling and thrombolysis procedures.
- Large catheters (between 2.0 and 3.0 Fr) are used to deliver large coils, particles, clot-retrieval devices, and intracranial stents.

Small Microcatheters

The smallest class of microcatheters has an outer diameter below 1.5 Fr (**Table 7.3**). They are used for liquid embolic materials, most commonly in the treatment of AVMs or vascular tumors. These small microcatheters are frequently referred to as "flow-guided" catheters, although most can be used in conjunction with a microwire for additional control.

Table 7.3   Flow-Guided Microcatheters

Catheter	Prox. OD	OD at tip	Length (cm)	Wire diameter	DMSO compatible?	Tip properties
Magic (Balt)	2.7 Fr	1.2 Fr*	165 or 180	.008	No	non-braided
Baltacci (Balt)	2.7 Fr	1.2 Fr*	165 or 180	.008	Yes	non-braided
Sonic (Balt)	2.7 Fr	1.2 Fr	165 or 180	.008	Yes	braided with non-braided detachable tip
Ultraflow (ev3)	3.0 Fr	1.5 Fr	165	.010	Yes	non-braided
Marathon (ev3)	3.0 Fr	1.3 Fr	165	.010	No	nitinol braid

*Olive tip available

Nonbraided Small Microcatheters
- They generally have the smallest tips available.
- They follow the direction of blood flow without wire guidance and essentially float to high-flow lesions, such as AVMs.
- Some of these catheters have a small "olive" at the tip to enhance their flow-guided properties. The olive will also arrest flow in the target vessel once it wedges into place to facilitate embolization.
- They can be damaged or perforated if used with a microwire.
- •Their low burst pressure may result in catheter rupture when injecting viscous embolic agents.

Braided Small Microcatheters
- They have a stainless steel proximally for support; some have a braided nitinol tip for flexibility.
- They can be safely guided over a microwire.
- They exhibit some flow-guided characteristics.
- They have higher burst pressure than non-braided microcatheters.

Hybrid Small Microcatheters
- The Sonic microcatheter (Balt) is a braided microcatheter with a 15 mm non-braided microcatheter fused to its tip. This hybrid construction allows the Sonic microcatheter to retain the small tip size of a non-braided catheter while maintaining the superior burst strength of a braided microcatheter. If the non-braided end is accidentally glued into place, it can be safely snapped off with gentle traction, allowing the rest of the catheter to be removed (**Fig. 7.10**).
- Ultraflow (ev3, Plymouth, MN) is also a hybrid microcatheter with a non-braided distal portion to allow for flow-guided navigation. This microcatheter is not designed to have a detachable tip.

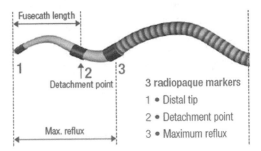

Fig. 7.10 Microcatheters, Sonic. The Sonic catheter (Balt) has a small unbraided catheter fused to the tip of a braided catheter. The unbraided portion can safely detach if the catheter is glued into place during AVM embolization.

Medium-sized Microcatheters (Table 7.4)
- They have tip diameters between 1.7 to 1.9 Fr.
- They are reinforced with a metal braid or coil for better stability and pushability.
- They are too stiff to be flow-guided in most circumstances, so they are usually steered using a guidewire.
- They hold their position better than small microcatheters to make it easier to deploy coils.
- Many have pre-shaped or shapeable tips.

Large Microcatheters (Table 7.5)
- They have a tip diameter between 2.0 and 3.0 French.
- They are large enough to accommodate intracranial stents, large embolic particles, and large aneurysm coils.
- Like the medium-sized catheters, large catheters have a reinforcing metal braid or coil to make them easy to advance over a wire and more burst resistant.
- They are used for intracranial stent delivery, large particulate delivery, mechanical thrombolysis, and deploying large coils.

Deflectable Microcatheters
The Courier Enzo (Micrus) has a deflectable tip that can be directly controlled from outside the patient. Deflection is accomplished with two microcontrol wires that are mechanically linked to a knob in the hub of the catheter. Turning the knob pulls on one of the wires, causing the tip to curl in one direction or the other (**Fig. 7.11**).

The additional mechanical components do add some bulk to the catheter (**Table 7.6**). The outer diameter of the smallest tip for the Enzo is 2.9 Fr, with a working lumen of 0.017". By comparison, the Echelon 10 (ev3) achieves the same working lumen with a 1.9 Fr tip.

Microcatheter Shaping
- A small malleable metal stylette is inserted into the tip of the microcatheter.
- The microcatheter is bent into the desired shape around the stylette.

Table 7.4 Medium-Length Microcatheters

Catheter	Company	ID	Prox OD	Dist OD	Length	Min. guide ID	Max wire	Construction	Shapes
Rebar 10	ev3	0.015"	2.3 Fr	1.7 Fr	153 cm	0.035"	0.012"	stainless steel coil	0
Prowler 10	Cordis	0.015"	2.3 Fr	1.7 Fr	150/170 cm	0.035"	0.012"	stainless steel braid, distal platinum coil	0,45,90,J
Prowler 14	Cordis	0.0165"	2.3 Fr	1.9 Fr	150/170 cm	0.035"	0.014"	stainless steel braid, distal platinum coil	0,45,90,J
Prowler Select	Cordis	0.0165"	2.3 Fr	1.9 Fr	150 cm	0.035"	0.014"	stainless steel braid, distal platinum coil	0,45,90,J
Excelsior SL-10	Boston Sci	0.0165"	2.4 Fr	1.7 Fr	150 cm	0.038"	0.014"	stainless steel braid, distal coil	0,45,90,J,S,C
Tracker Excel-14	Boston Sci	0.017"	2.4 Fr	1.9 Fr	150 cm	0.038"	0.014"	stainless steel braid	0
Echelon 10	ev3	0.017"	2.1 Fr	1.7 Fr	150 cm	0.035"	0.014"	nitinol braid	0,45,90
Echelon 14	ev3	0.017"	2.4 Fr	1.9 Fr	150 cm	0.050"	0.014"	nitinol braid	0,45,90
Rebar 14	ev3	0.017"	2.4 Fr	1.9 Fr	153 cm	0.035"	0.014"	stainless steel coil	0
Courier 170	Micrus	0.017"	2.3 Fr	1.8 Fr	150 cm	0.035"	0.014"	stainless steel braid	0,45,90
Concourse 14	Micrus	0.0165"	2.3 Fr	1.9 Fr	150 cm	0.035"	0.014"	stainless steel braid	0

Table 7.5 Large Microcatheters

Catheter	Company	ID	Prox OD	Dist OD	Length	Min. guide ID	Max wire	Construction	Shapes
Courier 190	Micrus	0.019"	2.4 Fr	1.9 Fr	150 cm	0.042"	0.014"	stainless steel braid	0,45,90
Excelsior 1018	Boston Sci	0.019"	2.6 Fr	2.0 Fr	150 cm	0.038"	0.016"	stainless steel braid with distal coil reinforcement	0,45,90,J,S,C
Nautica 14XL	ev3	0.018"	2.8 Fr	2.2 Fr	150 cm	0.050"	0.016"	nitinol braid	0
Prowler Plus	Cordis	0.021"	2.8 Fr	2.3 Fr	135, 150 cm	0.042"	0.018"	stainless steel braid and distal platinum coil	0,45,90,J
Prowler Select Plus	Cordis	0.021"	2.8 Fr	2.3 Fr	150, 170 cm	0.042"	0.018"	stainless steel braid and distal platinum coil	0,45,90,J
Rapid Transit	Cordis	0.021"	2.8 Fr	2.3 Fr	150, 170 cm	0.042"	0.018"	stainless steel braid with distal platinum coil	0
Rebar-18	ev3	0.021"	2.8 Fr	2.3 Fr	130, 153 cm	0.035"	0.018"	stainless steel coil	0
Renegade 18	Boston Sci	0.021"	3.0 Fr	2.5 Fr	150 cm	0.042"	0.018"	fiber braid	0

Table 7.6 Deflectable Microcatheters

Catheter	Company	ID	Prox OD	Dist OD	Length	Min. guide ID	Max wire	Construction	Shapes
Enzo-170	Micrus	0.017"	3.0 Fr	2.9 Fr	150 cm	0.050"	0.014"	stainless steel braid	deflectable
Enzo-190	Micrus	0.019"	3.1 Fr	3.0 Fr	150 cm	0.050"	0.014"	stainless steel braid	deflectable

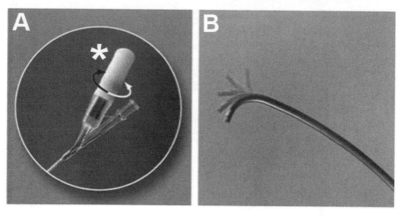

Fig. 7.11 Steerable microcatheter. The Enzo (Micrus) microcatheter has a deflectable tip that is controlled by a dial near the hub. (Image courtesy of *Codman Neurovascular*, Copyright © 2011 Codman Neurovascular.)

- The tip of the microcatheter is held in steam for 30–90 seconds.
- Saline is used to cool the tip prior to removing the stylette.
- Alternatively, the microcatheter can be shaped by very gently bending or running the tip of the microcatheter between the thumb and over a stiff metal stylette. Meticulous care must be taken to not collapse the inner lumen of the microcatheter. A stylette is normally provided with the microcatheter that is inserted into the lumen at the time of shaping.

Tips on Microcatheter Shaping
- The catheter will always straighten out a bit after the stylette is removed. Compensate by slightly over-angling the bend during the steaming process.
- Nitinol-reinforced catheters will need a longer time in the steam than catheters reinforced with stainless steel.
- A stylette is not used to shape the Magic (Balt) microcatheter.
- Factory pre-shaped tips will hold their shapes longer than steam-shaped tips.

Wires

Guidewires

Guidewires are wires used to select pre-cerebral vessels off the aortic arch. In most cases a regular stiffness 0.035″ angled wire is stiff enough to exhibit good torque and navigational control but gentle enough to be safe in the high cervical vessels. Stiff guide wires can be useful in tortuous anatomy or when pushing stiff guide sheaths/catheters such as the Cook Shuttle (Cook, USA). Hydrophilic wires tend to be easier to push and steer, particularly when used with a torque device (**Fig. 7.12**). Consider a non-hydrophilic wire for difficult exchanges to prevent the wire from slipping out of position.

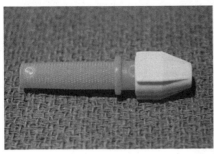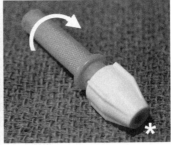

Fig. 7.12 Torque device. Small plastic device, which can be placed over (*asterisk*) glide or microwires and tightened down to allow the application of torque to the wire, thus facilitating navigation.

Microwires (Tables 7.7 and 7.8)

Microwires (with diameters from 0.007 inch to 0.021 inch) are used to steer microcatheters, balloons, stents, and other devices into distal pre-cerebral and intracranial vessels. All wires have soft tips that can be shaped on the table. Pre-shaped wires are also available from some manufacturers. Construction materials vary between manufacturers and include stainless steel, platinum, nitinol, and proprietary alloys. Each material confers subtle, subjective, unique handling properties.

Recommendations for Choosing a Microwire

- Most of the devices used for neurointerventional procedures are designed for use with a 0.014 inch microwire. Some notable exceptions include hyperballoons and some flow-guided microcatheters used for AVM embolization.
- Larger microwires (0.016 inch, 0.018 inch, or 0.021 inch) may help to straighten out tortuous anatomy or to manipulate through occluded vessels.
- Care must be taken when small microwires are used. They can be difficult to see and do not provide good support while passing devices.
- Choose one or two wires in each size and get to know them well rather than trying a new wire for every case. The differences between similarly sized wires are subtle and subjective.
- Nitinol wires generally have better torque control than platinum or stainless steel wires.

Balloons

Balloons used for neuroendovascular procedures can be divided into two categories, compliant and noncompliant. A compliant balloon is a soft, low-pressure balloon that conforms to the vessel wall as it is inflated. Compliant balloons are useful for temporary vessel occlusion and balloon-assisted aneurysm coiling because they are gentle on vessel walls. Noncompliant balloons, conversely, are stiffer balloons that attain a particular size and shape at a given pressure. These balloons will force the vessel to conform to their shape, making them better suited for angioplasty.

Table 7.7 Standard Microwires (0.014" to 0.016")

Wire	Vendor	Diameter	Length (cm)	Material	Options
Glidewire Gold 0.016	MV	0.016"	180	nitinol/tungsten	45/70 pre-shaped
Headliner 0.016	MV	0.016"	200	nitinol/tungsten	floppy,0,45,90,90/60/J
Traxcess	MV	0.014"	200	nitinol/SS	EX (Stiff)
Synchro-14	BS	0.014"	200/300	nitinol HT/SS	none
Synchro²	BS	0.014"	200	nitinol HT/SS	soft, pre-shaped
Synchro² 300	BS	0.014"	300	nitinol HT/SS	soft, pre-shaped
Transend EX	BS	0.014"	182	scitanium	soft, floppy, plat
Transend 300	BS	0.014"	300	scitanium	ES, floppy
Glidewire Gold 0.014	Ter	0.014"	180	nitinol/tungsten	45/70 pre-shaped
Agility	Cor	0.014"	205/350	SS/plat/tungsten	soft
Silverspeed 14	EV3	0.014"	175/200	SS/plat	none
X-Pedion 14	EV3	0.014"	175/200	SS/plat	none
X-Celerator	EV3	0.014"	300	SS/plat	none
Watusi	Mic	0.014"	205	SS/plat	none
Steel	Balt	0.014"	200	SS	
Sorcerer	Balt	0.014"	200	nitinol	n/a

Abbreviations: BS, Boston Scientific; MV, Microvention; Cor, Cordis; Mic, Micrus; SS, stainless steel; HT, hypotube; plat, platinum; ES, extra support.

Table 7.8 Small Microwires (0.007" to 0.012")

Wires	Vendor	Diameter	Length (cm)	Material	Options
Headliner 0.012	MV	0.012"	200	nitinol/tungsten	0,45,90,J,90/60
Sorcerer	Balt	0.012"	200	nitinol	n/a
Steel	Balt	0.012"	200	SS	n/a
Glidewire 0.011	MV	0.011"	180	nitinol/tungsten	0,45,70
Syncho 10	BS	0.010"	200/300	nitinol HT/SS	n/a
Transend 0.010	BS	0.010"	205	scitanium	n/a
Agility 10	Cor	0.010"	195	SS/plat/tungsten	soft
Silverspeed 10	ev3	0.010"	200	SS/plat	n/a
X-Pedion 10	ev3	0.010"	200	SS/plat	n/a
X-Celerator 10	ev3	0.010"	300	SS/plat	n/a
Sorcerer	Balt	0.009"	200	nitinol	n/a
Steel	Balt	0.009"	200	SS	n/a
Mirage 0.008	ev3	0.008"	200	SS/plat	n/a
Steel	Balt	0.008"	200	SS	n/a
Steel	Balt	0.007"	200	SS	n/a
Sorcerer	Balt	0.007"	200	nitinol	n/a

Abbreviations: BS, Boston Scientific; MV, Microvention; Cor, Cordis; Mic, Micrus; SS, stainless steel; HT, hypotube; plat, platinum; ES, extra support.

Compliant Balloons

Hyperform and Hyperglide

The Hyperform and Hyperglide (ev3, Plymouth, MN) are soft, compliant balloons that are mostly used for balloon-assisted aneurysm coil embolization and temporary vessel occlusion. Both balloons have a unique single-lumen wire-valve mechanism for inflation to keep them low profile (**Fig. 7.13**). As a result, these balloons can only be inflated over a wire. Typically, an Expedion 10 microwire (ev3) is used in conjunction with these balloons as they are packaged together. Inserting a smaller 0.008″ wire like the Mirage (ev3) will result in a slow "calibrated leak" of the balloon after inflation. This technique can be useful when treating vasospasm where only a transient, soft inflation is required.

- The Hyperform is the more compliant of the two balloons. Often the Hyperform balloon will assume a complex shape that will protect adjacent branches while coiling or embolizing near an eloquent branch (**Fig. 7.14A**).
- The Hyperglide balloon is less compliant, and will usually assume an oblong shape that is best suited for sidewall aneurysms and temporary vessel occlusions (**Fig. 7.14B**).
- These balloons have a reference inflation diameter of 4.5 mm but can be safely inflated in intracranial vessels with care.
- The manufacturer recommends inflating these balloons with a 1 cc syringe. For intracranial inflations, however, a 3 cc syringe on a 3-way stopcock will generate less force and reduce the risk of rupturing the balloon.
- If using a 1 cc syringe for inflation, fill the syringe with only enough contrast-saline mixture to inflate the balloon, to prevent inadvertent over-inflation. Alternatively, the 1 cc syringes can have a cadence or threaded design, so that each full rotation of the syringe administers a specified volume of contrast-saline mixture (for instance, 1 revolution is 0.1 cc). If the 3 cc syringe is used, it is best to fill it to 1.5 cc, recognizing that over-inflation may cause balloon rupture. Tactile sensation should warn the interventionist to stop any further force with inflation.
- For quick deflations, place a 20 cc syringe on the other hub of the stopcock. The larger syringe will allow for more rapid deflation with aspiration.
- It is important to always test the integrity of the balloon and to "negative prep" the balloon to ensure that no air is present prior to introducing it in the body. Keep the balloon submerged in saline or a contrast-saline mixture to avoid introducing air bubbles into the balloon.
- Hyperballoons are semipermeable to fluids, including blood. Over time, the contrast-saline mixture will be replaced with blood, making balloon inflations more difficult to visualize and deflate. When this occurs, the balloon can be purged of blood by removing the wire and flushing through a few milliliters of contrast-saline mixture.

Recommendations Regarding Using Balloon Occlusion
- The use of balloons increases the risk of cerebral ischemia by temporarily occluding blood flow to that particular vessel. Similar to aneurysm clipping, the balloon should be left deflated for 5 minutes before re-inflation to reduce the risk of cerebral ischemia/reperfusion injury.

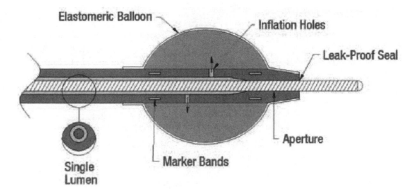

Fig. 7.13 Hyperballoons use a wire-valve mechanism for inflation. When the wire is in place it blocks the aperture at the tip, allowing inflation and deflation of the balloon via the inflation holes. When the wire is out, the fluid will flow through aperture rather than through the inflation holes. This will cause slow deflation of the balloon due to the intravascular pressure and prevent inflation at the hub.

- Consider electrophysiologic monitoring or keeping the patient awake during procedures for which balloon use is anticipated.
- Balloon-assisted techniques are associated with a higher rate of thromboembolic complications.[1] Systemic anticoagulation should be used, if possible, to maintain an ACT between 250–300 seconds. If their use is not contraindicated, consider antiplatelet medications in addition to systemic anticoagulation in high-risk cases.

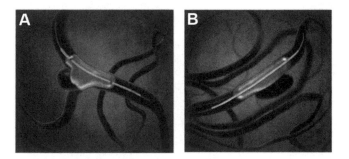

Fig. 7.14 Hyperform, Hyperglide balloons. **(A)** The Hyperform balloon is a very compliant balloon that will form multiple nodes to cover the neck of the aneurysm and any side branches. **(B)** The Hyperglide is slightly less compliant than that Hyperglide. It tends to form a cylindrical shape useful for temporary balloon occlusions and sidewall aneurysm embolizations.

Noncompliant Balloons

Noncompliant balloons force the vessel to comply with the shape of the balloon when it is fully inflated. This makes noncompliant balloons particularly well suited for dilating atherosclerotic plaque. On the other hand, noncompliant balloons are not ideal for temporary occlusion since they must often be oversized and inflated to relatively high pressure to be occlusive.

- Unlike compliant balloons, which are inflated freehand under fluoroscopic guidance, noncompliant balloons are inflated to a particular pressure (usually measured in atmospheres) using a mechanical insufflator. Each noncompliant balloon will come with a card that describes its pressure-volume response and its burst pressure.
- Noncompliant balloons do not use the wire-valve mechanism of the compliant balloons. Rather, these balloons are constructed with two lumens. One lumen is for the wire, to allow for navigation and placement of the balloon to the appropriate location, while the other lumen goes into the balloon, allowing for inflation and deflation of the balloon.
- Currently, the only noncompliant, FDA-approved intracranial balloon is the Gateway (Boston Scientific/Stryker, Natick, MA).
- Coronary balloons, such as the Maverick series (Boston Scientific/Stryker), have similar properties and are equally suitable for neurovascular intervention.
- Larger balloons, such as the Sterling (Boston Scientific/Stryker), are useful in carotid bifurcation and subclavian artery angioplasties. They have a higher crossing profile, so in very tortuous or stenotic vessels, these balloons may not perform as well.

Recommendations for the Use of Noncompliant Balloons

- Longer balloons are more difficult to push through turns than short balloons.
- The intracranial balloons should be sized to 80% of the vessel diameter to avoid vessel rupture. For this reason, noncompliant balloons are not recommended for temporary occlusion of nonstenotic vessels.
- For most intracranial procedures a 66% contrast/saline mixture is a good balance between high visibility and low viscosity. Consider a 50% contrast/saline mixture for carotid bifurcation angioplasties to shorten the balloon inflation/deflation time and to minimize the vagal response.
- Inflate slowly (over 5 minutes) in atherosclerotic intracranial vessels to avoid fracturing plaque and causing an embolus.

Monorail and Rapid Exchange Balloons

Monorail balloons (and other devices) are mounted inside a short 40 cm catheter attached to a pusher hypotube (**Fig. 7.15**). With this system, a device can be loaded and exchanged over a standard 180 cm microwire instead of a 300 cm exchange wire, allowing for faster, safer exchanges. For carotid or proximal interventions, monorail devices expedite the procedure considerably and are preferred. For intracranial procedures, over-the-wire devices provide better trackability and control.

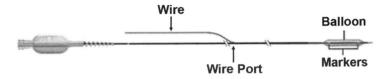

Fig. 7.15   Monorail balloons. Monorail and rapid exchange devices consist of a special short catheter that allows loading devices over a standard length microwire.

Stents

Vascular stents were initially created as an intravascular support structure to be placed after angioplasty to help prevent restenosis. These versatile devices have been adopted by neurointerventionists for various tasks, including:

- To repair a dissection flap (intimal tear)
- To provide a scaffolding for coiling wide-necked aneurysms
- To redirect flow away from an aneurysm as a primary treatment.
- To reconstruct the lumen of the cavernous carotid in an AV fistula
- To treat atherosclerotic disease and restore luminal patency
- To reopen occluded arteries with underlying atherosclerosis
- To treat venous occlusion or obstructions in sinus thrombosis or pseudotumor cerebri
- To treat other vascular conditions that lead to stenoses (fibromuscular dysplasia and moyamoya disease, to name a few).

Anatomy of a Stent (Vascular Reconstruction Device)

The walls of all stents are constructed from a latticework of thin metal struts. In some stents the latticework is created by weaving the struts together, while in others the latticework is cut from a solid piece of material. In either case, the spaces between the struts are referred to as cells. At the ends of the stent where the latticework ends, the struts will protrude from the body of the stents, forming the tines.

Cell Design

Stents can be constructed with either an open-cell or closed-cell design. The cells of closed-cell stents are completely surrounded by struts. The cells of an open-cell stent, conversely, are only partially surrounded by struts (**Fig. 7.16A**). As a result, closed-cell stents have more radial stiffness than comparably sized open-cell stents of similar construction. There is some evidence that closed-cell stents have a lower incidence of embolic complications during and after carotid stent placement procedures.

On the other hand, open-cell stents are more conformable. This makes open-cell stents ideal for spanning vessels with different diameters and easier to navigate through tortuous anatomy. Open-cell stents are also easier to cross during Y-stenting procedures or stent-assisted aneurysm coiling.

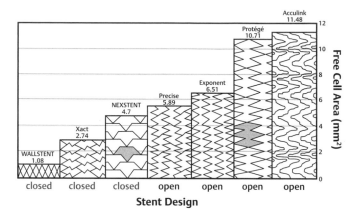

Fig. 7.16 Free cell area of different types of stents. The free cell area is the largest area in a stent that is completely surrounded by struts. In a closed-cell stent, each cell is completely surrounded by struts. In an open-cell stent, each cell is only partially surrounded by struts of the stent. The shaded area on the Nexstent and Protégé are examples of the free cell area within a closed- and open-cell stent.

Free Cell Area

Some investigators have described a measurement referred to as a free cell area in an attempt to quantify both closed and open cell designs. The free cell area refers to the largest area that is completely lined by struts. Assuming the strut width to be negligible, the free cell area of a stent is directly related to its porosity. For closed-cell stents, the free cell area is the area of an individual cell. For open-cell stents, the value will be the aggregate areas of multiple cells (**Fig. 7.16B**). In general, closed-cell stents will have a smaller free cell area and lower porosity than open-cell stents. In vitro and human studies suggest that stents with a smaller free cell area are less likely to allow embolic particles to pass through.[2]

Basics of Self-Expanding versus Balloon-Mounted Stents (Table 7.9)

Stents can be broadly classified as self-expanding or balloon-mounted, based on their mechanism of deployment. Balloon-mounted stents are crimped onto the outside of a noncompliant balloon. Inflation of the balloon simultaneously expands and deploys the stent (**Fig. 7.17A**). Most balloon-mounted stents are made from stainless steel or cobalt. These materials are strong but relatively stiff.

Self-expanding stents are made from a metal alloy with a memory (nitinol typically) and come preloaded in a catheter delivery system. Self-expanding stents are deployed by pulling back the delivery catheter while holding the stent in place with a pusher device. The memory metal alloy allows the stent to re-expand inside the vessel until it opposes the vessel walls (**Fig. 7.17B**).

Table 7.9 Comparison of Balloon-Mounted and Self-Expanding Stents

	Balloon-mounted	Self-expanding
Radial stiffness	Balloon-mounted stents generally have a higher radial stiffness than self-expanding stents. This makes balloon-mounted stents a good choice for calcified lesions, CCA origin lesions, and the vertebral origin.	The radial force of a self-expanding stent is lower than a balloon-mounted stent of similar size. Self-expandable stents, however, can be over-sized and may continue to expand in situ after they are deployed.
Foreshortening	Balloon-mounted stents generally do not exhibit significant foreshortening during deployment. This property allows BM stents to be accurately placed.	Self-expandable stents are sometimes significantly longer while constrained inside a catheter than they are when deployed. The amount the stent will foreshorten varies between stents but is predictable. Over-sized stents will foreshorten less because they are partially constrained after deployment.
Conformability	Balloon-mounted stents are deployed with noncompliant balloons that are not designed to conform to a vessel wall and should not be over-sized. Consequently, balloon-mounted stents are not recommended for spanning two vessels with a large discrepancy in diameters.	Self-expanding stents do not require a noncompliant balloon for deployment. When spanning two vessels of different diameter, the stent is sized to fit the bigger vessel while the part of the stent in the smaller vessel is slightly (and safely) over-sized. Some larger self-expanding stents are tapered to further improve the conformability of the stent across vessels of different diameters.
Kink resistance	Balloon-mounted stents that are subjected to bending or compression can be kinked.	Self-expanding stents are inherently kink resistant and are ideal for stenting vessels that might be subject to mechanical compression, such as the cervical vertebral or carotid arteries.
Crossing profile	Balloon-mounted stents tend to have a wider crossing profile that can make it difficult to get across a stenotic segment.	Tend to have a narrow profile, allowing them to navigate through stenotic lesions more easily.
Hyperplasia	Stent resides just under intima near vessel lumen and does not expand with time.	Stent resides near outside wall of vessel. This may result in less intimal hyperplasia and allow the vessel lumen to increase with time.
MRI	Compatible	Compatible, less artifact with nitinol.

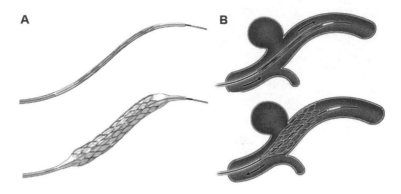

Fig. 7.17 Balloon-mounted stent. **(A)** A balloon-mounted stent is crimped onto the outside of a balloon. Inflating the balloon **(B)** opens the stent. The balloon can then be deflated and removed.

Radial Stiffness

Radial stiffness describes the ability of a stent to resist collapsing from the force imposed by the elasticity of the vessel walls.
- In general, a stainless steel stent has three times the radial stiffness of a similarly designed nitinol stent.
- Balloon-mounted stents have higher radial stiffness than self-expanding stents.
- The relatively low radial stiffness of a self-expanded stent can be overcome somewhat by over-sizing it.

Acute Recoil

Acute recoil refers to the narrowing that occurs in all stents immediately after deployment, due to the compressive force of the elastic vessel walls.
- The magnitude of acute recoil of a stent after deployment is inversely proportional to its radial stiffness.
- Self-expanding nitinol stents have relatively low radial stiffness and are therefore subject to more acute recoil than a similar-sized balloon-mounted stainless steel stent. This makes balloon-mounted stents more appropriate for heavily calcified lesions where the compliance of the vessel walls is low.

Hyperplasia

There are conflicting data about whether self-expanding stents incite more or less intimal hyperplasia than balloon-mounted stents. Over time, appropriately over-sized, self-expanding stents will migrate through the intimal layer of the vessel and support the vessel from the inside. Balloon-mounted stents, conversely, tend to remain close to the lumen of the vessel. There are few clinical data, however, to show that the location of the stent within the walls of a vessel has any bearing on long-term restenosis rates.

Radial Strength

The radial strength of a stent refers to its ability to withstand bending or external compression without being permanently damaged.

- In practice, radial strength is not relevant to self-expanding stents, as their nitinol "memory metal" construction allows them to snap back to their original shape once the deforming force is removed. This property makes self-expanding nitinol stents less likely to fracture or kink in vessels that are subjected to bending or compression, like the cervical carotid artery.
- Balloon-expandable stents are made of stainless steel. Since stainless steel is not a memory metal, compressive forces in excess of its rated radial strength can permanently deform it.

Cervical Carotid Stents (Table 7.10)

Currently, all carotid stents available in the United States are self-expanding stents. Off-label use of peripheral balloon-mounted stents has been described. Most carotid stents are constructed from nitinol, with only the Wallstent (Boston Scientific) constructed from a chromium-based alloy marketed as Elgiloy. All vendors have created their own distal protection devices, but many are cross-compatible with other stent systems.

- Nearly all carotid stents can be delivered via a rapid exchange or monorail system that is designed to simplify catheter exchanges. Most carotid stent delivery systems require a 6 Fr guide sheath (or 8 Fr guide catheter), but some 5 Fr systems are available. Exchanges are generally performed over a 0.014 inch wire, although the Precise stent (Cordis, Bridgewater, NJ) will accept up to a 0.018 inch wire.
- Carotid stents are typically classified as open-cell design or closed-cell design (**Fig. 7.18**). Open-cell stents offer the advantage of better conformability and are typically easier to navigate through tortuous anatomy. They are also less likely to kink when deployed on a steep vessel turn.
- Closed-cell stents are stiffer than open-cell stents of similar size and construction. This makes them less able to conform to the vessel lumen than open-cell stents, particularly when spanning vessels of disparate diameter. Newer tapered stents have been manufactured to help address this problem. The advantage of closed-cell stents is that they offer more plaque coverage than open-cell stents. There is evidence that this increased coverage may offer better embolic protection than open-cell stents.[2,3]

Covered Stents

Covered stents are created by covering the cells of a metal stent with a fine woven synthetic fabric or Gore-Tex liner (W. L. Gore, Elkton, MD). The result is a stent that is nearly impermeable to both particles and blood. Covered stents are only rarely used in the supra-aortic circulation. A randomized controlled study to look at the outcome of covered stents for carotid disease was stopped due to a very high rate

Table 7.10 Comparison of Commonly Used Carotid Stents

Stent	Vendor	Cell design	Sheath req.	Material	Protection device	Special features
Protégé Rx	ev3	Open	6.0 Fr	nitinol	Spyder	No foreshortening. Can cross lesion with wire of choice in combination with Spyder EPD.
Precise	Cordis	Open	5.5/6.0 Fr	nitinol	Angioguard	Up to 0.018" guide ok
Precise Pro RX	Cordis	Open	5.0/6.0 Fr	nitinol	Angioguard	High radial stiffness
Acculink	Abbott	Open	6.0 Fr	nitinol	Accunet	Highest cell area
Xact	Abbott	Closed	5.7 Fr	nitinol	EmboShield	Can cross lesion with wire of choice in combination with EmboShield EPD.
Nexstent	Boston Sci	Closed	5.0 Fr	nitinol	Filterwire EZ	Self-sizing
Wallstent	Boston Sci	Closed	5.0/6.0 Fr	Elgiloy	Filterwire EZ	Reconstrainable if less than 90% deployed
Cristallo	Invatec	Both	5.0 Fr	nitinol	Fibernet	Dual cell design

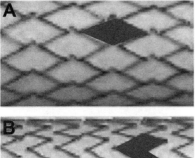

Fig. 7.18 The free cell area is the largest area in a stent that is completely surrounded by struts. In a closed-cell stent like the Nexstent **(A)**, the free cell area is the area of a single cell. In an open-cell stent like the Protégé **(B)**, the free cell area is the combined area of multiple cells. In general, closed-cell stents will have a lower free cell area.

of restenosis—38% at 6 months.[4] Covered stents are also much stiffer than bare stents of similar size, making them more difficult to deliver.

Still, there are some indications for the use of covered stents in the supra-aortic circulation, including:

- Excluding a pseudoaneurysm, extravasation, or dissection
- Performing an endolumenal repair of a carotid perforation
- Closing an arteriovenous fistula, such as a carotid-cavernous fistula

Some examples of covered stents suitable for use in the carotid artery include the Jostent (a balloon-mounted platform, Abbott Laboratories, Abbott Park, IL) and the Wallgraft (self-expanding) (Boston Scientific).

Intracranial Self-Expanding Stents

Stents for Intracranial Atherosclerosis

Wingspan Stent (Boston Scientific)

- Currently the Wingspan stent is the only intracranial stent approved for the treatment of intracranial atherosclerosis.
- The open-cell design of the Wingspan makes it more flexible, allowing it to navigate through tortuous anatomy.
- Struts are relatively short and thick to give it greater radial stiffness than aneurysm stents like the Neuroform (Boston Scientific) and Enterprise (Cordis, Bridgewater, NJ). The Wingspan has nearly five times the radial stiffness of the Neuroform stent.
- Despite its high radial stiffness, it is recommended that an angioplasty using the Gateway intracranial balloon (or equivalent) be performed prior to stent deployment.

Delivery of the Wingspan Stent
The Wingspan stent is packaged preloaded into a 3.5 Fr over-the-wire, dual catheter delivery system (**Fig. 7.19**). Both the inner and outer catheters can be connected to a continuous heparinized saline flush. Prior to stent placement, the lesion must be crossed with a 300 cm 0.014 inch microwire, either primarily or after an exchange. The stent delivery system is back-loaded onto the 0.014 inch exchange wire and advanced until it is just distal to the lesion. The stent is deployed by pulling back the outer catheter while holding the inner "pusher" catheter in place at the groin.

Aneurysm Stents

Enterprise Stent
- The Enterprise is a closed-cell nitinol stent designed for stent-assisted aneurysm coiling.
- Unlike the Wingspan or Neuroform stents, the Enterprise is prepackaged in a delivery system over a specialized delivery wire. The advantage of this delivery system is that it is very flexible, allowing for excellent trackability despite its closed-cell design.
- The customized delivery wire allows the stent to be recaptured as long as it is less than 75% deployed (**Fig. 7.20**).

Deployment of the Enterprise Stent
Position a Prowler Plus Select (Codman, Miami, FL) 0.021 inch microcatheter on a continuous heparinized saline flush approximately 1.5 cm distal to the deployment zone over a standard 0.014 inch microwire. Choose a stent long enough to extend 5 mm proximal and distal to the aneurysm. The stent is loaded into the hub of the microcatheter like a coil and pushed into position using its delivery wire. To deploy the stent, the microcatheter is gently pulled back while holding

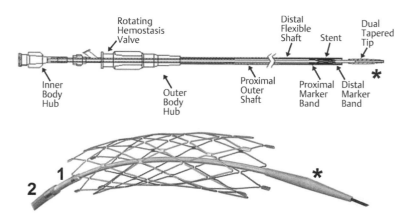

Fig. 7.19   Wingspan. The Wingspan delivery system consists of two catheters. The outside delivery catheter constrains the stent until delivery. The stent is mounted on the inner catheter, which doubles as a pusher catheter. (Image courtesy of Stryker, Copyright © 2011 Stryker.)

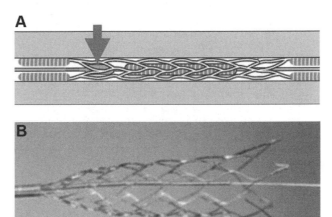

Fig. 7.20 Enterprise. The Enterprise stent comes preloaded on a proprietary delivery and is delivered through a Prowler Plus Select microcatheter. The wire has small knobs (*arrow* in **A**) that allow the catheter to be held in position during deployment or even recaptured if less than 75% deployed **(B)**. (Image courtesy of *Codman Neurovascular*, Copyright © 2011 Codman Neurovascular.)

the delivery wire in place. The stent can be recaptured and deployed (once) as long as 25% of the stent remains in the catheter. To maintain access after deployment, re-advance the microcatheter through the stent over the delivery wire. The wire is straight so it is not a good wire for navigation in the intracranial circulation.

Note that the Prowler Plus Select is the only catheter recommended by the manufacturer for use with the Enterprise stent.

Neuroform Stent
- The Neuroform is a self-expanding stent specifically designed for stent-assisted coiling.
- Its open-cell design makes it more flexible and maneuverable than the Wingspan stent, although at the expense of decreased radial stiffness.
- Re-accessing the aneurysm with a microcatheter through the tines of this stent is made easier due to its large open cells.

Delivery of the Neuroform Stent
The delivery of the Neuroform stent is unique. Like the Wingspan, the Neuroform can be deployed with the aid of a pusher catheter while maintaining wire access through the stent. Alternatively, the Neuroform can be deployed by removing the 0.014 inch microwire and advancing a 0.018 inch wire through the delivery catheter to deliver the stent, acting like a pusher catheter. Without the pusher catheter in the delivery system it becomes much more flexible, allowing the stent to be navigated more easily through tortuous anatomy. Wire access is not maintained with the Neuroform 2 and 3 systems; however, the newer Neuroform EZ stent is similar to the Enterprise stent system and has the ability to maintain distal wire access.

Flow-Diverting Stents

Pipeline (ev3, Chestnut Medical)

The Pipeline is a self-expanding stent with very fine cells. This stent is purported to be able to occlude an aneurysm without coils by diverting flow around the aneurysm like a covered stent. Often multiple overlapping stents must be used to achieve this result. The advantage of this technique is that no device is placed inside the aneurysm, minimizing the risks of either aneurysm rupture or an increase in aneurysmal mass effect. The Pipeline device received FDA approval in March 2011.

Leo Plus (Balt)

- The Leo Plus is a fine-celled stent similar in principle to the Pipeline.
- Its relatively high radial stiffness makes it suitable for treating atherosclerosis and aneurysms.
- It can be recaptured as long as 10% of it remains undeployed.
- It is not yet available in the United States.

Pharos (Micrus) Balloon-Mounted Intracranial Stent

- The Pharos is a balloon-mounted stent under investigation for use in the treatment of intracranial atherosclerosis and cerebral aneurysms.
- It has similar characteristics to a cobalt chromium coronary stent but is thinner for better deliverability. Angioplasty and stent placement are performed in one step.
- It does not shorten during deployment like a self-expanding stent, for improved positioning accuracy.
- It is not yet available in the United States.

Drug-Eluting Stents

- A drug-eluting stent has a sustained-release coating of an immunosuppressive drug like Everolimus to help prevent neointimal hyperplasia.
- Drug-eluting stents were designed and FDA approved for use in the coronary circulation, but there are several small series by investigators demonstrating safe and effective use in vessels supplying the brain.[5]
- Heparin-coated stents are no longer available in the United States.

Peripheral Stents

Treating lesions in the innominate or subclavian arteries requires larger peripheral stents. These stents are usually between 6 and 10 mm in diameter and are available in either balloon-mounted or self-expanding delivery systems.

- Self-expanding stents are less easily kinked by mechanical compression or movement.
- Self-expanding stents also conform better when spanning vessels of different diameters.

- When greater radial force and/or more precise positioning is required, such as when stenting an ostial lesion, a balloon-mounted stent may be appropriate.

Aneurysm Coils

Coils used for brain aneurysms[6] are generally made of very thin platinum wires wound in a tight helix called the primary wind. The coil can then be supercoiled into either a helix or other three-dimensional shape called the secondary wind (**Fig. 7.21** and **7.22**). Some manufacturers have incorporated other materials, such as nitinol, hydrogel, and polyglycolic-polylactic acid (PGLA), to enhance thrombosis, and/or promote endothelialization. Coil manufacturers have now focused on making their coil lines more resistant to stretching, that is, they have increased the force necessary to unwind the primary coil. The most common technique is to have a filament, wire, or suture around which the primary coil is wound.

Coil nomenclature is problematic. The conventional naming system of coils usually involves either the 10 or 18 system. However, these numbers are meaningless with regard to the size of the primary coil. Most manufacturers provide charts that list the true sizes of the primary coils or they may be listed on the box in which the coil is provided. To maintain consistent properties of the coils, the size of the primary coil will change with different sizes of the secondary coil and the lengths offered. Further, one must be aware of the pusher wire size, as this may also be a barrier to using a particular coil in a particular microcatheter.

Some standard numbers to know are that 18 coils are not 0.018 inch, but usually 0.015 inch, although not always, and 10-coil systems usually have pusher wires that are either 0.014 inch or 0.012 inch, not 0.01 inch. As such, attention

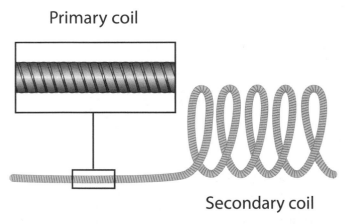

Fig. 7.21 Coil design. All aneurysm coils have a primary wire that is wound around a mandrel giving the primary wind. The coil is then shaped to form helical (pictured), spherical, or complex shapes.

360 Coil   **Helical Coil**

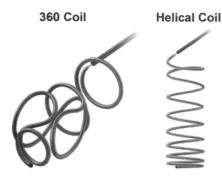

Fig. 7.22 360 Coil design. The combination of secondary wind and shaping can lead to several different coil designs. (Image courtesy of Stryker, Copyright © 2011 Stryker.)

must be paid to these measurements so that the situation does not arise where a coil you expect to use cannot be passed within the selected microcatheter. In addition, Codman and Micrus produce coils with either 0.012 or 0.014 inch diameters, and Penumbra produces their 0.02 inch diameter primary coils, so careful attention to coil and microcatheter compatability is important prior to beginning the procedure. Remember, choosing a microcatheter that is too large may result in the coil folding within the catheter itself, thus preventing deployment. The variation in primary coil sizes is often a result of altering the softness of the coil or the ability to increase the packing density of the aneurysm per unit length of coil used. However, increasing the diameter of the primary coil may result in a stiffer coil, making placement within the aneurysm potentially more difficult and dangerous.

Bare Platinum Coils

Guglielmi Detachable Coil (GDC) (Boston Scientific/Stryker)

- The Guglielmi detachable coil was the first coil to be FDA approved for the treatment of intracranial aneurysms.[5]
- It is made of platinum and attached to a stainless steel pusher wire.
- It is electrolytically detached.
- It is available in a wide range of sizes and shapes, including 3-D framing coils.
- Soft versions of GDC coils using thinner platinum wires are also available.

Target Coils (Boston Scientific/Stryker)

- Target coils have a shorter, softer junction than GDC coils and a flexible distal delivery wire segment that are intended to minimize microcatheter movement during coil deployment.
- The proximal delivery wire includes Fluoro-Saver marker bands, allowing the ability to track the coil through the majority of the microcatheter without using fluoroscopy. Marker bands are also available on Terumo coils (see below).
- The coils have improved stretch resistance (4.5x stronger than GDC).

- Target coils have smaller initial coil loops (approximately 75%) before full size coil loops (a common feature on most framing coils from Codman, ev3, and Terumo) (**Fig. 7.23**).
- There are multiple kinds of coil winds with varying degrees of softness.

Microplex Coil System (Terumo)

The Microplex coil system is a family of four types of bare platinum coils specifically designed to frame, fill, and finish coil most cerebral aneurysms.

- The system utilizes a fluid injection detachment system that has a shorter and softer detachment zone than electrolytic detachment systems to help prevent the catheter from backing out during embolization.
- Fluoro-saving marker bands on the pusher wire allow for the coil to be safely advanced through the microcatheter to that band prior to using fluoroscopy.

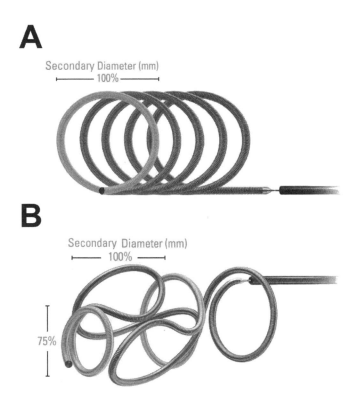

Fig. 7.23 Target coil. **(A)** Demonstration of equal helical loops in Target coils. **(B)** Demonstration of small initial coil loop in Target 360 coils. (Image courtesy of Stryker, Copyright © 2011 Stryker.)

- A self-contained, sterile electronic device along with a new delivery system called V-Tek make detaching the coils more convenient and nearly instantaneous.

MicroPlex Family (MicroVention)

- *Compass:* The Compass (MicroVention, Tustin, CA) spherical framing coil is designed to frame spherical and/or wide-necked aneurysms. It assumes a designated 3-D shape. Multiple compass coils can be used to fill spherical aneurysms concentrically with less chance of compartmentalization.
- *Cosmos:* The Cosmos is a conformable framing coil designed to treat non-spherical, complex aneurysms. It can also be used as a filling coil in larger aneurysms. This coil has a random wind that may improve packing density.
- *Helical:* Standard helical filling coils are available in both standard and soft versions.
- *HyperSoft:* The Hypersoft is a stretch-resistant, soft finishing coil with shorter detachment zone, minimizing deflection of catheter tip.

Axium Coils (ev3)

- The Axium coils are designed using a mathematical algorithm based on the premise that there is an optimal relationship between the wire diameter, the primary wind diameter, and the secondary wind diameter called the K-Factor.

$$K \propto \frac{(\text{wire diameter})^x}{(1° \text{ wind diameter})^y \ (2° \text{ wind diameter})^y}$$

- The coils are detached using a sterile, self-contained, proprietary device capable of near-instantaneous detachment on the field. It uses a mechanical detachment method and in cases of failure has a bailout technique that nearly always is effective at causing detachment.

Trufill DCS Orbit (Codman/Johnson & Johnson)

- The Trufill is a platinum coil available in both helical and complex shapes.
- Unlike a GDC coil, the distal coil of the Trufill is one-third smaller than the labeled 2 degree wind to reduce the incidence of the first loop exiting the aneurysm during deployment (**Fig. 7.24**).
- The loops of the coil are randomly oriented to improve conformability and reduce the incidence of sequestration.
- Coils are sized in half millimeter increments to make concentric framing easier.
- The coils utilize a hydraulic detachment system.
- The diameter of the primary wind (0.012 inch) of Cordis coils is larger than typical 10 coils from other companies. Studies have demonstrated that because of this larger primary wind and complex shape, a higher filling volume is possible.
- A softer "fill" version is also available.

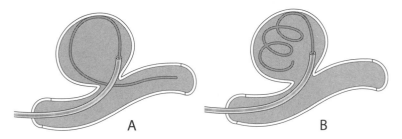

Fig. 7.24 Orbit coils. **(A)** In a standard coil the first loop of a large coil will sometimes exit the aneurysm during deployment. **(B)** Orbit coils have a small distal loop so that the first coil nearly always deploys inside the aneurysm.

Orbit Galaxy (Codman/Johnson & Johnson)

- The Orbit Galaxy is made of platinum with a polypropylene stretch-resistant suture and conformable shapes.
- The coils are available in an extrasoft (Xtrasoft), filling and framing version.
- The Xtrasoft and fill coils have a primary coil diameter of 0.012 inch, while the Frame coils have a primary coil diameter of 0.014 inch.
- It utilizes a hydraulic detachment system that may be more flexible than the electrolytic types of detachment system.
- The properties of the Xtrasoft coil (a primary wind done with a larger primary coil diameter (0.012 inch) than other finishing coils) allow filling of an aneurysm with a random loop design, which may lead to increased packing densities.

MicroCoil (Micrus)

- The MicroCoil is a bare platinum coil available in both spherical (Microsphere) and helical (Helipaq) configurations.
- Secondary wind coils are oriented at 90 degree angles to improve conformability.
- The system uses a low-temperature, resistive-heating detachment system that can detach the coil in less than 5 seconds.
- They are available in multiple shapes and diameters of coils, including Cashmere (filling type, 0.014 inch primary coil), Deltapaq/DeltaPlush (softer packing and finishing coils), and Presidio (framing 10 and 18 systems).

Penumbra Coil 400 (Penumbra)

- The Penumbra coils are stretch-resistant bare platinum coils.
- The system has a larger primary coil, approximately 0.02 inch.
- There is an increased packing density per unit length of coil, due to the larger primary coil.
- The coil is most often used with an accompanying catheter, the PX400, with an inner-diameter of 0.025 inch to accommodate the larger coils.

Bioactive Coils

Most aneurysms are completely embolized as the coil volume reaches 30–35% of the volume of the fundus, with the remainder of the volume filled with thrombus. If the thrombus is lysed prior to endothelialization, recanalization of the aneurysm may occur. To reduce the incidence of recanalization, various bioactive substances, such as gold, vitronectin, and various ion-planted proteins, have been added to coils to encourage thrombosis and prevent recanalization. Currently, the only bioactive material incorporated into coils is polyglycolic-polylactic acid (PGLA).

Polyglycolic-Polylactic Acid

- Polyglycolic-polylactic acid (PGLA) is a synthetic, biodegradable polymer that incites an inflammatory response within the aneurysm fundus to speed thrombosis and collagen deposition within the coil mass. This may lead to a reduction in recurrence rates.
- With exposure to blood, PGLA is broken down by hydrolysis within three months, avoiding long-term inflammatory effects.
- Currently, three PGLA coils are available—Matrix (Boston Scientific/Stryker), Cerecyte (Micrus), and Nexus (ev3).

Matrix Coils

- The Matrix coil (Boston Scientific) was the first bioactive coil to receive FDA approval (2002).
- A platinum core wire with a PGLA coating accounts for 70% of the volume of the coil. Some users report the coils are stiffer and stickier than bare platinum coils, making it more difficult to achieve a high packing density of coils within the aneurysm.
- The packing density decreases over time as the PGLA is reabsorbed. As a result, some clinical studies have suggested that aneurysms embolized with Matrix coils are more likely to recanalize than aneurysms treated with bare platinum coils.[7] Other studies suggest reduced recanalization rates with the current generation of Matrix coils.[8]
- The current generation of Matrix coils is currently under study in a randomized trial comparing them with bare platinum coils.

Cerecyte Coils

- The Cerecyte (Micrus) coils are platinum coils wound around a polyglycolic acid (PGA) filament. Blood is able to contact the inner core through small gaps intentionally incorporated into the primary wind (**Fig. 7.25**).
- Since the PGA is surrounded by platinum, these coils do not generate as much friction inside the microcatheter as PGLA-coated coils. Consequently, Cerecyte coils handle and pack more like bare platinum coils.
- Having the PGA inside the core of the coil also reduces the volume loss of the coil mass after reabsorption of the PGA and confers some degree of stretch resistance.
- Clinical data regarding the long-term recanalization rate of Cerecyte coils are sparse; however, recent randomized data suggest there is no difference in occlusion rates as compared with bare platinum coils.

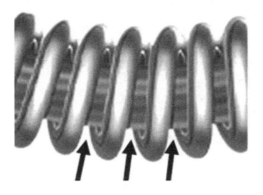

Fig. 7.25 Cerecyte coils. Cerecyte coils have a PGA filament. Spaces are deliberately incorporated into the primary wind to expose the PGA to blood. (Image courtesy of *Codman Neurovascular*, Copyright © 2011 Codman Neurovascular.)

Nexus Coils

- Nexus (ev3) coils are platinum coils with PGLA microfilaments interwoven into the primary wind that extend out like small hairs (**Fig. 7.26**).
- An inner nitinol core prevents compaction of the coil mass and confers stretch resistance.
- The nitinol core makes the coil mass less conformable, causing coils loops to be pushed into the parent vessel during embolization and making them resistant to balloon remodeling.
- The current Axium line no longer uses a nitinol core to improve handling. One line of these coils has the PGLA microfilaments interwoven to improve the healing response with embolization. This is also currently under study.

Hydrogel Incorporated Coils

Hydrogel Material

- Hydrogel is a highly absorbant polymer that expands when it contacts fluid such as blood (**Fig. 7.27**).
- The degree of expansion is specified for each coil diameter.
- Hydrogel does not incite inflammation but is supportive of the clotting cascade.
- Hydrogel does not degrade over time, minimizing volume loss over time.

HydroCoils (Microvention)

- HydroCoils are platinum coils coated in hydrogel.
- The working time of HydroCoils is also short, approximately 5 minutes before the coil becomes more difficult to recapture. As the hydrogel expands, depending on the type of HydroCoil, it may expand beyond the diameter of the microcatheter. If this occurs, then the coil cannot be retrieved by pulling it back into the microcatheter.
- There is a special overcoil to reduce (but not eliminate) the friction between the hydrogel and the microcatheter during deployment.

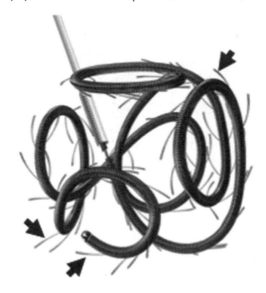

Fig. 7.26 Nexus coils. Nexus coils are bare platinum coils with PGLA fibers woven into the primary wind.

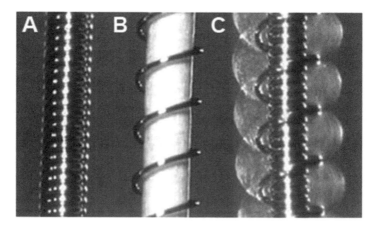

Fig. 7.27 HydroCoil. Comparison of bare platinum coil **(A)**, dry HydroCoil **(B)**, and expanded HydroCoil **(C)**. (With kind permission from Cloft HJ, HEAL Investigators. HydroCoil for Endovascular Aneurysm Occlusion (HEAL) Study: Periprocedural Results. AJNR Feb 2006;27:289.)

- Full expansion of the hydrogel occurs in 20 minutes.
- There may be a higher incidence of hydrocephalus with HydroCoil use compared with bare platinum coils in large or giant aneurysms.
- A randomized trial, HELPS, that was completed in 2010 demonstrated statistically significant reduction in recurrence rates with the HydroCoil arm compared with bare platinum coils. Though not statistically significant, there was 50% reduction in periprocedural thromboembolic events and retreatment rates in the HydroCoil arm compared with bare platinum. The rates of hydrocephalus were similar and not significantly different. At the time of publication, the final trial results have yet to be published.

Hydrosoft and Hydroframe Coils (Microvention)

- Hydrosoft and Hydroframe coils are platinum coils with a hydrogel core, similar in concept to Cerecyte coils.
- Upon exposure to blood, the hydrogel core expands, increasing the effective diameter of the coil from 0.010 inch to 0.014 inch.
- Although Hydrosoft coils do not expand as much as Hydrogel coils, they handle more like platinum coils and have an indefinite working time as the coil does not expand beyond the microcatheter diameter.
- Hydrosoft framing coils (marketed as Hydroframe) are also available with the Cosmos shape and the Hydrosoft technology.

Berenstein Coils

- Berenstein coils are pushable, bare platinum coils that are smaller and more flexible than detachable coils.
- They can travel through smaller microcatheters and into more distal vascular spaces than detachable coils. They are used primarily in AVMs to slow flow prior to using a liquid embolic.
- Pushable coils cannot be retrieved easily if their position is not ideal, so they are not commonly used in aneurysm coiling. These coils are currently not available for purchase.

Embolization Particles

Polyvinyl Alcohol (PVA) Particles

- Polyvinyl alcohol (PVA) particles are mixed with contrast for visibility.
- Heterogeneous particles come in various sizes, ranging from 45–150 to 1000–1180 microns.
- Vessels embolized with these particles tend to recanalize over time.[9]
- Particles can also cause an acute inflammatory process and even angionecrosis.[10]

Embospheres

- Embospheres are gelatin-coated particles made from acrylic polymer.[11]
- They are more uniform in size, and their spherical shape enables more precise application than traditional PVA particles.
- Sizes of 200–500 µm are most suitable for intracranial procedures.

Gelfoam

- Gelfoam is no longer commonly used for neurointerventional procedures.
- It causes an inflammatory reaction that leads to thrombosis.
- One potential benefit is that it reabsorbs over approximately four weeks, preventing a chronic inflammatory reaction.
- Its inability to adhere to the vessel wall lends toward recanalization.

Liquid Embolics

Liquid embolic agents are commonly used with arteriovenous malformations (AVMs)[12] and fistulae and are increasingly being used for preoperative embolization of tumors. There are several liquid embolics, but only Onyx[13] and n-BCA[14] are currently approved for use in the United States.

n-Butyl Cyanoacryl (n-BCA) (Table 7.11)

- The glue comes packaged with n-BCA, lipodal, and powdered tantalum. These agents can be mixed in variable concentrations to vary the radiopacity, viscosity, and rate of polymerization of the glue.
- The glue polymerizes when in contact with ionic solutions. Avoid contamination of the glue with blood, saline, and contrast during preparation.
- To prevent premature polymerization of the glue inside the catheter, the hub and the catheter should be flushed with copious amounts of 5% dextrose prior to introducing the glue.
- The glue should be administered immediately after flushing the catheter with dextrose, before blood has had a chance to back up the catheter.
- n-BCA is a strong adhesive. Significant reflux around the microcatheter cannot be allowed without risking catheter fracture or retention.
- The catheter must be removed swiftly to reduce the risks of glue embolizing into eloquent vessels during removal or of retention of the catheter itself.

Table 7.11 Advantages and Disadvantages of n-BCA

Advantages of n-BCA	Disadvantages of n-BCA
Less expensive.	May incite a chronic inflammatory reaction.
Short procedural time.	Radiopacity fades over time.
Recanalization is uncommon.	Glue embolization of AVMs prior to radiation may be less effective.

Tips on Mixing n-BCA

- The more concentrated the glue, the quicker it will polymerize when injected.
- Increasing the concentration of lipiodol increases the radiopacity, the time to polymerization, and viscosity of the glue. Increased viscosity may limit penetration of small vessels and requires more force with administration.
- The radiopacity of the glue can be increased by adding powdered tantalum, although this step is not necessary if lipiodol is used.
- Glacial acetic acid (GAA) is used by many interventionists to slow polymerization of the glue for better distal penetration. Unlike lipiodol, however, GAA decreases the viscosity of the glue. This may help improve distal penetration.
- For most embolizations, the authors use a mixture of 20 or 25% n-BCA to lipiodol plus of 2 drops of glacial acetic acid via a 27 or 30 gauge needle. Penetration of the glue is controlled by altering the rate of the injection.

Onyx (Ethylene Vinyl Alcohol Copolymer)

- Onyx is ethylene vinyl alcohol copolymer dissolved in dimethyl sulfoxide (DMSO).
- It comes pre-mixed with tantalum to provide radiopacity.
- It precipitates, not polymerizes, on contact with blood or saline.
- The number on the Onyx vial refers to its viscosity measured in centipoise (cP). Onyx-18 and Onyx-34 are used for vessel embolization, while the more viscous Onyx-500 is used for aneurysm embolization.[15]

Tips for Using Onyx (Table 7.12)

- To ensure radiopacity, the Onyx should be mixed on a shaker for 20 minutes prior to use to suspend the tantalum in the DMSO.
- It is necessary to use a DMSO-compatible catheter, usually one in the Rebar or Marathon microcatheter series.

Table 7.12 Advantages and Disadvantages of Onyx

Advantages of Onyx	Disadvantages of Onyx
Catheter likely to be retrieved even after a prolonged embolization.	Since it is not an adhesive, blood can sometimes flow by the Onyx cast after embolization, causing recanalizaztion.
Can flow down multiple arterial pedicles, allowing for treatment of the entire nidus from one or two feeding vessels.	Use of Onyx does prolong the procedural time and increases the amount of fluoroscopy with treatment.
Onyx emboli can be retrieved in some cases.	Injection of DMSO is painful, making it difficult to perform in awake patients.
	The Onyx cast results in substantial, permanent hardening artifact on subsequent CT scans.

- Once the catheter is in position, it should be flushed with saline to help purge blood from the catheter.
- It is paramount that the catheter then be flushed with DMSO just prior to administering the Onyx to prevent premature precipitation. The amount of DMSO injected during catheter preparation should be equal to the dead space of the microcatheter.
- DMSO should be flushed into the microcatheter at a rate of 0.1 mL/min. Remember that you are still injecting the DMSO in the dead space of the catheter at the beginning of the Onyx injection, so the rate of injection should be adjusted accordingly.
- Catheter removal should be done slowly to avoid breakage, vessel injury, and traction on cranial nerves. To remove a stubborn catheter, gently pull the catheter back until there is resistance and hold it there for 30–60 seconds by tightening the rotating hemostatic valve (RHV) located on the Touhy-Borst valve of the guide catheter. As the stretched catheter retracts it will slowly pull out of the Onyx cast. The process can be repeated multiple times, if necessary, until the catheter is loose.

Conclusions

Understanding the nomenclature and basic applications of the neuroendovascular armamentarium is fundamental to good clinical outcomes. In addition, this basis will provide a secure foundation for future technological advancements. Though this technology and its equipment are constantly evolving, many of the new instruments are variations on previous iterations of techniques and tools.

References

1. Sluzewski M, van Rooij WJ, Cloft H. Is the risk of balloon assistance underinflated? AJNR Am J Neuroradiol 2008;29:1777–1781
2. Bosiers M, de Donato G, Deloose K, Verbist J, Peeters P, Castriota F, et al. Does free cell area influence the outcome in carotid artery stenting? Eur J Vasc Endovasc Surg 2007;33:135–141, discussion 142–133
3. Hart JP, Peeters P, Verbist J, Deloose K, Bosiers M. Do device characteristics impact outcome in carotid artery stenting? J Vasc Surg 2006;44:725–730, discussion 730–731
4. Schillinger M, Dick P, Wiest G, et al. Covered versus bare self-expanding stents for endovascular treatment of carotid artery stenosis: a stopped randomized trial. J Endovasc Ther 2006;13(3):312–319
5. Qureshi AI, Kirmani JF, Hussein HM, et al. Early and intermediate-term outcomes with drug-eluting stents in high-risk patients with symptomatic intracranial stenosis. Neurosurgery 2006;59(5):1044–1051, discussion 1051
6. Eskridge JM, Song JK. Endovascular embolization of 150 basilar tip aneurysms with Guglielmi detachable coils: results of the Food and Drug Administration multicenter clinical trial. J Neurosurg 1998;89(1):81–86
7. Pierot L, Leclerc X, Bonafé A, Bracard S; French Matrix Registry Investigators. Endovascular treatment of intracranial aneurysms with matrix detachable coils: midterm anatomic follow-up from a prospective multicenter registry. AJNR Am J Neuroradiol 2008;29(1):57–61
8. Ishii A, Murayama Y, Nien YL, et al. Immediate and midterm outcomes of patients with cerebral aneurysms treated with Matrix1 and Matrix2 coils: a comparative

analysis based on a single-center experience in 250 consecutive cases. Neurosurgery 2008;63(6):1071–1077, discussion 1077–1079

9. Sorimachi T, Koike T, Takeuchi S, et al. Embolization of cerebral arteriovenous malformations achieved with polyvinyl alcohol particles: angiographic reappearance and complications. AJNR Am J Neuroradiol 1999;20(7):1323–1328

10. Germano IM, Davis RL, Wilson CB, Hieshima GB. Histopathological follow-up study of 66 cerebral arteriovenous malformations after therapeutic embolization with polyvinyl alcohol. J Neurosurg 1992;76(4):607–614

11. Rodiek SO, Stölzle A, Lumenta ChB. Preoperative embolization of intracranial meningiomas with Embosphere microspheres. Minim Invasive Neurosurg 2004;47(5):299–305

12. Velat GJ, Reavey-Cantwell JF, Sistrom C, Smullen D, Fautheree GL, Whiting J, et al. Comparison of N-butyl cyanoacrylate and Onyx for the embolization of intracranial arteriovenous malformations: analysis of fluoroscopy and procedure times. Neurosurgery 2008;63:ONS73–78, discussion ONS78–80

13. Cekirge HS, Saatci I, Ozturk MH, et al. Late angiographic and clinical follow-up results of 100 consecutive aneurysms treated with Onyx reconstruction: largest single-center experience. Neuroradiology 2006;48(2):113–126

14. n-BCA Trial Investigators. N-butyl cyanoacrylate embolization of cerebral arteriovenous malformations: results of a prospective, randomized, multi-center trial. AJNR Am J Neuroradiol 2002;23(5):748–755

15. Piske RL, Kanashiro LH, Paschoal E, Agner C, Lima SS, Aguiar PH. Evaluation of Onyx HD-500 embolic system in the treatment of 84 wide-neck intracranial aneurysms. Neurosurg 2009;64:E865–875

Endovascular Techniques for Aneurysm Therapy, Arteriovenous Malformation Treatment, and Carotid Artery Stent Placement

Alan S. Boulos and John C. Dalfino

Endovascular Aneurysm Therapy

Objectives

The goal of endovascular aneurysm embolization is to occlude the fundus of the aneurysm completely while maintaining the patency of the parent vessel. Partial embolization, both planned and unplanned, is a reasonable option in patients who are unable (or unwilling) to undergo surgery. Partial aneurysm embolization can be performed to protect the dome of wide-necked, ruptured aneurysms in patients who are elderly or critically ill, or who are within the vasospasm period. In some cases, more definitive treatment of a partially coiled, ruptured aneurysm can be performed after the patient recovers.[1] In rare cases, partial embolization is performed to make definitive clip reconstruction easier.

The ability to embolize an aneurysm fully is largely determined by its anatomy, in particular its dome-to-neck ratio (**Fig. 8.1**). A ratio greater than 2 is generally favorable for coil embolization. If the ratio is less than 2, adjunctive techniques should be considered, such as balloon-assisted coiling, stent-assisted coiling, dual microcatheter coiling, or surgical clipping.[2]

Medications

Anticoagulation

Stroke is the most common complication encountered in the endovascular treatment of unruptured aneurysms. In acutely ruptured aneurysms, the patient is in a hypercoagulable state as a result of the hemorrhage. In fact, it has been observed that the thromboembolic risk during angiography and interventions is higher in patients with ruptured aneurysms than in patients who undergo elective treatment.[3,4] Since patients with ruptured aneurysms often require external ventricular drainage or other supportive surgery, the use of aspirin and clopidogrel is avoided. Heparin is the most common agent used to prevent thromboembolic complications during the coiling of ruptured aneurysms. Other anticoagulants used during

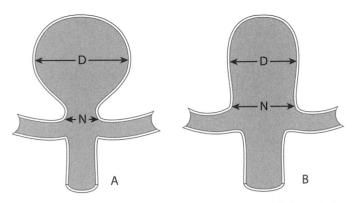

Fig. 8.1   The length of the dome (D) divided by the length of the neck (N) is the dome:neck ratio. **(A)** A favorable dome:neck ratio is 2 or greater. **(B)** A smaller dome:neck ratio may require adjunctive techniques like balloon or stent assistance for best results.

aneurysm coiling include bivalirudin, low-molecular weight heparin, and ketorolac (a reversible platelet inhibitor).

Heparin

The timing and amount of heparin administered during the coiling of a ruptured aneurysm varies between interventionists. One method is to give a standard bolus of heparin (70 units/kg) at the time the guide catheter is positioned, followed by 1000 units of heparin per hour. The target activated clotting time (ACT) is maintained at around 250 seconds.[5] A second method is to administer a half dose (or no dose) at the time the guide catheter is positioned and then to complete the bolus after deploying the first coil.[6] A third method is to give no intravenous heparin. Instead, 10,000 units of heparin per liter of saline are flushed intra-arterially through the guide catheter during the procedure. (John Barr, in a 2007 personal communication described this as the Kerber technique.)

Anti-aggregation

For elective treatment of unruptured aneurysms, an 81 mg dose of aspirin (in addition to intravenous heparin) has been advocated to reduce the risk of thromboembolic complications.[7] Others, including the authors, advocate the use of clopidogrel prior to the procedure, particularly if the placement of a stent is anticipated.[8] In the rare event of a rupture, however, the addition of a non-reversible antiplatelet drug will likely complicate efforts at surgical clot evacuation, clipping, or EVD placement.

Guide Catheter Selection

In younger patients with non-tortuous arch anatomy, the simplest method for obtaining access to the cervical vessels is to use a guide catheter. With standard diagnostic techniques, a 5 or 6 French (Fr) variable stiffness guide catheter can be used to select the cervical internal carotid artery or vertebral artery. Like diagnostic catheters, guide catheters are available in various shapes (Simmons-2, Headhunter, angled) to accommodate varying anatomy. A 6 Fr guide catheter has a large enough bore to accommodate two microcatheters, a critical feature for balloon-assisted coiling and other dual catheter techniques. A 5 Fr guide catheter will generally accommodate only one microcatheter but can be useful in smaller vessels, where a 6 Fr catheter is occlusive.

With a guide catheter alone, it may be difficult to obtain stable access in the carotid artery in patients with tortuous anatomy. In these patients, a stiffer 80–90 cm guide sheath can be used to straighten out the common carotid artery takeoff from the arch and prevent the system from herniating into the arch during catheterization and coiling of the aneurysm. A guide catheter can be coaxially passed through the guide sheath if more distal access to the internal carotid artery is desired. The combination of a guide sheath, guide catheter, and microcatheter into one system is often referred to as a "tri-axial" system.

Another option is to use an "intermediate" guide catheter. These relatively new guide catheters are softer and more flexible than traditional guide catheters. This allows them to be positioned intracranially while still providing a large enough working channel to accept a single microcatheter.[9] Positioning the guide catheter closer to the aneurysm may provide more stability and control of the microcatheter during embolization. Like traditional 5 Fr guide catheters, however, many of these small catheters will not accommodate dual microcatheter techniques.

Microcatheter Selection

In general, coil embolization requires placement of a microcatheter and microwire system into the fundus of the aneurysm. A multitude of microcatheters and microwires are available to catheterize aneurysms, each of which has unique properties that make it suitable (or unsuitable) for a particular treatment. It is important to understand the basic features each device so that the most compatible microcatheter/microwire combination is selected for a particular case. For smaller-necked aneurysms, we favor smaller microcatheters to make passing the catheter through the neck of the aneurysm easier. Conversely, for larger aneurysms, microcatheters with a larger inner diameter are preferred to allow for the use of larger coils.

Some microcatheters have a nitinol braid to stiffen them so that they are less likely to herniate out of the aneurysm during coil deployment. Stiffer microcatheters, however, may not track well through tortuous vessels. They may also be more likely to rupture the aneurysm if the tip comes into contact with the wall of the aneurysm.

The tip of the microcatheter should be shaped to mimic the vascular anatomy. Microcatheters pre-shaped at the factory are available in a variety of shapes and angles, but we prefer to custom shape our catheters. In general, a microcatheter will require 30 to 45 seconds in steam to maintain its shape. Shaping of the microcatheter should be done prior to its introduction into the guide catheter. Some interventionists flush the microcatheter continuously with heparinized saline, while others do not. We advocate having the microcatheter on a continuous heparinized saline flush at all times to help prevent thromboembolic complications and to keep the lubricious inner walls of the microcatheter well hydrated.

Microwire Selection

Microwire selection is similarly complex. Most interventionists use a 0.014" diameter wire to select the aneurysm. The 0.014" wire offers a good balance between softness, ability to be torqued, and visibility when compared with larger or smaller diameter wires. The wires most commonly used during neurointerventional procedures are made of nitinol, metal alloy, or platinum. Each of these materials has advantages and disadvantages. In general, the metal alloy and nitinol wires are more responsive to torque than platinum wires, but their tips are stiffer and therefore less delicate. We advocate getting comfortable with how one or two wires behave and using them regularly rather than changing the wire selection for each procedure depending on the anatomy. Some interventionists prefer smaller microwires and will use 0.012", 0.010," or even 0.008" diameter wires. In general, smaller wires are softer and may be less likely to injure a vessel or aneurysm inadvertently. Small wires are especially helpful when attempting to access distal mycotic or perinidal aneurysms. These smaller wires, however, may be less visible on fluoroscopy, so care must be taken when advancing them.

Another important consideration for microwires is the tip shape. Depending on the patient's anatomy, the tip of the microwire can make the catheterization of the aneurysm either simple or extraordinarily difficult. As with microcatheters, many manufacturers provide pre-shaped tips for purchase. Alternatively, the user can shape the tip of the wire by hand or with a stylette. In general, I use a "headhunter" shape, varying the length and severity of the distal and proximal curves depending on the anatomy to be catheterized (**Fig. 8.2**). I generally use a nitinol slot-machined microwire that is very responsive to torque (Synchro-2 soft 14 wire, Boston Scientific, Natick, MA). Because of its responsiveness to torque, it maintains a one-to-one relationship to small handheld movements during intervention and hence expedites intracranial navigation. Its tip also maintains its shape well during use.

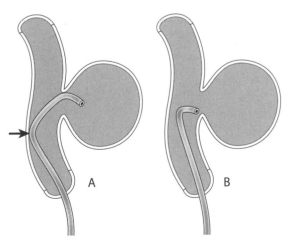

Fig. 8.2 The double-bend "headhunter" shape **(A)** will allow the body of the catheter to lean against the back wall of the parent vessel (*arrow*), providing more support than a simple curve **(B)**.

Microcatheterization Technique

It is extremely important to account for the built-up energy that occurs in a catheter/wire system after each turn in the vasculature. In straight vessels, advancing or withdrawing a device like a wire or catheter at the hub results in an identical movement at the tip. With increasing tortuosity within the vessels, advancing the tip of the device through the curves results in redundancy in the body of the device prior to tip movement. Once the device clears the turn, the stored energy will tend to straighten out the device and spring the tip of the device forward. Therefore, understanding the location of the aneurysm in relation to the vessel anatomy is critical to understanding the safest method of access.

For instance, if the aneurysm is either on or just distal to a turn, there is a high probability that the catheter/wire system will be propelled into the aneurysm during catheterization, with potentially catastrophic results. To avoid these uncontrolled movements, it is safest to advance the catheter and wire past the aneurysm first to release any stored energy, and then pull the system back more proximally to catheterize the aneurysm. In tortuous vessels, we prefer to cross the aneurysm first and then bring the microcatheter back slowly until it faces the aneurysm neck. The microcatheter/wire combination is then re-advanced into the aneurysm. In very small aneurysms I prefer to manipulate the microwire tip within the microcatheter while redirecting the microcatheter toward the aneurysm. Essentially, the microwire and microcatheter are advanced as one system into the aneurysm.

In general, the catheter should be positioned one-third to one-half the way into the aneurysm fundus to advance coils safely. If the aneurysm is small, it may be safer to position the catheter at its neck rather than in the fundus. In very small aneurysms, coils can even be deployed from the parent vessel across the neck of the aneurysm and into the fundus.

Coil Selection

A multitude of coil choices are available today. The core criteria for coil selection include its diameter, its length, and its 3-D shape. Other considerations include the diameter of the coil wire itself, the coil's intrinsic stretch resistance, and the specific properties of any "bioactive" coatings that have been applied. Newer framing coils are designed with smaller distal loops that are intended to tumble inside the aneurysm while the larger outer loops form a basket across the neck of the aneurysm. Without these smaller lead loops, the first loop of a large-diameter coil may exit the aneurysm instead of forming a basket inside it.

The 3-D shape of the coil selected should mimic the shape of the aneurysm as closely as possible. Aneurysms with a spherical shape tend to be framed well with "boxlike" coils. Dysmorphic, bilobed, or sausage-shaped aneurysms are better treated with alternative coil shapes.

The initial coils are selected to frame or "paint" the periphery of the aneurysm and cover the neck of the aneurysm. After placing several loops of coil across the neck, the subsequent coils are less likely to herniate through these loops and into the parent vessel. The diameter of the initial framing coil is selected to match the diameter of the aneurysm. Most aneurysms, however, are not spherical. In non-spherical aneurysms, some interventionists will use the mean value of the height, width, and depth of the aneurysm to size the first coil. A framing coil that is significantly over-sized may put excessive tension on the wall of the aneurysm and cause it to rupture. Over-sized coils also tend not to pack well and have a tendency to herniate into the parent vessel. If the diameter of the coil is significantly undersized, the coil will form its loops but may not apply any tension to the aneurysm wall. In this case, it is possible for the coil to move after detachment and embolize into the parent vessel.

After the framing coil is fully deployed, subtracted angiography should be performed to evaluate its position prior to detachment. It is better to remove a poorly sized framing coil (when possible) and look for a better fit than to struggle with the deployment of subsequent coils. An important improvement in coil design was increasing the length of the framing coils. A coil that is undersized in terms of its 3-D conformation but that is long may still generate adequate friction against the walls of the aneurysm to remain stable after deployment. Long, undersized coils are sometimes helpful in framing dysmorphic, bilobed, or sausage-shaped aneurysms that might otherwise be difficult to coil.

After the framing coil is placed, subsequent coils can either be filling coils or smaller framing coils. If a framing coil is used to fill the aneurysm, it should usually be smaller than the initial framing coil. With the use of additional framing coils, progressively smaller "baskets" are created inside the initial framing coil until the aneurysm is fully embolized. It has been suggested that the result of this technique is a coil mass analogous to Russian Matryoshka dolls[10] (**Fig. 8.3**). Alternatively, softer helical or complex shaped "filling coils" can be used to complete the embolization.

Coils are placed until either the aneurysm no longer fills with contrast during angiography or the microcatheter is pushed outside the aneurysm during coil placement and cannot be replaced after detachment. Most interventionists will perform an angiogram prior to detaching a coil to confirm patency of the parent vessel and to evaluate the efficacy of the coils that have already been deployed. This is often subtracted angiography, but other methods, such as subtracted fluoroscopy, are also acceptable. Another important consideration is to observe coil placement as it relates to the surrounding vessels. One of the earliest signs of coil impingement on a branch vessel includes a delay in emptying, so observation of this finding means that the vessel is compromised and that removal of the deployed coil should be considered. Often the delayed vessel (in emptying) will go on to thrombose on subsequent angiography if the coil is not repositioned.

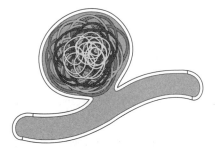

Fig. 8.3 Framing coils can be used to fill an aneurysm. The first coil (lightest gray) should be the same size as the dome of the aneurysm. Progressively smaller framing coils can then be deployed inside it until the aneurysm is filled. This has been referred to as the "Russian doll" technique.

Detaching Coils

Coils rely on one of three methods for detachment. Most vendors use an electrolytic method for coil detachment. During electrolytic detachment, a charge applied to the end of the coil heats up the material in the detachment zone, causing it to break and detach the coil (Boston Scientific, Micrus, ev3, Terumo).[11] Other detachment methods include mechanical (Cook, ev3) and hydraulic systems (Codman, Terumo). The hydraulic system relies on a hypotube attached to an insufflator for deployment. This system seems to have the softest detachment zone of the three systems, making it less likely to push the catheter out of the aneurysm during coil deployment. Care must be taken to avoid kinking or allowing air into the hypotube, as this may prevent the coil from detaching properly.

It is important to realize that the detachment zone of all of the coil systems is stiffer than the coil itself. As the relatively stiff pusher is advanced beyond the tip of the microcatheter during coil deployment, the catheter will often back out of the aneurysm. Many times the microcatheter can be carefully re-advanced into the aneurysm over the partially deployed coil. Other times, simply detaching the coil will allow the tip of the microcatheter to fall back into the aneurysm. If the stiff detachment zone is advanced quickly into the aneurysm, it may cause perforation of the aneurysm (**Fig. 8.4**).[12] Be aware of the interaction between the detachment zone and the microcatheter in small aneurysms (or when placing the last coils into a larger aneurysm) to avoid losing microcatheter access. Catheters that fall completely out of a partially coiled aneurysm are often difficult and potentially dangerous to reposition.

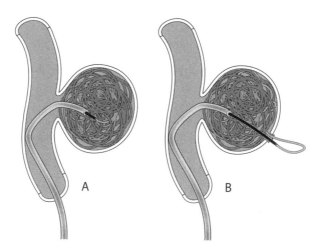

Fig. 8.4 (**A**) Ideally the pusher should extend just past the tip of the catheter during detachment. This is particularly important on the last coil, as deploying the coil inside the microcatheter will often leave a "tail" of coil in the parent vessel when the microcatheter is removed. (**B**) If the stiff detachment zone of the coil is deployed too far into the aneurysm, however, it may perforate the aneurysm.

Special Considerations for Very Large and/or Giant Aneurysms

Very large or giant aneurysms remain a significant challenge for cerebrovascular surgery. For endovascular treatment, the most important challenge is the high rate of recurrence.[13] To reduce the rate of recurrence, some interventionists (Jacques Dion, personal communication 2004) will advance the microcatheter around the fundus of the aneurysm until it is pointing toward the neck of the aneurysm. Then, if the aspect ratio is favorable, coils are deployed to form a latticework of coil loops across the neck of the aneurysm. This latticework acts like a stent to keep other filling coils from herniating through the neck of the aneurysm and into the fundus.

As a rule, coils will go where the catheter is not. This means that if the microcatheter is in the most distal part of the aneurysm, the coil loops will push off the wall of the aneurysm and deploy closer to the neck. If the catheter is in the neck, the coils will tend to deploy in the distal fundus of the aneurysm.

With very large or giant aneurysms, adjunctive therapy directed at preserving the parent vessel is important. To reduce recurrence, stent placement within the parent vessel can be performed.[14] Alternatively, balloon assistance to increase the density of coil embolization may help reduce recanalization. Lastly, dual microcatheter techniques can be used for wide-necked aneurysm treatment.[15,16]

Parent vessel occlusion should be considered when treating very large or giant aneurysms as it reduces the chance of recurrence considerably. An obvious risk to this strategy is ischemia or stroke. Only vessels that have undergone successful balloon test occlusion should be considered for sacrifice. Vessels that do not pass balloon test occlusion should be surgically bypassed prior to sacrifice.

Aneurysmal Mass Effect

Another important consideration is mass effect. The traditional dictum is that a third of patients with symptoms of mass effect (like a third nerve palsy or obstructive hydrocephalus) will worsen after coiling, another third will improve, and the last third will remain unchanged.[17] The risk of mass effect progression is increased in the setting of giant aneurysms, so periprocedural management of mass effect symptoms should be considered. Steroids (glucocorticoids) are usually the most effective adjunctive therapy for treating progressive mass effect from aneurysms. In patients who present with mass effect, steroids are generally recommended at the time of treatment and postprocedurally. Surgical clip ligation should be considered in patients with symptomatic mass effect, as clip ligation with evacuation of the aneurysm fundus does appear to reduce mass effect in a greater number of patients than does endovascular treatment.[18,19]

Adjunctive Endovascular Techniques for Coiling Aneurysms

Dual Microcatheter Technique

In the dual microcatheter technique, the aneurysm is catheterized and coiled as usual using a framing coil, but the coil is not detached. The aneurysm is then catheterized with a second microcatheter, and a second coil is deployed. If both coils are in good position, the coils are detached. If not, one coil or both coils can be recaptured and redeployed.

The dual microcatheter technique is useful in wide-necked aneurysms where the first coil might be pushed out of the aneurysm and into the parent vessel during deployment of the second coil. The use of two catheters simultaneously can also aid in the embolization of complex, multilobulated aneurysms, which can become compartmentalized using traditional single-catheter techniques. As with all multicatheter techniques, however, some level of complexity is added to the procedure, and there is an associated potential increase in thromboembolic events.

Balloon-Assisted Aneurysm Embolization

Balloon-assisted coil embolization refers to the positioning and inflation of a balloon in the parent vessel while coils are deployed within the aneurysm.[20–22] Once the coil or coils have been deployed, the balloon is deflated, and angiography is performed to verify that the parent vessel is patent. Some interventionists will deflate the balloon between each coil deployment to assess the stability of the coil mass and to shorten the vessel occlusion time. Others will deploy several coils prior to deflation of the balloon. Using the principles of aneurysm clipping with temporary clips, sufficient time should be allowed between balloon inflations to give the brain time to recover (usually 5 minutes between inflations).[23] Alternatively, rather than inflating the balloon routinely during coiling, a deflated balloon can be positioned at the aneurysm neck and inflated only as necessary.

Balloon-assisted coiling is especially useful for treating ruptured wide-necked aneurysms, because unlike stent placement, no antiplatelet agents are required. Once a few of the filling coils are in place, the coil mass will usually exert sufficient tension on the aneurysm wall that the balloon can be safely deflated and removed without dislodging the coil mass. A balloon can also slow subarachnoid hemorrhage if the aneurysm ruptures during the procedure.

There are some disadvantages to balloon-assisted coiling. First, balloon-assisted coiling is associated with ischemic complications. When inflated, the balloon blocks normal blood flow through the parent vessel to the brain, resulting in relative hypoperfusion. Stasis both behind and ahead of the balloon can lead to thrombus formation in the parent vessel, particularly if the patient has not received adequate anticoagulation treatment. Balloons can also damage the vessel wall and may cause a dissection.[24–27]

Technique

In most cases soft, compliant balloons are used for embolization assistance. These balloons are constructed with a wire-valve mechanism. As long as a wire is across the valve, the balloon will inflate and deflate. If the wire is withdrawn, the balloon cannot be inflated, and fluid administered through the hub of the microcatheter will escape through the center lumen. In preparing these balloons, it is important to evacuate any air from the balloon first. To do this, place the deflated balloon in a saline basin and attach a Tuohy-Borst valve connected to a three-way valve with 20 cc and 3 cc syringes. The insufflation solution is a two-thirds or three-fourths contrast-saline mixture. The air is evacuated from the lumen of the balloon by flushing the contrast-saline mixture through the balloon with the wire out. A 0.010″ wire is then passed into the lumen of the balloon, occluding the valve so the balloon can be inflated with a 3 cc syringe. The volume of the balloon is small (approximately

0.2 cc). One will receive tactile feedback through the syringe regarding the amount of pressure needed to inflate the balloon fully (R Chapot, personal communication, 2004). The balloon is semi-permeable, so balloon inflation should be done with the balloon fully submerged in saline (or contrast-saline mixture) to avoid pulling air into the balloon during deflation. A 20 cc syringe can be used to aspirate during deflation to reduce the likelihood of air entering the system. Once the balloon is prepared, it is advanced over the 0.010″ wire to the aneurysm neck, using a high-definition roadmap. The wire is advanced into a distal cerebral vessel to stabilize the balloon and to prevent it from inadvertently sliding into the aneurysm.

An inflated balloon will tend to "sail" forward with the arterial current, so it is often helpful to have an assistant hold the balloon in place while the operator deploys the coils. It will require patience and practice to inflate the balloon correctly and keep the balloon in a stable position across the neck of the aneurysm. Some interventionists will prepare the balloon using only saline to reduce friction between the wire and the balloon (A Molyneaux, personal communication, 2004). Once the balloon is in position, it can be inflated with a contrast/saline mixture. To remove the saline from the balloon, remove the wire and flush it with a contrast-saline mixture. The wire can then be reintroduced to inflate the balloon.

Though these balloons are soft, it is important to note that their reference diameter is usually 4 mm. In vessels less than 2 mm, try to position part of the balloon in a larger branch to allow the balloon to herniate into that branch if inadvertent over-inflation occurs. In a prospective trial examining prophylactic balloon inflation to prevent vasospasm, all of the vessel ruptures occurred in small vessels (less than 2 mm).[28-30]

Use of Liquid Embolics for Treatment of Aneurysms

Onyx HD 500 (ev3, Plymouth, MN), a liquid embolic agent, has been given conditional approval for treatment of cerebral aneurysms with balloon assistance. The method used for aneurysm embolization with Onyx is similar to balloon-assisted coil embolization: After catheterization of the aneurysm, a balloon is inflated over the aneurysm neck to isolate the aneurysm fundus from the parent vessel. With the balloon inflated, the Onyx is administered through the microcatheter and then allowed to precipitate over 2 minutes. The balloon can then be deflated. After a 5-minute reperfusion period, the process can be repeated if necessary to complete the embolization.

Stent-Assisted Aneurysm Coil Embolization

Stent placement for aneurysm coiling provides two important benefits. First, the stent tines help to prevent coils from herniating into the parent vessel. Second, the walls of the stent may help divert flow away from the aneurysm and act as a scaffold to promote endothelialization over the aneurysm neck. Several investigators have shown that stents with closed cells and less porosity promote aneurysm thrombosis and healing of the parent vessel better than more porous open-cell stents. Unfortunately, less porous stents tend to be stiffer, making them more difficult to maneuver through tortuous anatomy.

There is a small but significant thromboembolic risk with stent placement. As the stent composite rests within the artery itself, thrombus may form within the stent and embolize to normal cerebral vessels. A dual antiplatelet regimen (usually aspirin and clopidogrel) will reduce the risk of thrombus formation considerably. In ruptured aneurysms, the use of nonreversible antiplatelet agents is relatively contraindicated as they may affect the ability to manage hydrocephalus after the procedure. Alternatively, intravenous glycoprotein IIb-IIIa receptor antagonists can provide sufficient platelet inhibition to prevent stent thrombosis, and they have a short half-life, unlike oral agents like aspirin and clopidogrel.

There are four methods of stent-assisted coil embolization.

Staged Approach

Some interventionists will place a stent across the aneurysm first without coiling the aneurysm. After 4 to 12 weeks, the patient is brought back for coiling of the aneurysm through the stent. The advantage of this approach is that the stent has time to endothelialize along the parent vessel to prevent it from dislodging during coil deployment. One disadvantage of this approach is that the aneurysm is left unsecured for up to 3 months between stent placement and coil embolization. Another disadvantage is that re-accessing the aneurysm through the stent during the second procedure can be difficult or even impossible.

Stent-after-Coil Embolization

The initial description of the Neuroform (Boston Scientific, Natick, MA) technique was to perform balloon-assisted coil embolization and then, after coil embolization was complete, exchange the balloon for a stent. The stent would then be deployed across the neck of the aneurysm to prevent coil migration and reduce the likelihood of recurrence. Unfortunately, this procedure can be cumbersome. Balloons are designed for use with 0.010″ wires, while the stents tracks best over 0.014″ wires. This means that to exchange a balloon for a stent a two-step exchange must be performed. First, the balloon is removed over the 0.010″ wire and exchanged for a microcatheter large enough to accept a 0.014″ wire. The 0.010″ wire is then removed and replaced with an exchange length 0.014″ wire to accommodate the stent. Another disadvantage of the stent-after-coil technique is that the balloon must be deflated just prior to placing the stent, providing an opportunity for the coil mass to migrate.

Stent, Then Microcatheterize the Aneurysm

This is the most common method. First, the stent is deployed across the neck of the aneurysm. Next, a microcatheter is advanced through the cells of the stent and into the fundus of the aneurysm where the coils are deployed. Unlike balloon-assisted approaches, it is not necessary to stop flow through the parent vessel temporarily during the procedure, reducing the risk of ischemic complications. Essentially, the stent-then-microcatheterize technique is the same as in the staged approach except that the stent placement and coil embolization procedures are performed during the same session. The trade-off is that the stent is more likely to be dislodged during coil deployment and microcatheter manipulations than in the staged approach.

Dual Microcatheter Approach

In this method, a large microcatheter for stent deployment is placed across the neck of the aneurysm while a second microcatheter is placed within the aneurysm fundus. After the two catheters are in place, the stent is deployed, pinning the coiling microcatheter between the wall of the parent vessel and the stent. Only the tip of the coiling microcatheter will extend into the aneurysm fundus. This technique avoids the need to manipulate the freshly deployed stent except when withdrawing the coiling microcatheter after embolization. Another advantage of this technique is that the stent also helps to stabilize the coiling microcatheter during coiling and thus reduces the risk it will back out of the aneurysm.

In most cases, the dual catheter technique is our preferred treatment approach. This technique allows the stent and the coils to be placed in the same session while avoiding the sometimes tedious task of re-accessing the aneurysm through the stent. Jailing of the coiling microcatheter in the aneurysm also helps to stabilize it during coil deployment. Care must be taken with the dual microcatheter technique that the microcatheter in the aneurysm does not shoot forward into the wall of the aneurysm while the stent is deployed. If this situation is ignored, the movement of the coiling catheter could rupture the aneurysm. This situation can be avoided by applying a little negative tension on the coiling microcatheter during stent deployment to help maintain its position. In addition, either a wire or coil should be placed within the coiling microcatheter to help stabilize it while the stent is deployed. Be aware that the coiling microcatheter will be partly constrained by the stent. This may make it difficult to reposition the microcatheter in the fundus of the aneurysm if the coils compartmentalize during embolization.

Other Considerations during Stent-Coiling Procedures

Most stents are radiolucent except at the ends. This means that where the stent crosses the aneurysm, it is "invisible" to the user. Sometimes during coiling a loop of coil can herniate between tines of the stent and re-enter the parent vessel. Complete reliance on the stent to maintain the integrity of the parent vessel can result in parent vessel occlusion or thromboembolic complications. Another important consideration with this method is that during coil embolization, the microcatheter may back out into the parent vessel, resulting in coils being deployed across, rather than outside, the stent. A coil deployed in this manner will have a tail extending into the parent artery that will act as a nidus for thrombus.

Choosing a Stent for Aneurysm Embolization

Several self-expanding stents are available for aneurysm treatment. These include, as of this writing: Neuroform (Boston Scientific), Enterprise (Codman), Leo (ev3), Solitaire (Balt), and Pipeline (ev3, Chestnut Medical). The last three are not FDA approved but have CE marks in Europe. All of these stents are deployed through a microcatheter. Some, like the Leo (ev3), are fully retrievable, while others are only partially retrievable (Enterprise, Codman). Some have closed cells (Enterprise, Pipeline) while others are open-celled (Neuroform, Leo, Solitaire) (**Fig. 8.5**).

In general, balloon-expandable stents are not used for aneurysm treatment. In fact, there is only one balloon-expandable stent designed for aneurysm coiling, the

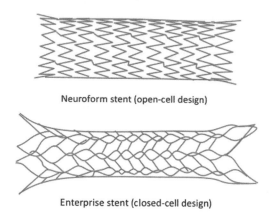

Neuroform stent (open-cell design)

Enterprise stent (closed-cell design)

Fig. 8.5 Open-cell stents offer better conformability, making them especially suitable for tortuous anatomy or when spanning two vessels of different caliber. Closed-cell stents have a higher radial force, making them ideal for calcified lesions. Closed-cell stents may also protect against emboli better than open-celled stents in friable plaque.

Pharos (Micrus), and it is not yet FDA approved. Although a balloon-expandable stent can be accurately placed across an aneurysm neck, the balloon inflation required to deploy it is more likely to damage smaller vessels than the deployment of a self-expanding stent. Self-expanding stents also contour better than balloon-expandable stents when it is necessary to span two vessels with a large difference in diameter. These properties make self-expanding stents less likely to migrate than balloon-expandable stents if the stent is inadvertently undersized.

Troubleshooting Complications during Aneurysm Coiling

Stretched Coils

The term "stretched coils" refers to coils that have detached prior to being fully deployed. When this occurs, the coil no longer moves in a one-to-one relationship with the user's hands. A stretched coil often will not advance fully within the aneurysm, so a decision must be made either to withdraw the coil or to try to complete the deployment. To help avoid this situation, one should inspect the coil in a basin of saline before advancing into the microcatheter to make sure it has not been damaged in storage.

When a stretched coil is identified and the interventionist decides to remove it, two strategies may be considered. If most of the coil is still in the catheter, simply pulling out the microcatheter may carry the coil out with it. In cases where most of the coil is outside the catheter, simply pulling out the catheter may leave the coil behind. One option is to advance a 0.010″ diameter microwire next to the partially deployed coil to wedge the damaged coil into place as the microcatheter is withdrawn. Alternatively, the hub of the microcatheter can be removed with scissors, and a 2 or 4 mm loop snare inside a second microcatheter can be advanced over the cut microcatheter and coil. Once it is positioned over the coil, the snare is closed, trapping the coil. The whole system, including the snare, the coil, and both microcatheters, is then removed under direct fluoroscopic guidance (**Fig. 8.6**).[31] Care must be taken not to dislodge previously detached coils into the parent vessel with this technique.

If the coil cannot be retrieved using the above methods, there are three alternatives. The first is to leave the coil in place and use antiplatelet agents and/or anticoagulants to prevent thromboembolic complications. The second is to stent the partially deployed coil against the wall of the vessel. Lastly, one can advance a loop or Alligator (ev3) snare through the parent vessel and retrieve the coil.

Herniated or Protruding Coils

Coils that protrude only slightly into the parent vessel are best treated medically. Treatment with antiplatelet agents, anticoagulation agents, or both will usually suffice to prevent thromboembolic sequelae. Consider long-term aspirin use to avoid late ischemic complications.

Coil Migration

If the entire coil exits the aneurysm after detachment and goes into the parent vessel, retrieval should be attempted. A loop or Alligator snare can be deployed to retrieve the coil. The Alligator is best used by deploying it just proximal to the coil and then advancing it to engage the coil. A loop snare, conversely, should be deployed distal to the coil and withdrawn while closing the loop to engage the

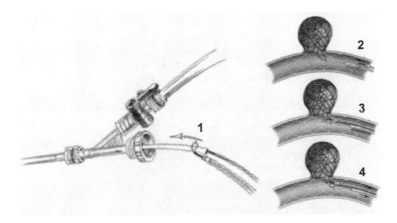

Fig. 8.6 (1) Illustration of insertion of goose neck snare over the coil apparatus. (2) The snare is navigated over the coil apparatus toward the stretched coil. (3) The snare is placed around the non-stretched coil. (4) The snare is retracted into its catheter, pulling the coil with it. (With kind permission from Fiorella D, Albuquerque F, Deshmuk V, et al. Monorail snare technique for the recovery of the stretched platinum coils: Technical case report. Journal of Neurosurgery Jan 2005;57(1):E210.)

coil. Size the snare slightly larger than the parent vessel for best results. If the coil cannot be retrieved, anticoagulation and/or antiplatelet agents can be used. Stent placement or even open surgical removal might also be considered.

Thromboembolic Complications

When thromboembolic complications occur, intra-arterial treatment with thrombolytics or antiplatelet agents can be used safely to restore vessel patency. Glycoprotein IIb-IIIa inhibitors are particularly effective in this setting and appear to be more effective at treating "clot on coil" than thrombolytic agents like tissue plasminogen activator (tPA).[32,33] Unlike tPA, GP IIb-IIIa inhibitors do not seem to increase the risk of aneurysm rupture, even when they are used in patients presenting with a ruptured aneurysm. If the clot is resistant to treatment or a major branch occlusion has developed, mechanical thrombolysis should be considered.

Aneurysm Rupture

If the aneurysm ruptures during coil deployment or during microcatheterization, do not back out the coil, as it is helping to plug the hole. Rather, finish deploying the coil completely, even if the coil protrudes into the subarachnoid space. Continue to fill the aneurysm with coils until extravasation of contrast stops. Reversal of anticoagulation is imperative and can be achieved rapidly with protamine and/ or recombinant factor VIIa. If there are changes in vital signs or neurophysiological markers, an emergent external ventricular drain can be life saving. Consider using a compliant intra-arterial balloon to tamponade bleeding from a ruptured aneurysm, particularly if it is already in place. Inflation for five minutes may help thrombus to form at the site of rupture. It should be noted that all of these adjuncts, including balloons, external ventricular drains, and protamine, should be ready in the interventional suite when treating any aneurysm.

Arteriovenous Malformation Embolization

Basic Tenets of Arteriovenous Malformation Embolization

Arteriovenous malformation (AVM) embolizations carry a fairly significant risk of neurological deficits from cerebral ischemia or hemorrhage. For this reason, AVM embolization procedures need to have clear goals. In some cases, angiographic cure is attempted. This includes embolization of the arterial feeders, the nidus, and the venous compartment of the AVM. Historically, this has been very difficult to achieve.

Selective embolization of an AVM, focusing on vessels that are difficult to reach surgically, helps make excision easier and reduces blood loss. Preoperative embolization is especially helpful in embolizing the deep arterial feeders of the AVM that are associated with poor outcomes in surgical series. Embolization can also help to decrease arteriovenous shunting within the AVM, thereby reducing the risk of normal perfusion pressure breakthough syndrome.

Partial embolization can also be used prior to radiosurgery, but the efficacy of this strategy has been questioned in the literature. In fact, it has been suggested that AVMs pretreated with n-butyl cyanoacrylate (n-BCA) have a lower cure rate with radiosurgery than AVMs of the same size that have not been treated with n-BCA. This finding has not been replicated with ethyl-vinyl alcohol copolymer (EVAL). Nonetheless, if embolization is tried in preparation for radiosurgery, then the goal should be to reduce the nidus near eloquent brain structures where radiation will be less tolerated (for example, near the optic nerve). Embolization should include not only the arterial feeders but also the nidus. If the feeders are embolized but the nidus is not, preradiation planning scans may not fully visualize the nidus, leading to an incomplete treatment. In large AVMs, embolization of the peripheral portions of the nidus may allow the central portion to be radiated more effectively. Conversely, embolization may further compartmentalize the AVM, necessitating a more complicated radiosurgical plan.

Partial AVM embolization can also be used for palliation. For instance, some large AVMs will cause fluctuating neurological deficits due to arterial steal. Partial embolization, by reducing the size of the AVM, can improve perfusion to surrounding brain areas and ameliorate symptoms. Partial embolization can also be used to treat dangerous features of the AVM, like prenidal and intranidal aneurysms, to reduce the risk of subsequent intracranial bleeding.

Periprocedural Medications Used during AVM Embolization

Anticoagulation

Since the risk of intracerebral hemorrhage is higher with AVM embolization than it is with other endovascular interventions, most investigators use a lower dose of periprocedural heparin. The risk of thromboembolic complications during AVM embolization may be lower than during other endovascular procedures, since any thrombus that forms on the catheter will usually embolize to the AVM itself rather than to normal brain areas. In fact, ischemic events during AVM embolization are more likely to occur from the embolic material itself rather than from thrombus formation on the catheter, a problem that will not likely be mitigated by anticoagulation alone.

Anticonvulsants

Periprocedural anticonvulsants should be considered for all AVM embolization cases, particularly if the patient has had a seizure in the past. The changes in blood flow patterns after AVM embolization can be epileptogenic, particularly in cortical AVMs. Some interventionists use anticonvulsants only if the AVM is located in an epileptogenic area, such as the medial temporal lobe.

Antihypertensives

Avoidance of hypertension is critical to prevent perioperative intracerebral hemorrhage. Some interventionists will use hypotension during the embolization in an attempt to reduce the risk of embolic material passing into the draining veins. Close monitoring and control of blood pressure in the immediate postprocedural period are also important to prevent bleeding from hyperperfusion.

Adjunctive Measures Used during AVM Embolization

During partial AVM embolization, it is important to prevent embolic material from migrating into the venous compartment, as this will cause congestion within the AVM and increase the risk of subsequent bleeding. Some interventionists will use a Valsalva maneuver during the administration of the embolic agent to transiently reduce flow through the venous system. By increasing the resistance of the venous outflow path, embolic material is more likely to fill the nidus than to exit via a draining vein. Others have used adenosine to cause brief, reversible asystole during embolization with similar effect (B Bendok, personal communication, 2006). It is important to note, however, that if a cure is to be achieved, all of the portions of the AVM must be treated, including the arterial feeders, the nidus, and the venous compartments. It is unclear if treatment of the arterial pedicles and nidus alone would result in cure, since patent venous channels may allow for arterial recruitment afterwards.

Guide Catheter Selection for AVM Embolization

There are multiple techniques for proximal catheter access when treating arteriovenous malformations. The traditional technique involves using a variable-stiffness 5 French or 6 French guide catheter positioned in the distal pre-cerebral cervical vessel of choice. The 5 French guide catheter is smaller, resulting in less risk of iatrogenic vasospasm, and may allow for more distal access but will not accommodate multiple microcatheters. In a tortuous arch, a 6 French guide sheath can provide good proximal support while providing a working channel large enough to support the use of a coaxially inserted 6 French guide catheter or intermediate guide catheter. Often the pre-cerebral vessel feeding an AVM is large, making the use of larger guide catheters more feasible than in aneurysm or atherosclerosis interventions.

Microcatheter Selection for AVM Embolization

Several microcatheters are available for AVM embolization, and they can be divided into three categories: flow-directed, braided, and hybrid.

Flow-Directed Catheters

Flow-directed microcatheters are not braided; therefore, they are thin and soft. Some are designed with a small "olive" at the tip to enhance their flow-directed properties. These catheters are advanced along with blood flow, allowing them to track quickly through the high-flow arterial feeders of an AVM. Flow-directed catheters are available in various sizes, ranging from 0.007″ to 0.012″ in diameter. Flow-directed microcatheters are particularly effective at getting distal access within the AVM in an atraumatic manner. All microcatheters are compatible with the use of n-BCA, but only a few are compatible with EVAL. Since they are small and unbraided, flow-directed catheters have a lower burst pressure, so the risk of rupture with this type of microcatheter is higher.

The use of a wire with these microcatheters is not necessary but is generally recommended by most interventionists. The wire selected must be compatible with the microcatheter selected. At different points in the procedure, the microwire can lead the microcatheter to ensure proper selection of a cerebral vessel. Once the vessel of choice has been selected, the microwire is withdrawn a few centimeters from the tip of the microcatheter to take advantage of the flow-directed properties of the microcatheter as it is advanced into the AVM. It is important not to remove the wire completely, however. Without the wire in place, the proximal shaft of the microcatheter may herniate into large side branches as it is pushed, making it difficult to advance. The wire can also help to enhance the fluoroscopic visibility of these small catheters.

Over-the-Wire Microcatheters

Standard braided microcatheters compose the second class of microcatheters used to treat AVMs. These catheters, which are also used for treating aneurysms, are usually larger and stiffer than non-braided catheters. They are not flow-directed and must therefore be directed to the nidus over a microwire. Consequently, braided microcatheters can be more difficult to navigate distally than flow-directed catheters. Over-the-wire microcatheters, however, do offer some advantages over their flow-directed counterparts. For example, braided catheters have a higher-rated bursting pressure than non-braided catheters, making them less likely to rupture while injecting a viscous embolic agent like EVAL. The inner lumen size is also larger, allowing for better vessel opacification during microcatheter angiography. Finally, braided catheters are less likely to fracture when removed from the embolic cast.

Hybrid Microcatheters

The Marathon microcatheter (ev3) is a small braided catheter with flow-guided characteristics. It is compatible with EVAL. This catheter offers a good compromise between the strength and stability of a braided catheter and the trackability of a flow-directed catheter. While it is not as flexible as other flow-guided catheters, the Marathon has higher burst and tensile strength and is therefore less likely to rupture or fracture during embolization.

Microwire Selection for AVM Embolization

Usually small microwires are chosen for AVM embolization procedures, because the feeding vessels become small as they approach the nidus. Most interventionists will use either the 0.008″ diameter Mirage microwire (ev3), the 0.007 Sorcerer (Balt, France), or one of the many available 0.010″ diameter microwires. Others will use larger microcatheter/microwire systems that are compatible with PVA particles or embospheres, although it should be noted particle embolization of AVMs is associated with a high rate of recanalization.

Personal Techniques and Experience with AVM Embolization

Microcatheter and Microwire Choice

In general, my preference for AVM embolization is to use a Marathon microcatheter with a Mirage microwire to access the feeding vessels as distally as possible. This is the smallest braided microcatheter/microwire system presently available. The microwire is given a headhunter shape, but the microcatheter tip is kept straight so it is easier to remove at the end of the case.

Catheterization Technique

The system is advanced coaxially under a high-definition road map until the feeding vessel of interest has been catheterized. Next, the microwire is withdrawn into the microcatheter until the tip of the wire is a few centimeters proximal to the tip of the microcatheter. Under a high-definition road map, the microcatheter (with the microwire inside) is advanced toward the nidus. This allows for improved visibility and stability of the catheter, while decreasing the likelihood that it will herniate into a more proximal branch point. It is important to note one-to-one movement of the hand to the microcatheter system. If this is not the case, inspect the catheter along its intracranial course to make sure it has not herniated into a side branch. Access to the nidus of the AVM is important, particularly with n-BCA embolization. With EVAL embolization, a more proximal position may allow multiple feeders to be treated at the same time. If the microcatheter is too proximal, then embolization may allow embolic material to enter eloquent branches.

Anticoagulation

In general, a low dose of intravenous heparin (30 units/kg) is administered after arterial access is obtained. If the AVM is small and the catheterization time will be long, a higher dose of heparin (50–60 units/kg) is given to reduce the risk of thromboembolic complications.

Provocative Testing

Once the microcatheter is in the appropriate position, provocative testing can be performed by injecting short-acting barbiturates (sodium amytal or methohexital sodium) or lidocaine through the microcatheter. In patients who are awake during the procedure, the results of provocative testing are obtained by neurological examination. SSEP, MEP, and electroencephalogram (EEG) recordings can be monitored in patients under general anesthesia. If a neurological deficit occurs after the administration of these agents, it should be assumed that the branch is eloquent. Caution is required in the interpretation of a negative result. Prior to treatment, large AVMs may shunt the flow of drug away from an otherwise eloquent branch, causing a false-negative result. After embolization of the AVM, the flow pattern changes may allow the embolic agent to flow into the previously "silent" eloquent branch, causing a stroke.

Microcatheter Angiography

Microcatheter angiography of the feeding vessel from the microcatheter helps to define the angioarchitecture of the AVM in more detail. The transit time from the arterial phase to the venous phase is important to note, as the concentration of the embolic agent can be altered to match the rapidity of the blood flow. Take note of the distance between the last eloquent artery and the microcatheter tip, as this is the maximum distance of reflux that can be tolerated. The ideal working projection for administration of embolic agent should elongate the AVM so that the arterial pedicle, nidus, and vein are visualized separately. In addition, visualization of the distal microcatheter at a perpendicular angle will elongate the vessel and allow for accurate visualization of embolic reflux. Poor visualization of this portion of the catheter may delay the visualization of reflux and increase the risk of microcatheter retention or fracture upon its removal (**Fig. 8.7**).

AVM Embolization with Glue

The choice of embolic material is controversial. Each agent has its benefits. With n-BCA, there is a long history of effectiveness. The n-BCA is mixed at different concentrations, depending on the transmit time of the arteriovenous malformation as well as user preference. In general, the n-BCA is mixed with lipiodol in at least a 1:1 ratio. Decreasing the concentration of n-BCA by mixing it with more lipiodol will lengthen the polymerization time of the glue, allowing it to travel farther into the nidus and venous compartment before solidifying. Remember, however, that lipiodol is more viscous than n-BCA, so that the more the glue is diluted, the more viscous it becomes. The glue itself is radiolucent, but lipiodol is radiopaque, allowing the glue to be visualized by fluoroscopy. In addition, one can mix barium particles with the n-BCA to improve visualization.

In my experience, I use either 1:4 parts n-BCA to lipiodol or on occasion, 1:3 parts n-BCA to lipiodol. I try to keep the n-BCA mixture consistent and fluctuate or vary the pressure that I use to administer the glue with my hand rather than changing the concentration of the glue. This allows me to understand how the glue will behave more consistently.

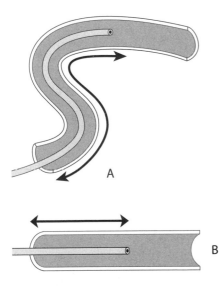

Fig. 8.7 Determining the amount of reflux depends on selecting the proper working angle. **(A)** At the correct working angle, the end of the feeding vessel is elongated, showing that there has been a great deal of reflux. **(B)** At a poor working angle, the turns of the vessel are superimposed. This may lead to underestimating the degree of reflux.

Glacial acetic acid can also be mixed with n-BCA glue to delay its polymerization by changing its pH. Unlike lipiodol, glacial acetic acid lowers the viscosity of the glue, making it easier to inject. I typically use 1–2 drops of glacial acetic acid from a 27-gauge syringe in a 3:1 lipiodol n-BCA mixture for this purpose. It is important to mix the n-BCA well. I do not use particulate barium to enhance visualization because it affects the fluidity of the embolic agent and makes it more difficult to control. Once the n-BCA is mixed, the microcatheter system must be fully flushed with 12 mL of D5W to remove any blood, saline, or contrast in the catheter that might cause the glue to prematurely polymerize. After the microcatheter is fully flushed with dextrose, the glue can be administered. Injecting the glue under a negative roadmap (a roadmap acquired without injecting contrast) will aid in visualizing it. As mentioned previously, the induction of hypotension and Valsalva maneuvers will increase venous pressure and promote stasis within the AVM to aid in embolization.

It is important to watch the n-BCA as it fills the AVM nidus and the arterial pedicles. Avoid embolization of the venous compartment of the AVM. If a small amount of glue flows into the venous compartment it is best to stop embolization. If, however, the venous side appears to have been occluded by the n-BCA, then it is best to continue to embolize the nidus to reduce inflow into the AVM and reduce the risk of hemorrhage. If there is reflux of n-BCA along the catheter, embolization should be stopped, and the catheter should be removed. When n-BCA is used, the microcatheter is generally removed in a rapid fashion to prevent retention of the microcatheter. Aspirate on the microcatheter prior to its removal to make sure glue is not still extruding from the catheter during removal to avoid embolizing eloquent branches.

Some interventionists will change the guide catheter flush to dextrose while administering n-BCA. This is particularly useful during external carotid artery embolizations, because the dextrose solution allows the n-BCA to penetrate further into the lesion. In the intracranial circulation, the D5W likely would be diluted with blood flow from the circle of Willis, limiting its utility. In addition, D5W in the intracranial circulation may promote brain edema.

AVM Embolization with EVAL (Onyx, ev3)

If EVAL is used, the administration technique is slightly different. The EVAL comes pre-packaged in different concentrations. EVAL-34 is twice as concentrated (and viscous) as EVAL-18. In both cases, the EVAL is dissolved in dimethyl sulfoxide (DMSO) while tantalum opacifies the solution. The tantalum will settle out of the solution if it is left standing, so it is recommended that the EVAL be shaken for 20 minutes prior to administration.

As with n-BCA glue, the microcatheter must be flushed prior to administration of EVAL. In this case, the microcatheter is flushed with 12 mL of saline to remove any blood. Next the catheter hub is filled with DMSO, and approximately 0.3 mL of DMSO is infused into the catheter at 0.1 mL per minute. The exact amount of DMSO will depend on the dead space of the microcatheter, which is approximately 0.23 mL in the case of the Marathon microcatheter. DMSO is irritating to blood vessels, so it is important not to inject more DMSO than necessary to fill the dead space of the microcatheter.

Once the microcatheter is filled with DMSO, the EVAL can be injected at the rate 0.1 mL per minute. As with glue administration, a negative road map is used to visualize the EVAL as it fills the nidus. The rate of injection can be varied, depending on where the EVAL is going in the AVM. Like n-BCA, EVAL will often flow far distal into the nidus before refluxing. Unlike n-BCA, however, EVAL will sometimes even flow retrograde from the nidus to other feeding arteries that supply the AVM. Therefore, it is important that when you do EVAL embolizations you understand fully the AVM architecture. In some cases, the EVAL can travel retrograde into vessels that were not visualized on prior angiograms. This can result in neurological deficits if the EVAL enters eloquent branches. For this reason, some investigators will demarcate the AVM on guide catheter angiography from both the selected artery as well as from a second pre-cerebral branch via a second diagnostic catheter (personal communication, Robert Mericle, 2005). Once the edges of the AVM are demarcated, EVAL can be administered. By defining the perimeter of the AVM from multiple vessels, you can avoid inadvertent embolization of "en passage" vessels.

One potential advantage of EVAL over glue is that it is non-adhesive, so recurrent embolization is feasible for many minutes. If the EVAL is noted to be heading in the wrong direction, the infusion can be stopped for 45–60 seconds and then restarted. This will often result in the EVAL taking a different (and hopefully better) route. All of this can be done without changing out the microcatheter, simplifying the procedure.

The objectives with EVAL must be carefully delineated prior to beginning embolization, just as with glue. If there is significant reflux and it occurs for a prolonged period of time, removing the microcatheter can be quite difficult and may result in a fractured or retained catheter. It is important to observe the degree of reflux and the length of time the microcatheter has been inside the reflux cast, so the catheter is not left in too long. As with n-BCA, care should be taken to avoid embolizing the venous compartment of the AVM with EVAL early in the procedure to avoid periprocedural intracranial bleeding.

Removal of the microcatheter usually involves some strain on the microcatheter. An intermediate guide catheter may help in removal of the microcatheter by redirecting the force of the pull in line with the feeding vessel. It is recommended that the microcatheter be removed slowly. Once the catheter begins to straighten, it should be held in tension for a minute or more to allow the stretch of the catheter to ease the catheter out of the cast. Once the tension in the catheter dissipates, the process can be repeated until the catheter tip is out of the cast. The more reflux is tolerated, the more difficult it will be to remove the catheter. Excessive reflux and/or embolization time may result in fracturing of the catheter during removal.

After removal of the microcatheter, guide catheter angiography is recommended to understand the anatomy of both the AVM and the surrounding vasculature to make sure no inadvertent embolization of normal branches has been performed and to assess for residual nidus. The patient should be assessed by clinical exams or neurophysiological monitoring for signs of hemorrhage. Further embolizations can be performed with repeat microcatheterizations if desired. It is important to manage blood pressure during extubation and in the postoperative period (72 hours) to avoid normal perfusion pressure breakthrough bleeding or bleeding from residual nidus. Consider keeping high-risk patients under anesthesia with neurophysiological monitoring for 24–72 hours after the procedure to maintain hypotension during this period.

Some interventionists with extensive experience embolizing AVMs with EVAL will start embolizing with EVAL-34 to form a cast around the tip of the microcatheter deliberately. Embolization of the AVM is then performed with EVAL-

18 for better nidal penetration. In this technique, the initial cast formed by the EVAL-34 is designed to prevent reflux of the less viscous EVAL-18 as it is injected into the nidus (A Evans, personal communication, 2008; technique ascribed to Dr. Prior).

A simultaneous dual catheter technique has also been described. In this technique, two microcatheters are positioned in different arterial feeders (D Lopes, personal communication, 2008). Embolization is started in one microcatheter. If reflux occurs or if EVAL is going into an undesired area, embolization is stopped. Embolization can then proceed from the other microcatheter. The process can be repeated as necessary until embolization is complete. This technique reduces the length of the procedure and minimizes reflux, both of which reduce the risk of fracturing the microcatheter upon removal.

Interventional Technique of Carotid Stent Placement

Carotid artery stent placement has been approved at this time for symptomatic patients with greater than 70% stenosis and risk factors that put the patient at high risk of procedural complications from endarterectomy. These risk factors can be neurological, systemic, or anatomical. A patient's decision to have a carotid stent procedure should come after a balanced discussion with a specialist that outlines the benefits and risks associated with medical, surgical, and endovascular treatment.

The major risks of carotid stent placement include cardiovascular events (myocardial infarction related to periprocedural hypotension), neurological events (transient ischemic attack [TIA], stroke, or intracerebral hemorrhage), or access site events (groin hematoma, peripheral arterial occlusion). Avoidance of these complications requires good interventional technique as well as careful monitoring and management of the patient's vital signs. Both hypotension and hypertension carry risk in this patient population, so it is important that blood pressure is monitored and controlled closely.

Preprocedural Medications for Carotid Stent Placement

All patients undergoing carotid stent placement should be treated with two antiplatelet agents—usually aspirin and clopidogrel. Aspirin can be started within 24 hours of stent placement, as its onset of action is short. Clopidogrel at a dose of 75 mg/day should be started at least 4 days from an elective procedure for maximal effect. Higher doses of clopidogrel can be used for urgent procedures. For example, a 300 mg load of clopidogrel will reach maximum efficacy within 12–18 hours, while a 600 mg dose will work within 6 hours.

Other options in the case of emergent or urgent stent placement include intravenous medications to achieve platelet inhibition. Glycoprotein IIb-IIIa receptor inhibitors, such as abciximab or eptifibatide, are commonly used in this setting. Abciximab has a longer half-life, but unlike clopidogrel it can be reliably reversed by platelet infusion. Eptifibatide has a very short half-life, so cessation will result in reversal of platelet inhibition within hours. Transfused platelets, however, will be ineffective to reverse eptifibatide as long as enough drug is freely circulating to inhibit the transfused platelets.

Technique for Carotid Stent Placement

Diagnostic angiography of the arch, cervical vessels, and intracranial vessels is commonly performed for planning prior to a stent placement procedure. Once initial angiography is completed, a 6 Fr 125 cm Simmons II catheter and a 6 Fr sheath are used to access the common carotid artery. An armored sheath is used when the arch is sharply angled or there is proximal common carotid tortuosity that would kink a standard sheath. Note, however, that the armored sheath has a larger outer diameter and may increase the likelihood of either access vessel injury or occlusion.

The 6 Fr Simmons II diagnostic catheter is reconfigured in the descending aorta or subclavian artery and then used to access the carotid artery of interest. If it is amenable, the external carotid artery on that side is selected with a stiff Terumo glide wire. The sheath is then advanced over the stiff Terumo glide wire and the 6 Fr Simmons II catheter, allowing for appropriate placement within the common carotid artery. This technique works with both bovine as well as Type C aortic arch configurations.

If the anatomy does not allow a stiff wire to be advanced into the carotid far enough to advance the sheath, an 8 Fr Cordis H1 guide catheter is used with the Simmons II diagnostic catheter to gain access to the common carotid. Alternatively, an 8 Fr Cordis Simmons 2 guide catheter can be used. These two approaches have been successful, particularly in cases of increased tortuosity or common carotid artery stenosis that made advancing a stiff glide wire into the common carotid artery or ECA impossible.

In cases of carotid origin stenosis, the guide sheath or guide catheter must remain in the descending aorta. An unconfigured 6 Fr Simmons II Envoy guide catheter works well for this purpose. A filter wire can be passed through the guide catheter and into the carotid artery to obtain access. To stabilize the catheter, a second 0.014 or 0.018-inch diameter microwire can be passed through the sheath or guide catheter and into the carotid artery next to the filter wire. This second stabilizing wire is often referred to as a "buddy wire." The use of a buddy wire should be considered for any intervention when the proximal catheter is unstable. Usually, larger balloon-expandable peripheral stents are required to treat stenosis with a common carotid artery origin. In these cases, a larger access catheter is required (usually a 6 Fr sheath or 8 Fr guide catheter).

For cases of carotid artery stenosis in which distal filter protection appears difficult, we have used a proximal balloon catheter occlusion technique. Most commonly, we use this approach in patients with long, severe blockages through which a filter wire will not pass. Once the catheter is in position in the common carotid artery, the balloon is inflated to cause flow arrest, and the procedure is performed. In addition, a second balloon is placed in the external carotid artery to prevent retrograde ECA to ICA flow. Once both balloons are inflated, flow reversal is applied to the guide catheter, further protecting against embolism and stroke. In some cases, the blood is filtered and reintroduced into the venous side so that blood loss is minimized (Gore Flow Reversal System, Gore, PA). The intervention is performed on the stenotic carotid artery, and then the balloons are deflated and removed. It is important to check for collateral flow when using proximal protection techniques. The balloon occlusion technique may precipitate seizures or hypoperfusion of the hemisphere if collateral cerebral circulation is poor. Patients with contralateral carotid occlusions are probably better treated with alternative strategies to prevent emboli.

Anticoagulation during Carotid Artery Stenting

During carotid artery stenting (CAS), we administer 80 to 100 units/kg of heparin intravenously after placing the sheath to attain an activated clotting time (ACT) of 250 to 300. Heparin is rebolused hourly to maintain this value during longer procedures. It is also acceptable to use intravenous bivalirudin to achieve an ACT around 300. One advantage of bivalirudin over heparin is that its shorter half-life lowers the risk of groin hematoma after removing the sheath. Bivalirudin can also be safely used in patients with a history of heparin-induced thrombocytopenia and thombosis (HITT) syndrome. The literature suggests that bivalirudin is equivalent, but not superior, to unfractionated heparin in safety.

Pre-Stenting Balloon Angioplasty during Carotid Artery Stenting

In nearly all cases, we perform balloon angioplasty prior to stent placement to allow for smoother delivery of the stent. In general, a small cardiac balloon with a low crossing profile is used, such as a 2.5 mm × 30 mm Maverick balloon. A monorail system is more convenient for a single operator than an over-the-wire system, but either is acceptable. Hemodynamic instability is extremely uncommon with the inflation of these small balloons.

Stent Deployment

After pre-dilation of the lesion, the stent is deployed. A 30–40 mm stent is usually long enough to extend a few millimeters proximal and distal to the lesion to ensure adequate coverage. We commonly use a self-expanding nitinol stent 1 to 2 mm larger in diameter than the common carotid artery to treat a carotid bifurcation lesion. There are both closed-cell and open-cell nitinol stents for use in the carotid artery. Increasing evidence suggests that the closed-cell design carries less risk of postprocedural neurological complications. There may also be a lower incidence of re-stenosis with closed-cell stents. One disadvantage of closed-cell stents is that their delivery systems tend to be stiffer than those of comparably sized open-cell stents. This makes them less suitable for tortuous anatomy. Therefore, in tortuous anatomy or in a sharply angulated carotid artery, an open-cell stent is used, while in straighter vessels we prefer to use a closed-cell design.

Post-Stent Angioplasty

After stent deployment, a post-stent placement angioplasty is often performed. The angioplasty balloon should be sized appropriately for the diameter of the vessel, usually around 4–5 mm. A balloon shorter than the stent should be used, so that the angioplasty occurs only inside the stent. This recommendation is based on the observation that angioplasty of coronary vessels outside a previously placed stent has been found to increase the incidence of re-stenosis. Usually a 20 mm balloon is long enough to span the lesion without protruding from the stent and is short enough to deflate quickly should bradycardia or asystole occur due to stimulation of the carotid sinus. A less viscous mixture for balloon angioplasty of one-third contrast and two-thirds saline will improve deflation times even further, at the cost of decreased visualization. Pretreatment with atropine (0.6 mg) is occasionally used in patients with severe coronary artery disease or recent myocardial infarction, but in most cases atropine is used only if needed. Other interventionists use glycopyrrolate, as this provides the cardiac effects of atropine but avoids the potential central nervous system side effects. One might consider undersizing the balloon in high-risk patients (such as those about to undergo coronary artery bypass grafts) to prevent hypotension and bradycardia during balloon inflation.

Nevertheless, some patients will experience postprocedural hypotension requiring intravenous pressors. Depending on the heart rate, either neosynephrine (heart rate >65) or dopamine (heart rate <65) is used. Prolonged hypotension can be treated with midodrine, an orally administered α-agonist. Since midodrine is available as a pill, patients with mild but persistent postprocedural hypotension can be sent home on it, potentially decreasing the length of their hospital stay.

Retrieval of the Filter Device

Retrieval of the filter device can sometimes be difficult. The retrieval catheter has a relatively high profile, and as it passes through, it tends to get caught on the proximal tines of the stent. Angling the tip of the catheter can sometimes allow it to be maneuvered within the stent. In addition, simply having the patient turn his or her head can rotate the carotid artery slightly to facilitate safe passage of the retrieval catheter. If neither of these maneuvers is successful, advancing the sheath or guide catheter into the stent over a balloon or dilator will allow the retrieval catheter to subsequently advance to the filter.

As the filter is removed, it is important to make sure the distal tines of the stent do not damage the device and release any captured emboli into the carotid circulation. Once the device has been pulled into the guide sheath, it can be safely removed without fluoroscopy. Inspection of the filter after removal will identify any debris captured by the device.

It is common practice to perform a carotid ultrasound the day after carotid artery stent placement. The ultrasound confirms the patency of the stent and also provides an angiographic correlation to the velocities obtained on ultrasound. By performing a postprocedural ultrasound, new baseline velocities can be established for comparison to future ultrasound exams. If velocities are significantly higher than expected, additional testing to rule out in-stent thrombus formation or dissection should be considered.

References

1. Brisman JL, Roonprapunt C, Song JK, et al. Intentional partial coil occlusion followed by delayed clip application to wide-necked middle cerebral artery aneurysms in patients presenting with severe vasospasm. Report of two cases. J Neurosurg 2004;101(1):154–158
2. Debrun GM, Aletich VA, Kehrli P, Misra M, Ausman JI, Charbel F. Selection of cerebral aneurysms for treatment using Guglielmi detachable coils: the preliminary University of Illinois at Chicago experience. Neurosurgery 1998;43(6):1281–1295, discussion 1296–1297
3. Qureshi AI, Luft AR, Sharma M, Guterman LR, Hopkins LN. Prevention and treatment of thromboembolic and ischemic complications associated with endovascular proce-

dures: Part II–Clinical aspects and recommendations. Neurosurgery 2000;46:1360–1375, discussion 1375–1376

4. Qureshi AI, Mohammad Y, Yahia AM, et al. Ischemic events associated with unruptured intracranial aneurysms: multicenter clinical study and review of the literature. Neurosurgery 2000;46(2):282–289, discussion 289–290

5. Viñuela F, Duckwiler G, Mawad M. Guglielmi detachable coil embolization of acute intracranial aneurysm: perioperative anatomical and clinical outcome in 403 patients. J Neurosurg 1997;86(3):475–482

6. Qureshi AI, Suri MF, Khan J, et al. Endovascular treatment of intracranial aneurysms by using Guglielmi detachable coils in awake patients: safety and feasibility. J Neurosurg 2001;94(6):880–885

7. Qureshi AI, Luft AR, Sharma M, Guterman LR, Hopkins LN. Prevention and treatment of thromboembolic and ischemic complications associated with endovascular procedures: Part I—Pathophysiological and pharmacological features. Neurosurgery 2000;46(6):1344–1359

8. Yamada NK, Cross DT III, Pilgram TK, Moran CJ, Derdeyn CP, Dacey RG Jr. Effect of antiplatelet therapy on thromboembolic complications of elective coil embolization of cerebral aneurysms. AJNR Am J Neuroradiol 2007;28(9):1778–1782

9. Hurley MC, Sherma AK, Surdell D, Shaibani A, Bendok BR. A novel guide catheter enabling intracranial placement. Catheter Cardiovasc Interv, 2009

10. Slob MJ, van Rooij WJ, Sluzewski M. Coil thickness and packing of cerebral aneurysms: a comparative study of two types of coils. AJNR Am J Neuroradiol 2005;26(4):901–903

11. Guglielmi G, Viñuela F, Sepetka I, Macellari V. Electrothrombosis of saccular aneurysms via endovascular approach. Part 1: Electrochemical basis, technique, and experimental results. J Neurosurg 1991;75(1):1–7

12. Lim YC, Kim BM, Shin YS, Kim SY, Chung J. Structural limitations of currently available microcatheters and coils for endovascular coiling of very small aneurysms. Neuroradiology 2008;50(5):423–427

13. Sluzewski M, Menovsky T, van Rooij WJ, Wijnalda D. Coiling of very large or giant cerebral aneurysms: long-term clinical and serial angiographic results. AJNR Am J Neuroradiol 2003;24(2):257–262

14. Jahromi BS, Mocco J, Bang JA, Gologorsky Y, Siddiqui AH, Horowitz MB, et al. Clinical and angiographic outcome after endovascular management of giant intracranial aneurysms. Neurosurgery 2008;63:662–674; discussion 674–675

15. Kwon OK, Kim SH, Kwon BJ, et al. Endovascular treatment of wide-necked aneurysms by using two microcatheters: techniques and outcomes in 25 patients. AJNR Am J Neuroradiol 2005;26(4):894–900

16. Kwon OK, Kim SH, Oh CW, et al. Embolization of wide-necked aneurysms using three or more microcatheters. Acta Neurochir (Wien) 2006;148(11):1139–1145, discussion 1145

17. Malisch TW, Guglielmi G, Viñuela F, et al. Intracranial aneurysms treated with the Guglielmi detachable coil: midterm clinical results in a consecutive series of 100 patients. J Neurosurg 1997;87(2):176–183

18. Chen PR, Amin-Hanjani S, Albuquerque FC, McDougall C, Zabramski JM, Spetzler RF. Outcome of oculomotor nerve palsy from posterior communicating artery aneurysms: comparison of clipping and coiling. Neurosurgery 2006;58(6):1040–1046

19. Heran NS, Song JK, Kupersmith MJ, et al. Large ophthalmic segment aneurysms with anterior optic pathway compression: assessment of anatomical and visual outcomes after endosaccular coil therapy. J Neurosurg 2007;106(6):968–975

20. Aletich VA, Debrun GM, Misra M, Charbel F, Ausman JI. The remodeling technique of balloon-assisted Guglielmi detachable coil placement in wide-necked aneurysms: experience at the University of Illinois at Chicago. J Neurosurg 2000;93(3):388–396

21. Lefkowitz MA, Gobin YP, Akiba Y, et al. Balloon-assisted Guglielmi detachable coiling of wide-necked aneurysms: Part II—clinical results. Neurosurgery 1999;45(3):531–537, discussion 537–538

22. Moret J, Cognard C, Weill A, Castaings L, Rey A. Reconstruction technic in the treatment of wide-neck intracranial aneurysms. Long-term angiographic and clinical results. A propos of 56 cases. J Neuroradiol 1997;24(1):30–44

23. Taylor CL, Selman WR, Kiefer SP, Ratcheson RA. Temporary vessel occlusion during intracranial aneurysm repair. Neurosurgery 1996;39:893–905

24. Bendszus M, Chapot R. Balloon-assisted coil embolization. "Surgical clip application should be considered as a first treatment option in large and wide-necked aneurysms." J Neurosurg 2007;106(4):734–735, author reply 735

25. Brooks NP, Turk AS, Niemann DB, Aagaard-Kienitz B, Pulfer K, Cook T. Frequency of thromboembolic events associated with endovascular aneurysm treatment: retrospective case series. J Neurosurg 2008;108(6):1095–1100

26. Ross IB, Dhillon GS. Complications of endovascular treatment of cerebral aneurysms. Surg Neurol 2005;64(1):12–18, discussion 18–19

27. Sluzewski M, van Rooij WJ, Beute GN, Nijssen PC. Balloon-assisted coil embolization of intracranial aneurysms: incidence, complications, and angiography results. J Neurosurg 2006;105(3):396–399

28. Muizelaar JP, Zwienenberg M, Mini NA, Hecht ST. Safety and efficacy of transluminal balloon angioplasty in the prevention of vasospasm in patients with Fisher Grade 3 subarachnoid hemorrhage: a pilot study. Neurosurg Focus 1998;5(4):e5

29. Muizelaar JP, Zwienenberg M, Rudisill NA, Hecht ST. The prophylactic use of transluminal balloon angioplasty in patients with Fisher Grade 3 subarachnoid hemorrhage: a pilot study. J Neurosurg 1999;91(1):51–58

30. Zwienenberg-Lee M, Hartman J, Rudisill N, et al.; Balloon Prophylaxis for Aneurysmal Vasospasm (BPAV) Study Group. Effect of prophylactic transluminal balloon angioplasty on cerebral vasospasm and outcome in patients with Fisher grade III subarachnoid hemorrhage: results of a phase II multicenter, randomized, clinical trial. Stroke 2008;39(6):1759–1765

31. Fiorella D, Albuquerque FC, Deshmukh VR, McDougall CG. Monorail snare technique for the recovery of stretched platinum coils: technical case report. Neurosurgery 2005;57(1 Suppl):E210, discussion E210

32. Gralla J, Rennie AT, Corkill RA, et al. Abciximab for thrombolysis during intracranial aneurysm coiling. Neuroradiology 2008;50(12):1041–1047

33. Ries T, Siemonsen S, Grzyska U, Zeumer H, Fiehler J. Abciximab is a safe rescue therapy in thromboembolic events complicating cerebral aneurysm coil embolization: single center experience in 42 cases and review of the literature. Stroke 2009;40(5):1750–1757

Periprocedural Patient Evaluation

Randall C. Edgell and Justin Sweeney

Consent and Procedural Risks

Informed consent is a critical preprocedural task in today's medico-legal environment. This involves a detailed discussion between the neurointerventionist or designated physician and either the patient, the patient's family, and/or the person holding the patient's power of attorney regarding the disease process and the proposed treatment (**Table 9.1**).

Neurointerventional procedures carry the specific risks of anesthesia, stroke, kidney damage, bleeding, contrast allergy, vessel injury, and infection;[1] these are discussed in more detail in the sections below.

Cardiac Disease

Atherosclerosis

Atherosclerosis develops as oxygen free radicals oxidize low-density lipoproteins (LDLs) that in turn damage the intima, or inner lining of the arterial walls. This leads to a chronic inflammatory response involving macrophage accumulation and smooth muscle hyperplasia, with subsequent cholesterol and calcium deposition (**Table 9.2**).

Because atherosclerosis of the coronary and cerebral arteries is usually concomitant, it is important to obtain an appropriate preoperative work-up from a multidisciplinary point of view, and to incorporate this information in the context of perioperative management[2] (**Table 9.3**).

Difficulties with Anesthesia

Cardiac disease can often complicate cardiovascular and respiratory management for both the neurointerventionist and the anesthesiologist. A comprehensive preoperative work-up to define the extent of both cerebral and cardiac atherosclerotic disease is an imperative first step in this process. This allows both the interventional and anesthesia teams to stratify the risks involved in the procedure, particularly those with severe cardiac disease, and plan accordingly.

Postoperative myocardial infarction is a serious concern for patients with cardiac disease. It most commonly occurs 48 hours following anesthesia. Greater than

Table 9.1   Components of Informed Consent

1. Describe the problem.
2. Outline risks/benefits of procedure.
3. Describe alternative treatments/options.
4. Use layperson's terms.
5. Place documentation of consent in the medical record.

Table 9.2   Major Risk Factors for Atherosclerosis

1. Hypertension
2. Hyperlipidemia
3. Diabetes mellitus
4. Family history of atherosclerosis
5. Tobacco
6. Elevated or modified low-density lipoprotein
7. Genetic alterations

Table 9.3   Preoperative Considerations for the Patient with Severe Cardiac Disease[15]

Consider cardiology consultation.
Safest type of anesthesia—local, MAC?
Additional perioperative medications needed, e.g., antiplatelet agents or beta-blockade?
Continuous intra-arterial blood pressure and electrocardiographic monitoring?
Limits of fluid administration to avoid overload, e.g., CHF and pulmonary edema?
The need for cardiac pacing or disabling of cardiac defibrillator or pacemaker?

Abbreviations: CHF, congestive heart failure; MAC, monitored anesthesia care.

90% are silent, but symptoms may include chest pain, shortness of breath, and a fluttering sensation in the chest. Close monitoring with serial ECGs, telemetry and cardiac enzymes in high-risk patients is recommended.

Careful monitoring of respiratory status includes oxygen saturation (pulse ox monitoring), breath rate, and volume status. Aspiration, mucus obstruction, medication-induced bronchospasm, and sedation- or analgesic-induced respiratory depression are important causes of respiratory compromise in any patient undergoing anesthesia (**Table 9.4**).

Table 9.4 Important Factors Compromising Respiratory Status

Aspiration
Mucus obstruction
Medication-induced bronchospasm
Sedation-induced respiratory depression
Analgesic-induced respiratory depression
Volume overload

Peripheral Vascular Disease

Vascular Access

Atherosclerosis is a systemic disease affecting the length of the vascular tree and often presenting challenges to vascular access. Vascular access is frequently obtained through a transfemoral route with navigation of wires and catheters in the aorta; peripheral vascular disease (PVD) is often severe along this route and can be focal, circumferential, or run the length of the approach. This can lead to unsuccessful access or complications, such as dissection, distal thromboemboli, and vessel occlusion requiring further treatment (see Chapter 7).

Peripheral Vascular Injury

Dissection or thromboembolism leading to a distal vessel occlusion and an ischemic leg most often presents early after a procedure; however, delayed occlusion is possible. Serial evaluation of any attempted vascular access points with pulse, temperature, pain, and ankle-brachial indexes (ABIs), if necessary, is an important step in recognizing problems. If distal occlusion is suspected or discovered, anticoagulation with intravenous heparin is critical in these patients to prevent continued organization and propagation of the clot. Vascular surgery consultation for open repair or revascularization may be necessary in severe cases.

Stroke Risk

Patients with PVD undergoing routine diagnostic angiography have an increased risk of stroke of 1–2%, as compared with disease-free counterparts.[2] The more severe the disease, the more prevalent atherosclerotic plaques, which increases the risk of catheter-related complications, including stroke. Furthermore, catheters, wires, stents, and coils all have the possibility to form clot on and around them, potentially leading to thromboemboli. The judicious use of wires and roadmap technology, while minimizing catheter contact with the vessel walls, usually decreases this risk.

Renal Disease

Contrast-Induced Nephropathy

Contrast-induced nephropathy (CIN) is one of the most common iatrogenic causes of kidney injury. In most cases, it causes a benign and often transient form of acute renal failure, which is defined as having at least a 0.5 mg/dL or a 25% increase in the baseline serum level of creatinine. However, in patients with preexisting renal insufficiency with or without concomitant diabetes, it may be more severe and eventually require dialysis. The pathogenesis of this condition is complex and not completely understood; the available literature suggests direct free radical tubular injury and/or a hemodynamic imbalance leading to medullary ischemia as possible etiologies.[3] Patients with baseline creatinine concentrations above 1.5 mg/dL have an approximately 40% chance of developing CIN.[4] Preoperative screening for these risk factors is an important first step in prevention (**Table 9.5**).

Discontinuation of nephrotoxic medications 48 hours prior to angiography can help reduce the rate of CIN. Patients with glomerular filtration rates (GFRs) less than 60 mL/min may benefit from further preventative measures to reduce renal injury, such as preoperative hydration and bicarbonate or Mucomyst intravenous administration.

Prophylaxis

The most commonly used regimens for CIN prophylaxis include hydration with intravenous bicarbonate, saline, and/or the use of N-acetylcysteine (**Table 9.6**). These are discussed in more detail below. The effects of ascorbic acid, calcium channel blockers, dopamine, fenoldopam, furosemide, mannitol, and theophylline have also been studied; however, no clear benefit bears out in the literature.

Table 9.5   Risk Factors for Developing Contrast-Induced Nephropathy[4]

1. >70 years old
2. Chronic renal insufficiency
3. Volume depletion
4. Hypotension
5. Diabetes mellitus
6. Congestive heart failure
7. Anemia
8. Nephrotoxic drugs
9. High dose of contrast
10. Hyperosmolar contrast agents

Table 9.6 CIN Prophylaxis

Medication	Mechanism
Hydration (sodium chloride or bicarbonate)	Free radical attenuation
Mucomyst (NAC) 600 mg PO BID for 24 hours prior and 48 hours after procedure	Free radical scavenger

Abbreviation: NAC, N-acetylcysteine.

Hydration

The primary prophylaxis for CIN is hydration. However, caution should be exhibited in patients with preexisting renal impairment, as overzealous fluid administration can lead to pulmonary edema and respiratory compromise. There continues to be controversy in the literature regarding which type of hydration, i.e., sodium chloride or sodium bicarbonate, is more effective. Bicarbonate is a safe, readily available agent that alkalizes the tubular urine and is thought to attenuate free radical formation, thus preventing renal tubular injury. A randomized, controlled single-blinded study of 353 well-matched patients with baseline creatinine levels of 1.5 mg/dL and GFR of 48 mL/min found a rate of CIN of ~14% in both those pretreated with 0.9% saline and those pretreated with 150 mEq/L of sodium bicarbonate.[5] They concluded that there was no extra benefit in using sodium bicarbonate.

Mucomyst

The use of Mucomyst (N-acetylcysteine [NAC]) has been validated by recent studies.[6,7] The exact mechanism of nephroprotection provided by NAC is unclear, but it has been proposed to be a vasodilator via nitric-oxide pathways, a free radical scavenger by increasing available glutathione, which is effective in the prevention of apoptosis. The typical regimen given is 600 mg PO twice daily for 24 hours prior to the procedure and for 48 hours after the procedure. There is also evidence of a dose-dependent effect in patients without preexisting renal impairment whereby using a higher dosage protocol of 1200 mg may further reduce the risk of CIN.[6] A recent review of available studies by Stenstrom et al[7] found that the use of NAC is safe and inexpensive and will prove to be beneficial in prophylactic prevention of CIN.

The Diabetic Patient

Patients with diabetes and preexisting diabetic nephropathy provide unique challenges to the interventional team. Other common, coexisting comorbities frequently include HTN, hyperlipemia, and hypercholesterolemia, all major risk factors for the development of atherosclerosis and pathology requiring angiography. These patients often have a reduced GFR and are taking medications, such as ACE inhibitors that may predispose them to CIN. Diabetes has been found to be an independent risk factor for CIN and preventative measures should be taken to reduce renal insult.

Glucophage (Metformin)

Glucophage is an oral antihyperglycemic agent used in type 2 diabetics to reduce gluconeogenesis in the liver, glucose uptake in the intestines, peripheral glucose intolerance, and LDL levels in the blood. It is not metabolized by the liver, but is excreted primarily by the kidneys. Its most serious side effect is a rare condition called metformin-associated lactic acidosis (MALA), which can develop when exposed patients taking this medication undergo contrast angiography. Contrast media may reduce renal tubular excretion of metformin, leading to enhanced anaerobic metabolism. The incidence of MALA is 1 in 33,000/yr and has a mortality of 50%. Patients with preexisting kidney and liver disease, congestive heart failure, excessive alcohol use, or dehydration are at highest risk. Metformin should be discontinued 24 hours prior to the procedure and for 48 hours thereafter. It may be restarted when baseline creatinine levels are reached. Symptoms of lactic acidosis include irregular heartbeat, dizziness, fatigue, abdominal and muscle pain, and shortness of breath (**Table 9.7**). Treatment is usually supportive and directed at rapid correction of the acidosis with sodium bicarbonate. In extreme cases, hemodialysis may be required.

Gastrointestinal Bleeding

Neurointerventional procedures often require patients to undergo treatment with antiplatelet and/or anticoagulation therapies. Gastrointestinal (GI) bleeding may be exacerbated by these medications and is associated with a mortality rate of 1–13%.[8] Known risk factors for GI bleeding (**Table 9.8**) include old age, female sex, diabetes, chronic renal failure, congestive heart failure, history of GI bleeding, peptic ulcer disease, *H. pylori* infection, alcohol abuse, anticoagulation/antiplatelet combination therapy, supratherapeutic anticoagulation levels, and NSAID and corticosteroid use.[8] The majority of patients with GI bleeding are asymptomatic or have symptoms of chronic anemia: lethargy, fatigue, shortness of breath, or pallor. Patients on anticoagulation therapy should undergo routine monitoring of their coagulation parameters and cell blood counts to evaluate for large variations. Any patient suspected of, or at high risk for, a chronic GI bleed should undergo serial fecal occult blood tests. If positive, a formal upper or lower GI endoscopy to identify the cause is warranted. These patients are often placed on proton pump inhibitors, which have been shown to reduce upper GI bleeding risk. The use of

Table 9.7 Risk Factors and Symptoms of Lactic Acidosis Associated with Metformin

Risk factors	Symptoms
Preexisting renal and liver disease	Irregular heartbeat
Congestive heart failure	Dizziness
Excessive alcohol use	Fatigue
Dehydration	Abdominal and/or muscular pain
	Shortness of breath

Table 9.8 Risk Factors for GI Bleeding

Elderly
Female
Diabetes
Chronic renal failure
Congestive heart failure
History of GI bleeding
Peptic ulcer disease
H. pylori infection
Alcohol abuse
Combination antiplatelet/anticoagulation therapy
Supratherapeutic anticoagulation levels
NSAID use
Corticosteroid use

Abbreviations: GI, gastrointestinal; NSAID, nonsteroidal anti-inflammatory drug.

these agents prophylactically should be considered in high-risk patients who are placed on long-term antiplatelet regimens as a result of a neurointerventional procedure. However, recent studies on the interactions of proton pump inhibitors and antiplatelet agents demonstrated that PPIs can render antiplatelet agents ineffective. Therefore, it is recommended that patients use an alternative GI medication if the need of antiplatelet agents is part of the treatment paradigm. The decision to discontinue antiplatelet/anticoagulation often entails a complex weighing of risk given the potentially disastrous consequences to the central nervous system. Serious acute GI bleeding may present with hematochezia, melena, hematemesis, dizziness, hypotension, tachycardia, decreased urine output, and syncope, and may be life threatening. Patients may require fluid resuscitation, blood transfusions, and reversal of coagulopathy. Helical CT scan of the abdomen and pelvis is a first step in identification of the bleeding site. Endoscopy is also an essential tool in identifying the site of bleeding. Mesenteric angiography may be useful in cases of severe lower GI bleeding for identification, selective vasopressin administration, or supraselective embolization of bleeding sites. Surgical or endoscopic intervention may be required to control severe cases.

Platelet and Coagulation Disorders

Genetic coagulation disorders can be divided into those affecting primary hemostasis—platelet aggregation, and those affecting secondary hemostasis—coagulation factors. They vary in their inheritance patterns and severity.

Although many patients are asymptomatic, clinical signs can be solicited from the patient's history (**Table 9.9**). These patients carry an increased risk of both spontaneous and procedurally related hemorrhage.

Table 9.9 Symptomatic Concerns for Genetic Coagulation Disorders

Frequent gum and nose bleeds
Fatigue
Severe bruising
Menorrhagia
Hematochezia
Hematuria
Muscle or joint pain from internal bleeding

Hypocoagulable Disease States (Table 9.10)

Von Willebrand Disease (vWD)

The most common hereditary coagulation disorder is von Willebrand disease, which is involved in primary hemostasis. There are many different subtypes, but it most commonly arises from either a quantitative or qualitative defect in the gene, producing an overall deficiency of functional von Willebrand factor (vWF). Von Willebrand factor is a protein required for platelet adhesion. The most frequent inheritance pattern is autosomal dominant, but it is rarely acquired. It has a prevalence of 1 in 100 people and affects those with type O blood more severely.[9] Prophylactic treatment for neurointerventional procedures in patients with known vWD can be undertaken with desmopressin (DDAVP), which induces release of vWF from stores in Weibel-Palade bodies of endothelial cells or with Humate-P (vWF + purified Factor VIII).

Hemophilia A (Factor VIII Deficiency)

Hemophilia A, or factor VIII deficiency, is the most common type of hemophilia and is inherited in an X-linked recessive pattern. Females are carriers of the trait, and males express the phenotype with an incidence of 1 in 5000 in the general population. Factor VIII is a protein that is synthesized and released into the bloodstream by the intima and that binds to vWF. It is activated by thrombin and is involved in the propagation of the coagulation cascade, eventually leading to fibrin formation, crosslinking, and clot formation. Partial thromboplastin time (PTT) is

Table 9.10 Hypocoagulable Disease States

Disease	Deficiency	Replacement therapy
von Willebrand disease	von Willebrand factor	DDAVP
Hemophilia A	Factor VIII	Factor VIII or DDAVP
Hemophilia B (Christmas disease)	Factor IX	Factor VII
Hemophilia C	Factor XI	Factor XI

Abbreviation: DDAVP, desmopressin.

elevated in the setting of a normal prothrombin time (PT), and factor VIII levels can be measured directly. These patients require frequent routine factor VIII supplementation and can be given either factor VIII or DDAVP prophylaxis for surgical procedures.

Less Common Hereditary Coagulation Disorders

The less common hereditary coagulation disorders include hemophilia B (factor IX deficiency, a.k.a Christmas disease), hemophilia C (factor XI deficiency), and factor VII deficiency.

Hypercoagulable State

There are several disorders that cause a hypercoagulable state and lead to increased thromboembolic events. A helpful mnemonic is CALMSHAPES (**Table 9.11**).

Of these genetic disorders, the most common is the factor V Leiden mutation. It is present in 5–7% of the general population and is inherited in an autosomal dominant pattern.

Plavix

The thienopyridine-class drug Plavix, or clopidogrel, is a potent oral antiplatelet medication used for preventing platelet aggregation and the resulting formation of clots in patients with cerebral, coronary, or other peripheral vascular diseases. Patients requiring catheter-based intervention may already be taking this drug for a concomitant disease or may be loaded with this medication or another in its class in preparation for an intervention, such as intravascular stent placement. Clopidogrel works by irreversibly inhibiting ADP receptors on platelets, thus interfering with the conformational change necessary for the glycoprotein IIb/IIIa receptor to cross-link other activated platelets with fibrinogen. This medication has a slow onset, and often patients are loaded to decrease time to efficacy. Since it irrevers-

Table 9.11 Hypercoagulable States

C	Protein C deficiency
A	Antiphospholipid syndromes (anticardiolipin antibodies and lupus anticoagulant)
L	Factor V Leiden
M	Malignancy/medication
S	Protein S deficiency
H	Homocystinemia
A	Antithrombin III deficiency
P	Prothrombin G20210A mutation
E	Elevated factor VIII
S	Sticky platelet syndrome

ibly inhibits any platelets it binds, its effects last 5–10 days from discontinuing the medication until new circulating platelets can be produced. No routine method of monitoring plasma level or other functional level is currently available. However, there are several platelet function tests on the market, for example VerifyNow (Accumetrics, San Diego, CA), PFA-100, light transmission aggregometry (LTA), and multi-electrode aggregometry. There is currently no standard or agreed upon measure of platelet function. In the event that clopidogrel administration needs reversal, platelet transfusion has been the most frequently employed method. Investigation regarding the efficacy of this method is ongoing. Anecdotal evidence of clopidogrel reversal with desmopressin or DDAVP has emerged.[10] There is also evidence that GI prophylaxis may reduce GI bleeding seen with Plavix.[11]

Contrast Allergy

Anaphylactoid reactions to contrast material have been well described and encompass approximately 90% of contrast allergic reactions.[12] Unlike classical anaphylaxis reactions, which are IgE-mediated immune responses, anaphylactoid reactions involve direct release of mediators by basophils and mast cells in response to an eliciting agent. These mediators include histamine, leukotriene C4, prostaglandin D2, and tryptase, and their release can lead to rapid onset of increased secretion from mucous membranes, increased bronchial smooth muscle tone, decreased vascular smooth muscle tone, and increased capillary permeability. Most reactions to radiocontrast are usually mild and may include nausea, vomiting, increased mucous secretions, urticaria, and/or dyspnea. However, fatalities secondary to rapid-onset systemic angioedema, hypotension, and bronchospasm have been reported, with an overall risk of a fatal reaction estimated at 0.9 cases per 100,000 exposures. There is a linear, dose-dependent reaction curve. Patients with a previous history of asthma or adverse reaction to contrast agents have an increased risk of future events.

Contrast Material

There has been a trend toward nonionic contrast materials, with studies showing a decreased risk of adverse reaction; risks range anywhere from 6–8% with ionic contrast materials to 0.2% with nonionic contrast materials.[12] The use of gadolinium-based contrast angiography has suggested lower adverse reaction rates, in particular lower rates of nephropathy. However, new data suggest that gadolinium exposure may lead to a chronic, irreversible necrotizing fibrosing dermatopathy months to years after exposure.[13] However, this usually occurs in patients with already chronic renal disease. Current recommendations are to weigh the risks and benefits of this method in individual patients.

Prophylaxis

Pretreatment with antihistamines (diphenhydramine 50 mg per os [PO, by mouth]) and corticosteroids (hydrocortisone 100 mg IV) has shown clear benefits in lowering the rates of anaphylactoid reactions to IV contrast, especially when nonionic forms are used. Consider these measures for patients who have a prior history of reaction, because the rate of recurrence is estimated at 17–60%. Patients who are atopic and/or asthmatic also are at increased risk of reaction. In addition, allergic reactions are more difficult to treat in patients taking β-blockers, which may increase bronchospasm and vascular collapse. Patients who undergo preoperative prophylaxis with these agents usually continue their use with one to two doses in the postoperative period.

Treatment

If a contrast-induced allergic reaction is found, it is important to assess the severity and apply the ABCs of resuscitation as necessary. Bronchospasm can be treated with a fast-acting β_2-agonist, such as albuterol, and antihistamines. Severe respiratory distress, hypotension, or altered mental status should be addressed with intubation and mechanical ventilation. Fluid resuscitation should be tempered in patients with CHF or CRI. Subcutaneous, intramuscular, or intravenous epinephrine (0.3–0.5 mL 1:1000 solution subcutaneous or intramuscular [SC/IM] every 15 minutes, or 0.5–1 mL 1:10,000 solution intravenously [IV] administered slowly and repeated prn, respectively) or other vasocontrictors may be necessary in the setting of severe hypotension (**Table 9.12**).

General Concepts of Postprocedural Care

Complications arising from endovascular procedures may include, but are not limited to, stroke, vessel injury, bleeding, contrast allergy, myocardial infarction, nephropathy, and infection.[1] The key to a successful postprocedure course is the prompt recognition and treatment of these problems. This starts immediately after the procedure, often on the angiography table or in the recovery room, and continues in lessening degrees until discharge. Serial evaluations of the patient's vital signs, focused neurologic exams, and checks on vascular access points and distal pulses are the mainstays in detecting complications. Laboratory and imaging studies should be obtained in a focused manner to evaluate for specific problems.

Postprocedural Stroke

Stroke is probably the most important complication to recognize early because prompt detection may increase the possibility of a successful intervention. If a new neurological deficit does occur, it is important to distinguish between an occlusive process, such as an in-stent thrombosis or an arterial dissection, and an embolic process. The first step is to repeat catheter angiography to exclude treatable etiologies, followed by an MRI to evaluate the extent of injury. Supportive care, including ABCs and IV fluids, as well as antiplatelet and anticoagulation medications, are important treatment measures to reduce further injury.

Expanding Groin Hematoma

The vascular access point for catheter angiography most often requires entry through the femoral arteries. However, the recovery team must be aware that radial, brachial, or bilateral transfemoral access may have been attempted, and they must recognize the potential for incomplete hemostasis at each site.

Table 9.12 Treatment for Acute Contrast Allergy

Type of reaction	Comments
Mild reaction	1. Discontinue or slow injection of contrast. 2. Continue IV fluids. 3. Diphenhydramine 25–50 mg PO/IV. 4. Treat nausea/vomiting, if present. 5. Document in medical record.
Moderate reaction	1. Discontinue injection of contrast. 2. Continue IV fluids. 3. Place O_2 6–10 L/min via face mask. 4. If the reaction is progressive, administer 0.1–0.3 mg SC epinephrine 1:1,000 (contraindicated in severe cardiac disease). 5. If evidence of hypotension, give epinephrine 0.1 mg IV 1:10,000 slowly. Up to 1 mg may be given. 6. If bronchospasm occurs, administer β-agonist inhalers. May give 0.1–0.3 mg SC epinephrine 1:1,000. If the condition is progressive, may administer 0.1 mg IV epinephrine 1:10,000 slowly. 7. If patient is still not responding, call anesthesia. 8. Transfer to appropriate care unit. 9. Document in medical record.
Severe reaction/ anaphylaxis	1. Discontinue injection of contrast. 2. Notify the anesthesiologist Immediately. 3. Continue IV fluids. 4. Monitor all vital signs. 5. Place O_2 6–10 L/min via face mask. 6. If evidence of hypotension, raise the patient's legs up or put patient in Trendelenberg position. 7. If significant bradycardia, may administer 0.6–1 mg IV atropine. May give up to 2 mg in adults. 8. For severe hypertension, 5 mg phentolamine (1 mg in children) may be administered. 9. If anaphylactic reaction, administer 1 mL epinephrine 1:10,000 slowly over 1 minute. Also administer steroids. 10. Transfer patient to the ICU.

Abbreviations: ICU, intensive care unit; IV, intravenous; PO, per os (by mouth); SC, subcutaneous.

Signs and Symptoms (Table 9.13)

Pulsitile groin mass, femoral bruit, decreased peripheral pulses, and leg hypothermia, pallor, or pain are common symptoms in access point complications.

Work-up and Treatment

An expanding hematoma may require further treatment, with either manual compression or a FemoStop device (Radi Medical Systems, Uppsala, Sweden). Serial examinations and skin markings of hematoma size are important to document change. Close monitoring of vital signs for evidence of hypotension or tachycardia and serial complete blood counts (CBCs) are important to evaluation of the severity of blood loss. A CT scan of the abdomen and pelvis should be obtained if

Table 9.13 Signs/Symptoms of Expanding Groin Hematoma

Pulsatile groin mass
Femoral bruise
Diminished peripheral pulses
Leg hypothermia
Leg pallor
Leg pain

the patient is symptomatic or has a significant drop in hemoglobin or hematocrit levels. Transfusion of blood products may become necessary, and in some cases the patient will need endovascular or open surgical repair of the damaged vessel.

Contrast Allergy

If contrast allergy occurs, it should be recognized promptly and treated if necessary.

Postoperative Myocardial Infarction

Postoperative myocardial infarction (MI) most often occurs within 48 hours of the procedure but can occur up to a week following surgery. It is clinically silent in 90% of cases; however, symptoms of chest pain, shortness of breath, diaphoresis, nausea, lightheadedness, and a fluttering sensation in the chest may occur.

Signs and Symptoms

The signs and symptoms of myocardial infarction include congestive heart failure, hypotension, or arrhythmias on an electrocardiogram (ECG). Historically, the rate of postoperative MI in unselected patients undergoing noncardiac surgery is <2%, but it can carry a mortality rate of greater than 40%.[14] It is essential to remain vigilant for this disease in the postoperative period.

Work-up and Treatment

There are no clear guidelines for surveillance in the literature, but high-risk patients should undergo close observation, telemetry monitoring, cardiac enzyme evaluation, and ECG monitoring in the first two days following their procedure. Beta-blocker prophylaxis, if appropriate, has been shown to reduce the two-year mortality rate of cardiac events by 65%.[15] Patients who develop ischemia should be monitored in a critical care environment and managed similarly to the medical patient, with the caveat that not all may be appropriate candidates for aspirin or β-blockade. First-line therapies for MI include aspirin 325 mg per day, oxygen supplementation, pain control, heart rate management (usually with β-blockers), and nitroglycerin for preload and chest pain reduction. A cardiology consultation may be helpful regarding decisions involving heparin, thrombolysis, or percutaneous coronary interventions.

Contrast-Induced Nephropathy

In patients who have undergone a neurointerventional procedure, it is essential to monitor urine output as well as creatinine levels. Contrast nephropathy is often mild and treatable, especially when detected early (see **Table 9.5**).

Infection

Infection is usually rare; however, patients with fever, purulence, fluctuence, erythema, or pain at their vascular access point need further evaluation. Serial site exams and serial white blood cell counts (WBCs), erythrocyte sedimentation rates (ESR), and CRP may be helpful in following infection/inflammatory resolution. Even rarer than site infections are infected vascular implants (i.e., stents, coils, etc.). In these cases, the patients will exhibit signs and symptoms of systemic infection, often with positive blood cultures. This potentially devastating complication may be refractory to broad-spectrum antibiotics, and in some instances it requires surgical excision of the infected device.

Clinical Pearls

1. Make a careful patient selection by weighing the patient's overall health and the risk of the procedure against the natural history of the disease being treated (for example, an 80-year-old with severe coronary artery disease [CAD] and a 6 mm basilar tip aneurysm is very different from a healthy 35-year-old with the same lesion).
2. Perform thorough preoperative evaluation and planning. Minimize the risk of the most common complications by identifying patients with a high atherosclerotic burden, diabetes, chronic renal insufficiency, etc. Take proactive measures, such as pretreatment with N-acetylcysteine in patients with renal insufficiency.
3. Take a team approach to the disease. Ensure that all support personnel are aware of your treatment strategy and crucial points in the procedure.
4. Perform meticulous serial exams postprocedurally. The impact of inevitable complications can be minimized through early recognition of a neurological change or expanding hematomas, for example.
5. Possess the knowledge and ability to treat complications. Knowing the appropriate sequence of work-up and treatment is crucial in emergency situations. You may not have the luxury of time to consult a reference.
6. Re-catheterize as necessary to rule out treatable complications. When in doubt about the patency of a parent or branch vessel, re-catheterization often provides the most accurate modality for diagnosis as well as the most rapid mode of treatment.

References

1. Hessel SJ, Adams DF, Abrams HL. Complications of angiography. Radiology 1981;138(2): 273–281
2. Hass WK, Fields WS, North RR, Kircheff II, Chase NE, Bauer RB. Joint study of extracranial arterial occlusion. II. Arteriography, techniques, sites, and complications. JAMA 1968;203(11):961–968

3. Guzman LA, Costa MA, Angiolillo DJ, Zenni M, Wludyka P, Silliman S, Bass TA. A systematic review of outcomes in patients with staged carotid artery stenting and coronary artery bypass graft surgery. Stroke Feb 2008;39(2):361–365

4. Massicotte A. Contrast medium-induced nephropathy: strategies for prevention. Pharmacotherapy 2008;28(9):1140–1150

5. Brar SS, Shen AY, Jorgensen MB, et al. Sodium bicarbonate vs sodium chloride for the prevention of contrast medium-induced nephropathy in patients undergoing coronary angiography: a randomized trial. JAMA 2008;300(9):1038–1046

6. Marenzi G, Assanelli E, Marana I, et al. N-acetylcysteine and contrast-induced nephropathy in primary angioplasty. N Engl J Med 2006;354(26):2773–2782

7. Stenstrom DA, Muldoon LL, Armijo-Medina H, Watnick S, Doolittle ND, Kaufman JA, Peterson DR, Bubalo J, Neuwelt EA. N-acetylcysteine use to prevent contrast medium-induced nephropathy: premature phase III trials. J Vasc Interv Radiol Mar 2008;19(3):309–318, review

8. Barada K, Abdul-Baki H, El Hajj II, Hashash JG, Green PH. Gastrointestinal bleeding in the setting of anticoagulation and antiplatelet therapy. J Clin Gastroenterol 2009;43:5–12

9. Castaman G, Federici AB, Rodeghiero F, Mannucci PM. Von Willebrand's disease in the year 2003: towards the complete identification of gene defects for correct diagnosis and treatment. Haematologica 2003;88(1):94–108

10. Leithäuser B, Zielske D, Seyfert UT, Jung F. Effects of desmopressin on platelet membrane glycoproteins and platelet aggregation in volunteers on clopidogrel. Clin Hemorheol Microcirc 2008;39(1-4):293–302

11. Ibáñez L, Vidal X, Vendrell L, Moretti U, Laporte JR; Spanish-Italian Collaborative Group for the Epidemiology of Gastrointestinal Bleeding. Upper gastrointestinal bleeding associated with antiplatelet drugs. Aliment Pharmacol Ther 2006;23(2):235–242

12. Cochran ST, Bomyea K, Sayre JW. Trends in adverse events after IV administration of contrast media. AJR Am J Roentgenol 2001;176(6):1385–1388

13. Wertman R, Altun E, Martin DR, et al. Risk of nephrogenic systemic fibrosis: evaluation of gadolinium chelate contrast agents at four American universities. Radiology 2008;248(3):799–806

14. Eagle KA, Berger PB, Calkins H, et al.; American College of Cardiology/American Heart Association Task Force on Practice Guidelines (Committee to Update the 1996 Guidelines on Perioperative Cardiovascular Evaluation for Noncardiac Surgery). ACC/AHA guideline update for perioperative cardiovascular evaluation for noncardiac surgery—executive summary: a report of the American College of Cardiology/American Heart Association Task Force on Practice Guidelines (Committee to Update the 1996 Guidelines on Perioperative Cardiovascular Evaluation for Noncardiac Surgery). Circulation 2002;105(10):1257–1267

15. Mangano DT, Layug EL, Wallace A, Tateo I; Multicenter Study of Perioperative Ischemia Research Group. Effect of atenolol on mortality and cardiovascular morbidity after noncardiac surgery. N Engl J Med 1996;335(23):1713–1720

10

Endovascular Complications

Christopher S. Eddleman, Stacey Quintero Wolfe, Roham Moftakhar,
and Mohammad Ali Aziz-Sultan

Cerebrospinal angiography is a set of invasive procedures that can result in significant morbidity and (very rarely) even in death. While the risks of complications are generally low, it is the effects of the complications that matter most, for example, blindness, quadraparesis, limb ischemia, etc. Some complications may occur irrespective of the preparations; however, most endovascular complications can be avoided with meticulous and careful angiographic technique. In this chapter, we discuss the most common complications, techniques to avoid them, and finally the steps that must be taken when complications occur. Just remember, angiography and endovascular management may have low complication risks and fewer days in the hospital, but they also have a great potential to hurt someone if every procedure is not taken seriously.

Vascular Access and Closure Device Complications

Vascular access and closure complications are important considerations, given that they may become involved in every diagnostic and interventional procedure. Vascular access complications, which are reported in roughly 2% of those undergoing femoral artery catheterization (both diagnostic and interventional), include groin hematomas (1.3%), retroperitoneal hematomas (0.4%), pseudoaneurysms (0.1%), and arterial dissections (0.3%).[1] The rates of complication are higher in patients receiving anticoagulation or antiplatelet therapy during interventional procedures.

Retroperitoneal hematomas can be life threatening, in rare cases leading to shock and cardiovascular collapse. Patients with abdominal or flank pain should immediately be screened with a CT of the abdomen, have hematocrits checked every 4–6 hours until stable, and receive transfusion accordingly. Additionally, antiplatelet and anticoagulation therapy should be stopped and reversed with platelets and protamine sulfate if there is a significant decrease in the hematocrit and the endovascular procedure allows for reversal. A decrease in hematocrit can be a late finding in retroperitoneal hematoma. Often, the first sign is relative hypotension that is unresponsive to intravenous fluid administration. This should prompt an emergent CT of the abdomen and pelvis.

Pseudoaneurysms can be prevented with proper closure technique and prevention of hip flexion for 24–48 hours following the procedure. In the case of a patient presenting with an enlarging, pulsating groin mass following angiography, an ultrasound should be performed immediately, and the patient should be referred to a peripheral vascular surgeon for evaluation. In the case of small pseudoaneurysms (approximately <2 cm), manual compression or thrombin injection may be sufficient, while in larger ones (>2 cm), open or endovascular treatment is required, and it is usually performed by a vascular surgeon or interventional radiologist. Another complication of a pseudoaneurysm may be an arteriovenous fistula, requiring close follow-up and potentially an intervention to correct the fistula. The risk of fistula formation is much higher when the patient is anticoagulated during the procedure.

Vessel wall injury or dissection may occur as the vessel is cannulated with the wire or sheath, creating a false lumen within which blood flows. This risk can typically be lowered by performing a single-wall puncture with slow advancement of the wire in a twisting motion under fluoroscopy. As a result, some advocate use of a micropuncture needle. In the case of dissection, angiography should be performed to assess limitation of flow, and there should be consultation with vascular surgery and interventional radiology to assess the potential need for stent placement.

There is excellent collateral circulation in the lower extremities, usually allowing for the loss of one arterial branch; however, the loss of the common femoral artery can result in vascular claudication and even profound ischemia requiring revascularization. Most thromboembolic events that occur with vascular access are due to distal showering of calcified plaque in patients with significant peripheral atherosclerosis. Loss of distal pulses requires an emergent ultrasound of the leg to evaluate the level of occlusion. If there is flow below the popliteal artery, this condition can usually be managed with intravenous heparin; however, more proximal thromboses typically require endovascular or surgical intervention. Stenosis of the common femoral artery is almost always due to failure of a closure device. Closure devices are not recommended in arteries with significant atherosclerosis.

Closure Devices

Closure devices are being used more often in neuroendovascular procedures in an attempt to prevent potential complications associated with anticoagulation and antiplatelet therapy. In a single-center study of 1,443 neurointerventional procedures, AngioSeal (St. Jude Medical) was used for 745 diagnostic procedures and 670 neurointerventions.[2] The procedural success rate was 99.7%. Major complication rates related to closure were 0.13% in the diagnostic group and 1.4% in the interventional group. Angioseal did not appear to enhance inflammatory response when compared with mechanical compression.[3]

In a large meta-analysis of coronary angiography (30 studies, 37,066 patients), no difference between Angioseal or Perclose and mechanical compression was seen in diagnostic procedures.[4] There was a trend toward fewer complications with AngioSeal in the interventional setting.

In another study examining lower extremity ischemia after cardiac catheterization in patients with peripheral vascular disease, neither AngioSeal nor Perclose was associated with a reduction in the ankle-brachial index when compared with manual compression.[5]

Two of the more recent closure devices on the market, namely the StarClose and the Mynx closure device, have recent studies regarding efficacy. McTaggart et al. reviewed their institutional experience with StarClose and reported a 0.7% and 0.4% rate in minor and major complications with a 95% success rate in patients with an attempt.[6] However, Chiu et al. reported increased minor complications with the Starclose closure device as compared with others, but all were managed with additional manual compression.[7] The Mynx closure, which involves deployment of a sealant plug, was reported by Fields et al. to be associated with an increased presence of intravascular sealant and pseudoaneurysms (11%) without major complications.[8]

Procedure-Related Complications

While vascular access and closure complications are probably the most common due to their presence in every endovascular procedure, several complications exist that are procedure specific. These complications can typically be classified into equipment/implant and/or post-procedure related. All of these complications must be vetted with the patient and their family to truly obtain and maintain informed consent for any procedure.

Equipment- and Implant-Related Complications

Radiation

As stated in Chapter 5, enough cannot be said regarding radiation safety. The effects of radiation are often taken for granted, especially given its invisibility and potential for long-term effects. Despite this, awareness of the complications of excessive radiation is imperative, both to the patient as well as to the interventionists and those in and around the immediate working area. Obviously, quantification of radiation to the patient and interventionist involves many factors, so that every situation will be different. A diagnostic angiogram should involve a significantly lower amount of radiation than embolization of an intracranial arteriovenous malformation (AVM). However, procedures can be instituted that significantly reduce the risks of prolonged radiation exposure in every case. The reported complications of excessive radiation exposure tend to be delayed malignancy, growth retardation, lenticular opacities, premature atherosclerotic disease, and mental retardation after in utero exposure.

More short-term effects of radiation exposure or concentration can be local skin reactions, edema, hair loss, and changes in constitution, such as nausea and headache. Furthermore, the tissues being treated can also exhibit both short- and long-term local changes that may produce tissue or tumoral edema, leading to other physical manifestations like increased intracranial pressure (ICP), seizures, and various neurological deficits. Although these potential complications are rare in patients who undergo several diagnostic procedures, they can become significant in patients who undergo repeated embolization procedures. In general, reducing and/or limiting the amount of radiation exposure to both the patient and the interventionist can avoid or minimize complications of radiation exposure. The importance of proper radiation shielding and reduction of radiation scatter cannot be stressed enough; this reduction can be accomplished by several maneuvers, including moving the radiation source closer to the patient, reducing the number of frames per second, and avoiding unnecessary contrast injections.

Contrast

Contrast agents also pose potential complications. Although most institutions now use nonionic preparations of contrast, which allow the use of lower effective concentrations and provide a marginally safer usage profile, similar complications have been reported. While ionic preparations are still available at some institutions, they should not be used in patients with contrast allergies, asthma, diabetes mellitus, sickle-cell anemia, renal dysfunction, cardiac dysfunction, or known compromise of the blood-brain barrier (**Table 10.1**). The most common complications from contrast are systemic reactions and acute or worsening renal failure. Patients with known allergies can often be prepped for receiving contrast with steroids and Benadryl for 24 to 48 hours before the procedure; the same treatment can be continued several days afterwards, depending on the significance of the allergy. If by chance a patient has a contrast reaction, without having prior knowledge of a contrast reaction, several management schemes can be undertaken, depending on the severity of reaction. Methods of preventing or minimizing the systemic effects of contrast are the use of low-osmolar contrast agents, adequate hydration, N-acetylcysteine (Mucomyst) administration, and sodium bicarbonate infusions (**Table 10.2**).

Microcatheters and Microwires

Once vascular access is obtained and a sheath is placed, the placement of either a diagnostic or guide catheter follows. Any time a wire or catheter, micro or otherwise, is passed into and through a vascular channel, there is the possibility of either injury to that vessel or thromboembolic complications. Injury to the vessel can lead to dissection, with or without a resultant pseudoaneurysm. To avoid such complications, catheters are most frequently passed over wires in the setting of anticoagulation (activated clotting times [ACTs] >200) and manipulated with careful movements under fluoroscopic visualization. When wires may not be used, intermittent "puffing" of contrast can keep the catheter from impinging on the vessel wall. Thromboembolic complications can occur in older individuals with a significant amount of atherosclerotic plaque either along the vessel walls or at points of curvature (aorta) or bifurcations (common carotid). In addition, continuous heparinized flush or intermittent "puffing" of contrast on catheters can often prevent accumulation of blood inside the tips, thereby reducing the formation of thrombus in this location. Keeping the ACT in the appropriate range can also reduce the risk of distal thromboembolism from vessel-related atherosclerosis. Obviously, this risk

Table 10.1 Risk Factors for Contrast Reactions

Factor	Contribution
Age	Infants, elderly
Sex	Female
Medical comorbidities	Asthma, cardiac disease, DM, dehydration, renal disease, BBB disruption
Hematologic comorbidities	Myeloma, sickle-cell disease, polycythemia
Medications	NSAIDs, IL-2, β-blockers, biguanides
Contrast	>20 mg iodine, fast injection rate, intra-arterial injection, previous/documented contrast reactions

Abbreviations: DM, diabetes mellitus; NSAID, nonsteroidal anti-inflammatory drug.

Table 10.2   Treatment for Acute Contrast Allergy

Type of reaction	Comments
Mild reaction	1. Discontinue or slow injection of contrast 2. Continue IV fluids 3. Diphenhydramine 25–50 mg PO/IV 4. Treat nausea/vomiting, if present 5. Document in medical record
Moderate reaction	1. Discontinue injection of contrast 2. Continue IV fluids 3. Place O_2 6–10 L/min via face mask 4. If progressive reaction, administer 0.1–0.3 mg SC epinephrine 1:1,000 (contraindicated in severe cardiac disease) 5. If evidence of hypotension, give epinephrine 0.1 mg IV 1:10,000 slowly. Up to 1 mg may be given 6. If bronchospasm, administer β-agonist inhalers. May give 0.1–0.3 mg SC epinephrine 1:1,000. If progressive, may administer 0.1 mg IV epinephrine 1:10,000 slowly. 7. If still not responding, call anesthesia 8. Transfer to appropriate care unit 9. Document in medical record
Severe reaction/ anaphylaxis	1. Discontinue injection of contrast 2. Notify anesthesia immediately 3. Continue IV fluids 4. Monitor all vital signs 5. Place O_2 6–10 L/min via face mask 6. If evidence of hypotension, raise legs up or put patient in Trendelenberg position 7. If significant bradycardia, may administer 0.6–1 mg IV atropine. May give up to 2 mg in adults 8. For severe hypertension, 5 mg phentolamine (1 mg in children) may be administered 9. If anaphylactic reaction, administer 1 mL epinephrine 1:10,000 slowly over 1 minute. Also administer steroids 10. Transfer patient to the ICU

is higher in older individuals and those with significant atherosclerotic risk factors. Lastly, when a wire is used to navigate through the vasculature, it should never rest just outside the tip of the catheter, as this may render the wire very stiff and make it act as a piercing device. Further, during navigation through vessels of smaller caliber, the shape of the wire tip should be somewhat curved and moved with constant rotation, because this reduces the chance of vessel injury or perforation.

Stent/Balloon/Coil/Embolics

Even though complications can occur when only diagnostic catheters are used, the risks of potential problems most certainly increase when endovascular equipment is used in addition to catheters and wires. The most commonly encountered endovascular equipment includes coils, balloons, stents, and liquid embolics. Each of these endovascular tools has its own inherent set of potential complications. It is important that the interventionists take precautions to select carefully the properly indicated and size device, especially since the recipient vessels for these tools are only millimeters in diameter, making vascular injury highly possible.

Coils

Endovascular coils have been significantly transformed since their initial FDA approval in 1991, going from bare helical coils to ones with complex folding patterns and various biological coatings. As the coil family becomes more diverse, so do the complications that accompany them. In general, bare platinum coils, when placed carefully and sized appropriately, do not result in significant complications and are highly tolerated by patients. However, in large amounts, platinum coils can cause localized reactions, resulting in swelling, surrounding edema and potential headaches, eye pain, delayed cranial nerve palsies, and increased ICPs. For controlling these potential complications when a large amount of coils are placed, a short course of steroids may also be administered. Biologically coated or bioactive coils can also result in similar reactions. Hydrogel-coated coils have been reported to be associated with some cases of hydrocephalus (at a reported rate of 1%), while other coil types appear to have lower risks of this complication. Coils can also herniate out of the aneurysm dome and into the parent artery, leaving a surface that is a potential source of thrombus formation. Therefore, an antiplatelet agent, frequently aspirin, is often administered for several months postprocedure. Infrequently, if the coils deployed into the aneurysm are undersized with respect to either the neck or the remaining dome, the coils can embolize to distal locations. This can lead to thromboembolic complications and even significant ischemia. Increasing coil packing density beyond 24% has been associated with decreased rates of recurrence, but this reduction likely depends on the type and characteristics of coils used as well as the amount of coil compaction over time. Therefore, overpacking the aneurysm, if desired, should be done with caution, as it could lead to the possible rupture of the aneurysm. Underpacking can also lead to coil compaction if the inflow zone of the aneurysm is hemodynamically significant, and such compaction leads to a higher incidence of aneurysm recurrence and remnant rupture. Sometimes coils can be prevented from embolizing by placing an intracranial vascular reconstruction device (stent). Lastly, when coil deployment is not satisfactory, an attempt to retract the coil could lead to "stretching" the coil, that is, losing its folding or helical properties. Due to the design and construction of most coils, stretched coils can extend for several yards. In such a case, there is no way to pull the catheter back far enough to retrieve all of the coil length. In these cases, a stent may need to be placed to tack the stretched coil against the vessel wall. Otherwise, the coil can serve as a persistent source of thrombus formation. These patients are also treated with dual antiplatelet therapy for at least three months.

Stents

The FDA has only recently approved self-expanding nitinol stents for intracranial use; however, balloon-mounted cardiac stents have been used in some cases for many years. The intracranial stents have been significantly improved with respect to their navigation abilities, designs, and retrievability. Complications that can result from the use of intracranial stents include undersizing the stent (resulting in post-deployment migration), jailing of smaller vessels emanating from the parent artery, acute or delayed in-stent stenosis, and vessel injury by the stent tines when it is placed on a significantly curved vessel. If the stent is placed early in a procedure, movement of catheters through and between the tines of the stent can lead to catheter fractures. Because deployment of a stent requires the coordinated effort of not only the interventionist but also the equipment, premature or partial deployment can occur that may render the device useless, thus requiring its removal. These maneuvers can lead to vessel injuries or perforations.

Balloons

Intravascular balloons are used for a variety of endovascular procedures and are available in a variety of sizes and shapes, with different inflation techniques and pliability. Whether it is balloon test occlusions, distal protection during CAS, balloon-remodeling for aneurysm embolization, or intracranial angioplasty, intravascular balloons can lead to many potentially devastating consequences if not carefully applied. Possible complications include vessel injury/rupture from overinflation, navigation through tortuous vessels, or ischemia from prolonged inflation.

Embolics

The use of embolics for the treatment of vascular pathological entities has been around for decades. The most common embolics used for treatment of vascular disease are particles, liquid or push microcoils, cyanoacrylates (n-BCA), sclerosing agents, and precipitated polymers (Onyx).

Particles are solid-state entities that come in a variety of shapes and sizes. Determination of the target site is very important when particles are used. They are not recommended for high-flow fistulae or AVMs, simply because occluded vessels can recanalize over time and the particles can travel more distally due to their small size and non-adherent properties, which can lead to other complications. Because most particles are flow directed, smaller particles have the risk of traveling to other vessels. Oversizing particles compared with the target vessel is the best strategy to ensure minimal embolization of undesired vessels. Particles also tend to clog the microcatheter if they are too large or injected in too large of a quantity.

Microcoils are small, sometimes present with thrombogenic fibers, and are pushable, that is, they do not have a detaching mechanism. Given the larger sizes than particles, the microcatheter through which these coils are pushed is often larger and can often become occluded by the coils. The destination of the coils is also unpredictable and somewhat uncontrolled. Vessels occluded using coils may still recanalize at a later time.

Cyanoacrylates, such as n-butyl cyanocrylate (n-BCA), are acrylic agents that polymerized in the presence of an ionic environment and are generally thought to provide a permanent occlusion. The rate of polymerization is very fast but can be altered with different mixtures. Despite this, the polymerization is highly dependent on many other factors, which tend to create situations for complications. Given the highly adhesive nature of these agents, it is highly possible to "glue" the catheter in place, thus making it necessary to leave the catheter behind. If the mixture is such that the polymerization is delayed more than anticipated, the liquid nature of the mixture can result in the deposit of embolic material in undesired locations, possibly causing embolic complications related to occlusion.

Sclerotic agents are used to occlude vessels by facilitating thrombosis. Common agents are thrombin and ethanol. Patients may complain of extreme pain when injections are done near a meningeal surface. Further, ethanol has been shown to permeate outside and be accompanied by contrast extravasation, often leading to neurological complications and even death. Given the difficulty of knowing when to stop injections, due to the delayed onset of occlusion, and the numerous reports of neurological complications, ethanol is not often recommended for intracranial use. However, it still has a role in extracranial vascular lesions and tumors.

Nonhydrophilic polymers have only been approved for intracranial use and have proven to be very useful in vascular or tumor embolization procedures. These nonadhesive precipitated polymers, such as Onyx (ev3, Irvine, CA), precipitates when exposed to a hydrophilic environment after their solvent (dimethyl sulfoxide, DMSO) disperses. As a result, this requires DMSO-compatible catheters, which often do not have the same physical properties as other microcatheters. However, newer catheters are being manufactured as DMSO compatible (for example, Marathon, ev3, Irvine, CA) and offer similar distal navigation abilities. DMSO can be toxic to the vessels and therefore should not be injected too quickly. If injected too quickly, the polymer can also result in reflux of the agent and either occlude undesired vessels or (although very rarely) the catheter itself, despite being a nonadhesive agent.

Postprocedure Complications

Even though the immediate risks from angiography end with the procedure, postprocedure complications have been known to occur. These complications can be organized into groups: contrast-related, catheter/wire-related, pathology-related, device-related, and systemic comorbidity-related. The most common complications usually result from catheter angiography itself and rates vary from 0.4% to 12.2%. The types of complications are usually minor, involving complications related to access, transient thromboembolic effects, and/or transient global amnesia. The most common major complications involve permanent neurological changes, resulting from either large thromboembolic complications or acute occlusion, whether from dissection, thrombosis, or stent occlusion. Most cases of major thromboembolic complications are taken back to the angiography suite for intra-arterial thrombolytics or mechanical thrombolysis. Most patients with significant medical comorbidities are at risk for cardiopulmonary complications, especially myocardial infarction (MI) after general anesthesia. Despite the fact that risk of MI after angiography is exceptionally low (<1%), cardiovascular disease is associated with a higher complication risk, approximately 2.3%. Given the possibility of major complications after either a diagnostic or interventional procedure, close monitoring of the patient should always be done after these procedures, including vital signs, neurological exam, and assessment of the access site.

Summary

Although the risks of complications related to neuroendovascular procedures, whether diagnostic or interventional, are normally low, the operator should always consciously anticipate them. Intimate knowledge of the possible complications can help the operator to avoid complications and to manage them successfully when they occur. The combination of dedication to patient safety and expert technical skill can lead to successful treatment, not only of vascular pathology but also of the patient.

Clinical Pearls

1. Complications can be expected to happen. The key factor is not the complication itself but how you handle it, i.e., always anticipate and prepare for them.
2. If a complication occurs, always be honest about it.
3. Complications can create stressful situations. Always try to take a deep breath and relax, as this will make the next several steps easier than getting tense and angry, which never helps the situation.
4. Handling technical complications involves two main parts: (1) not making it worse and (2) doing what is best for the patient and not the pictures.

References

1. Cox N, Resnic FS, Popma JJ, et al. Managing the femoral artery in coronary angiography. Heart Lung Circ 2008;17(Suppl. 4):S65–S69
2. Geyik S, Yavuz K, Akgoz A, et al. The safety and efficacy of the Angio-Seal closure device in diagnostic and interventional neuroangiography setting: a single-center experience with 1,443 closures. Neuroradiology 2007;49(9):739–746
3. Applegate RJ, Sacrinty M, Kutcher MA, et al. Vascular complications with newer generations of angioseal vascular closure devices. J Interv Cardiol 2006;19(1):67–74
4. Nikolsky E, Mehran R, Halkin A, et al. Vascular complications associated with arteriotomy closure devices in patients undergoing percutaneous coronary procedures: a meta-analysis. J Am Coll Cardiol 2004;44(6):1200–1209
5. Kälsch HI, Eggebrecht H, Mayringer S, et al. Randomized comparison of effects of suture-based and collagen-based vascular closure devices on post-procedural leg perfusion. Clin Res Cardiol 2008;97(1):43–48
6. McTaggart RA, Raghavan D, Haas RA, Jayaraman MV. StarClose vascular closure device: safety and efficacy of deployment and reaccess in a neurointerventional radiology service. AJNR Am J Neuroradiol 2010;31(6):1148–1150
7. Chiu AH, Coles SR, Tibballs J, Nadkarni S. The StarClose vascular closure device in antegrade and retrograde punctures: a single-center experience. J Endovasc Ther 2010;17(1):46–50
8. Fields JD, Liu KC, Lee DS, et al. Femoral artery complications associated with the Mynx closure device. AJNR Am J Neuroradiol 2010;31(9):1737–1740

Intraoperative Neurophysiological Monitoring

Blair Calancie, Amit Singla, and Eric M. Deshaies

The intraoperative identification of neural structures by electrophysiologic means (i.e., "mapping") has been used for many years in a provocative manner to guide the surgical procedure. Much of our understanding of the functional role played by specific regions of the cerebral cortex in humans came from examining the effects of electrical stimulation applied to the exposed cerebral cortex in awake humans.[1] However, intraoperative monitoring is also developing an important niche in neuroendovascular procedures, particularly in patients requiring general anesthesia during provocative testing for arteriovenous malformation (AVM) embolization and occlusive procedures such as balloon angioplasty or balloon-assisted aneurysm coiling. Intraoperative monitoring allows the proceduralist to detect changes in neurological function when an exam cannot be obtained, and it can also be used to prevent permanent neurological injury in some situations.

In the broadest sense, intraoperative neurophysiological monitoring (IOM) has two main applications: (1) mapping, both to identify structures and to evaluate the proximity of certain implants to nearby neural structures and (2) neuroprotection, to guard against inadvertent (i.e., iatrogenic) injury to neural structures as a direct consequence of surgical or interventional activities.

In its arguably more widely practiced role, IOM is also used for neuroprotection, to provide information about the functional status of central nervous system (CNS) structures during procedures that place these structures at risk. Should a surgical or endovascular action, such as provocative Brevital testing prior to AVM embolization, lead to a change in IOM-specific waveforms, the surgical team is alerted to this change, giving them the opportunity to undo or avoid that action. This second role of IOM—to provide immediate feedback about CNS functional integrity in the anesthetized (or comatose) patient—will serve as the focus of the remainder of this chapter.

It is important at the earliest stage of this discussion to point out that an assumption at the heart of IOM for neuroprotection is that a changed waveform reflects functional deterioration within the neurologic pathway mediating that waveform. Thus, if the IOM test being used does not utilize that portion of the CNS at risk from the procedure, then the test will not be useful in predicting injury. In the following sections, we will provide an overview of the types of IOM tests that are now considered standard in the field, and the pathways and relevant vascular supplies that are monitored by these tests.

Electroencephalogram (EEG)

EEG—Signal Generators and Pathways

The electroencephalogram (EEG) reflects the spontaneous and time-varying post-synaptic activity of large populations of neurons within the cerebral cortex. In the healthy individual, there is an inverse relationship between the frequency of EEG activity and its amplitude, as summarized in **Table 11.1**. A reduction in mean EEG can be perfectly normal (e.g., in a person shifting from waking toward sleep), or it may reflect a more sinister cause, such as inadequate cortical oxygenation due to hypoperfusion or diminished oxyhemoglobin.

For IOM, either raw or processed (fast-Fourier transformed) EEG is continually sampled from multiple recording sites on the scalp. Sudden changes in this spontaneous activity may reflect the consequences (usually vascular in nature) of some surgical action and serve as one of the primary outcome measures for this type of monitoring.

The EEG originates from populations of neurons in cortical and subcortical regions, hence this approach examines functional activity within gray matter rather than projection tracts. For extracranial electrodes (that is, those on or just under the scalp), the most superficial 3–5 mm of cortex contributes most of the signal power. For IOM applications, a minimal series of electrodes would include sites over the frontal, temporal, and parietal lobes bilaterally.

EEG—Vascular Considerations

The distinctions between regional arterial blood supply are highly relevant to this review, as it means that regions giving rise to upper-limb versus lower-limb motor and sensory cortices have dissimilar blood supplies. These vascular distributions are reviewed in Chapter 1 and summarized in **Table 11.2**.

Table 11.1 Summary of EEG Characteristics

Frequency name	Frequency range (Hz)	Relative amplitude	Associated with
Delta	<4	high	deep anesthesia, hypoxia
Theta	4–8	high	anesthesia, sleep
Alpha	8–13	intermediate	quiet wakefulness; resting
Beta	13–30	low	awake and alert
Sigma	14–15	high	sleep; sometimes called "sleep spindle"

Table 11.2 Key Aspects of Different IOM Modalities Used

Test name	What is monitored?	Key blood vessels	Anesthesia influence	Alarm criteria	Strengths (S) and weaknesses (W)
EEG	Spontaneous neuron activity, cerebral cortex	ACA; MCA; PCA	Deep levels suppress EEG	Reduction in frequency (raw) or power (processed)	S: Easy to perform; low risk. W: recording sites may be suboptimal if craniotomy is used.
SEP	Dorsal columns and DC nuclei, med lemniscus, thalamus, int capsule, post-central gyrus	Posterior spinal artery; BA; PCA	Amp decreases at >1 MAC, otherwise OK with all major agents	For supramaximal stimuli: >50% reduction in amp, >10% in latency, after BP and anesthesia ruled out	S: Accurate for predicting postprocedure sensory loss; minimal to low risk. W: delays due to averaging; prone to noise; very sensitive to pre-existing conduction problems (myelopathy; diabetic neuropathy)
BAEP	Brainstem auditory pathways	AICA; PICA; BA; PCA; MCA	Limited; very resistant to major agents	Latency and/or amp increase in waves I, III, and V	S: Robust response with normal hearing; low risk; samples multiple brainstem blood vessels. W: technical/mechanical errors in sound delivery can easily lead to incorrect interpretation of nerve damage
VEP	Retina, optic nerve and radiations, LGN, occipital cortex	ICA; ophthalmic artery; ACA; AChA; PCA	Very sensitive (too sensitive?) to major agents	Not well-defined, because test failure is common	S: Should provide unique means to monitor critical sensory pathway and occipital cortex. W: prone to noise, anesthesia. Not considered reliable enough for regular use.
MEP	Neuromuscular junction, both lower and upper motor neurons, corticospinal tract (including internal capsule)	ACA; MCA; AChA; PCA; BA; anterior spinal artery	Very sensitive to sevo/des/isoflurane; these should be avoided. Best with intravenous infusion of propofol and opioid; avoid NM block.	Maximum stimulation intensity needed to elicit minimal muscle response (i.e., the "threshold"). Others say do not warn until signal is lost; we disagree. Literature shows controversy.	S: Extremely accurate for predicting postoperative motor weakness, if used properly; very sensitive to both mechanical and vascular compromise; immediate feedback (i.e., averaging not required); can localize between arm/leg, and left/right changes. W: risk of movement/bite and (rarely) seizure; will fail (sooner or later) if even low levels of sevo/des/isoflurane are used.

Abbreviations: ACA, anterior cerebral artery; AChA, anterior choroidal artery; AICA, anterior inferior cerebellar artery; BA, basilar artery; EEG, electroencephalogram; ICA, internal carotid artery; LGN, lateral geniculate nucleus; MCA, middle cerebral artery; NM, neuromuscular; PCA, posterior cerebral artery; PICA, posterior inferior cerebellar artery.

EEG—Methods

EEG is used during IOM in one of two ways. One can look for changes in stable levels of EEG activity as an indicator of potential insult to the cerebral cortex. Alternatively, one can deliberately depress EEG activity pharmacologically, thereby lowering cortical metabolic demand in anticipation of, or in response to, an interruption of cortical blood flow.

During induction of anesthesia, the EEG will demonstrate a characteristic pattern of progressively lower mean frequency content, with superimposition of brief, larger-amplitude spikes, bearing some resemblance to certain stages of sleep. At even deeper levels of anesthesia, the EEG will begin to oscillate between prolonged periods of very limited activity (isoelectric) and shorter periods (or "bursts") of activity. This stage is known as burst-suppression.

Virtually all general anesthetics will reduce EEG frequency and its total amount (that is, its power) once a steady-state has been achieved; at higher concentrations, some can even cause an isoelectric state. Given this, it is important that in the event of a significant EEG change, anesthetic considerations are ruled out before the endovascular team is alerted to this change. Note that some anesthetic agents, including etomidate and propofol, may result in a brief stage of increased cortical spiking activity during induction, which may be accompanied by myoclonic-like jerks or tremors in the extremities. Such activity can be confused with a seizure, but it is thought to reflect a transient imbalance between the anesthetic depth of cortical versus subcortical motor areas.[2]

EEG—Indications

The establishment of EEG burst-suppression via thiopental renders cortical neurons less susceptible to ischemic injury.[2] Not all hypnotic agents are equal in this neuroprotective role.[2] Burst-suppression is routinely called for by many physicians as a prophylaxis during procedures in which the patient's cerebral oxygenation might be compromised, such as when the common carotid artery is cross-clamped during endarterectomy (**Fig. 11.1**).[3]

EEG changes associated with cortical ischemia during neurovascular procedures are often unilateral. In contrast, a major change in systemic physiology, like the delivery of a bolus of anesthetic agent or profound hypothermia, will affect both cortical hemispheres in parallel. A unilateral change in EEG normally serves as a reliable signal that neuronal injury might be underway, necessitating a warning to the surgical team (**Table 11.2**).

Prophylactic use of burst-suppression prior to initiation of a high-risk procedure may mask important changes in the EEG that reflect compromised cerebral perfusion. We recommend against the use of burst-suppression unless there is evidence of an acute change in the EEG that is suggestive of altered (that is, diminished) oxygenation of the cortical tissue giving rise to that EEG signal. This way, the sensitivity of the EEG to change would be maintained at its highest level, yet the neuroprotective effects of burst-suppression could be implemented shortly after a detection of a change in EEG characteristics.

A different circumstance in which one looks for a brief and total abolishment of EEG activity is encountered during procedures to treat vascular malformations (pial arteriovenous malformation or dural arteriovenous fistula) of the brain. In this case, cortical tissue and the malformation may share a common arterial sup-

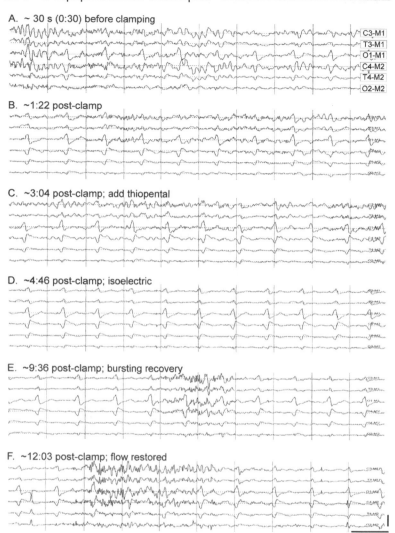

Fig. 11.1 Multiple EEG records sampled at different times **(A)** before and **(B–F)** after clamping the common carotid artery. Within each panel, the top three traces show activity under left-side leads positioned over the hand motor area (C3), temporal lobe (T3), and occipital lobe (O1), each referenced to the left mastoid process (M1). The bottom three traces of each panel show activity under corresponding right-side leads. Each panel heading lists the time relative to clamping (approximately 30 seconds in A, in minutes:seconds otherwise). The clamp had been removed approximately 30 seconds prior to the activity shown in panel F. Rhythmic waveforms evident across all six leads that are especially prominent in panel D originate from the EKG. Horizontal calibration bar = 1 second; vertical bar = 30 μV.

ply, so that one would not normally choose to embolize the malformation because of a concern for a worsening of neurologic function. To establish the functional link—if any—between the vascular malformation and cortical tissue, an endovascular catheter can be placed with its tip at the malformation's nidus. A bolus of relatively short-acting barbituate (typically sodium amobarbital or methohexital) is injected into the arterial feeding pedicle of the malformation. If the level of EEG power from nearby electrodes shows a marked decline, this indicates that the malformation includes a branch to the cerebral cortex, and it should therefore be left intact to prevent an ischemic complication. This approach takes its origins from the Wada test, which is used to localize eloquent cortex for speech and memory during craniotomy procedures when the patient is awake.[3]

EEG—Strengths and Weaknesses

One great strength of EEG as a monitored outcome measure for IOM techniques— its simplicity—also serves as a weakness, in that the EEG provides a sense of the neurologic status of just the cerebral cortical layers of the CNS, primarily from those gyri that are adjacent to the skull (**Table 11.2**).

EEG—Risks

The risks directly associated with EEG monitoring are relatively low (**Table 11.2**).

EEG—Anesthesia

Several reviews cover many aspects of neuroanesthesia, including intraoperative monitoring.[4,5] We will simply remind the reader that virtually all agents used to sedate or induce general anesthesia in patients will cause a reduction in EEG power once a steady state has been established. Several commercially available devices (such as the BIS monitor) have been developed to quantify EEG to predict various stages (or "depths") of sedation. More in-depth examinations of these technologies can be found elsewhere.[6]

Evoked Potentials

General Comments

A variety of different evoked potentials are available to the monitoring specialist (see **Table 11.2**). In general the idea is to activate nerve cells on one side of the surgery ("upstream"), causing electrical signals within these nerve cells to conduct through and beyond the region at risk from the surgery, and then to record the response to this activation from the same (rarely) or a different (usually) population of nerve (or muscle) fibers that are "downstream" from the surgery site. If the signals downstream from where surgery is taking place are unchanged, this indicates that the nerves conducting that signal have not been affected by the surgery. Provided certain confounding factors have been ruled out (examples to follow), the team is immediately alerted and will attempt to undo surgically whatever led to that signal change, to reduce the risk of permanent neural injury.

Somatosensory Evoked Potential (SEP)

SEP—Signal Generators and Pathways

Somatosensory evoked potentials typically use electrical stimulation of the median or ulnar nerves at the wrist or of the posterior tibial nerve at the ankle. A single stimulus activates large sensory fibers, whose action potentials are conducted proximally to the spinal cord and up the dorsal columns to the brainstem nuclei (gracile or cuneate). After synapsing, second-order fibers decussate at the level of the medulla as internal arcuate fibers and travel via the medial lemniscus to the ventroposterolateral thalamus, the site of a second synaptic relay. Finally, a third group of fibers from the thalamus transmits this nerve volley via the internal capsule to the postcentral gyrus of the parietal lobe's primary somatosensory cortex, which forms the final destination of these nerve signals.

SEP—Vascular Considerations

In the spinal cord, the dorsal columns and related neuronal structures are supplied by the posterior spinal arteries (PSA) arising from the vertebral arteries (VA) and are reviewed in Chapter 2 and **Table 11.2**.

SEP—Methods

With appropriately placed electrodes, one can follow the SEP signal from its origin (the wrist or ankle) all the way to the contralateral cerebral cortex. While surface EEG cup-type electrodes can be used for recording, it is far more common in the operating room setting to use needle electrodes for EEG and evoked potential applications (usually corkscrew electrodes, because they are virtually impossible to dislodge accidentally).

Stimulation to the nerve must be of sufficient intensity to cause action potentials in the large myelinated fibers within that mixed nerve. Adequate stimulation can be confirmed by brisk contractions of intrinsic muscles in the hand and foot, provided that neuromuscular blockade is not in place. Despite the fact that the stimulus intensities suggested above typically exceed the maximum needed to activate all large myelinated fibers in that nerve (that is, it is supramaximal), the resultant SEP is too small to see, so that signal averaging is necessary to generate a reliable SEP reading. In practice, one typically averages 200 to 500 individual trials (the actual number depends on the amount of background noise). This means that the results of an SEP test will be delayed one to three minutes. We will warn the procedural team if the major component of the waveform amplitude declines by more than 50% (peak-to-peak) of the baseline or if the latency to the initial peak/trough in that waveform increases by more than 10%.

SEP—Indications

Any procedure (surgical or endovascular) that places the pathways outlined earlier at risk is a candidate for SEP monitoring (see **Table 11.2**). For vascular cases, SEPs are useful for establishing the functional consequences of vascular perturbations. Often this testing can be done in a provocative manner, whereby application of a temporary clip or provocative intra-arterial testing can be used and the SEPs evaluated for change. If no change in waveforms develops over the next four to eight minutes, this indicates that the neural pathways mediating that SEP either are not perfused by the blood vessel in question or are receiving adequate flow from collateral sources.[7]

SEPs can be used to confirm that the somatosensory pathway to the cerebral cortex is still functional, even during periods of deep anesthesia, as demonstrated by a burst-suppression pattern (as illustrated in **Fig. 11.3B**). However, further depression of cortical activity, either through still-deeper anesthesia or because of ischemia, will soon lead to the loss of even the SEP.

SEP—Strengths and Weaknesses

The SEP test procedure is relatively quick and simple to administer, and is well tolerated by most awake subjects (**Table 11.2**). It is a very good predictor of normal proprioceptive function. That is, a person with a large-amplitude and short-latency SEP is not expected to have significant sensory dysfunction. Note that the converse is not necessarily true: persons may have relatively normal sensation, yet the SEP might be poorly defined. This is because anything that interferes even slightly with nerve conduction along the pathway taken by an SEP may cause the waveforms at the scalp to be either abnormally small or absent altogether. Pre-existing problems with peripheral nerve conduction, such as diabetes or alcohol-related neuropathy, can make it difficult to obtain an SEP response from a patient, particularly after he or she has been anesthetized (anesthesia typically depresses cortical SEP response amplitudes but has less of an effect on potentials of subcortical origin). Advanced cervical myelopathy also virtually ensures that SEP responses, either from subcortical or cortical generators, will be of low amplitude or absent altogether.[8]

SEP—Risks

The risks associated with SEP monitoring are listed in **Table 11.2**.

SEP—Anesthesia

The actions of general anesthetics on EEG as described in earlier sections will also apply to SEPs. If neurologic function is normal, typical cortically recorded SEPs will persist at anesthetic concentrations just adequate to perform spinal or cranial surgery (that is, 1 MAC or MAC-equivalent), but response amplitudes will rapidly decline with even modest increases in general anesthetic levels beyond these amounts. Nitrous oxide will cause a further diminution in SEP response amplitudes, in a dose-dependent manner. Subcortical potentials are more resistant to the effects of anesthetic agents. Analgesic agents (for example, fentanyl) at typical surgical doses have little effect on SEP response properties. The intravenous agents ketamine, propofol, and etomidate are all associated with preservation of SEP responses relative to any of the halogenated agents (for example, iso/des/sevoflurane).

Brainstem Auditory Evoked Potential (BAEP)

BAEP—Spinal Generators and Signal Pathways

Brainstem auditory evoked potentials (BAEPs; also frequently referred to as brainstem auditory evoked responses) are used to monitor the function of the ear, cochlear nerve, and brainstem auditory pathways up to the level of the mesencephalon. BAEPs utilize sound stimulation to excite hair cells in the cochlea, initiating a volley of action potentials within axons of the cochlear portion of cranial nerve VIII. The signal generators for the BAEP are within the brainstem, so that the response amplitude is much smaller than that of a typical cortically recorded SEP response. Because of the short conduction distances, BAEP response latencies are extremely short, with the entire waveform complex typically ending within 10 milliseconds of the stimulus. Waveforms making up the BAEP are complex, with multiple peaks. Responses are strictly unilateral, so each ear should be tested independently.

BAEP—Vascular Considerations

As with other evoked potentials, damage to the blood supply anywhere along the pathway taken by BAEP signals can result in a reduction or complete loss of responses (**Table 11.2**).

BAEP—Methods

Sound stimuli are introduced to the ear via a foam earpiece, which is compressed and inserted into the external auditory meatus. Within this earpiece is a narrow silicon tube, the end of which lies close to the tympanic membrane. The other end of this tube is connected to a small electronic device that converts controlled electrical pulses into sound clicks that can be adjusted for intensity (typically 90 to 95 dB). This sound pressure wave perturbs the tympanic membrane, initiating the mechanical transmission that leads to activation of a relatively large proportion of hair cells in the cochlea.

Because the signal source lies deep in the brainstem, the BAEP response magnitude is only around one-tenth that of the SEP. This means that a larger number of trials need to be averaged to achieve an acceptable signal-to-noise ratio. From 1,000 to 2,000 individual trials might be averaged for a typical BAEP.

Another form of monitoring that is often used in conjunction with BAEPs is spontaneous and stimulus-evoked EMG from muscles innervated by cranial nerve VII. This combination of monitoring modalities first emerged for vestibular schwannoma resection, in efforts to preserve innervation of facial musculature.[9]

BAEP—Indications

Procedures placing the brainstem or its vascular supply at risk are obvious choices for BAEP monitoring (**Table 11.2**). Obliteration or resection of a vascular malformation within the posterior fossa is also a prime candidate for inclusion of BAEP monitoring, as is microvascular decompression of cranial nerves V and VII.[10]

BAEP—Strengths and Weaknesses

The BAEP is very reliable in persons with normal hearing. It serves as the only practical test based on evoked potential for pathways restricted to the brainstem (**Table 11.2**). For the BAEP, both waveform amplitude and response latency are very sensitive to irritation of the nerve or its blood supply (for example, from retraction of the cerebellum), and sustained deterioration in waveforms is highly predictive of postoperative hearing loss.[11]

BAEP—Risks

Compared with other tests used for IOM, the risks associated with testing of BAEPs are low (**Table 11.2**). The sound intensity typically used for a BAEP (90 to 95 dB) is approaching the limits recommended to avoid permanent hearing loss, but to our knowledge there have been no reports of hearing damage caused specifically by the sound intensity used in a typical BAEP examination. Fluid accumulation in the external auditory canal can attenuate the sound stimulus, leading to loss of the BAEP entirely. Steps to minimize fluid incursion can include placing a wad of bone-wax over the ear insert, conforming to the contours of the ear, or the more effective method of covering the ear with a waterproof skin dressing (for example, Tegaderm, 3M).

BAEP—Anesthesia

Waveforms making up the BAEP tend to be more resistant to the depressant effects of general anesthetics than those of any of the other procedures typically used for intraoperative monitoring. This is likely due to the very short conduction distances and the paucity of GABAergic inputs to the brainstem nuclei mediating the main components of the BAEP waveform,[12] so that the potentiation of the GABA receptor that is thought to be a common mechanism of most general anesthetics[2] will have less effect on the BAEP.

Visual Evoked Potential (VEP)

VEP—Synopsis

For visual evoked potential (VEP) testing, a light flash or pattern is presented to the orbit, and the resultant potentials are recorded with EEG electrodes over the occipital lobes. In patients who are awake, the cortically recorded VEP is a large, widespread potential. The fact that this signal is dominated by low-frequency components would suggest considerable divergence in the time of arrival of neuronal volleys to the visual cortex. One could therefore predict that the VEP would be especially susceptible to the effects of general anesthetics, and this is indeed the case.[13]

In theory, this test should be able to monitor activity within neural pathways extending from the retina through the optic chiasm to the lateral geniculate nucleus, and, after synapsing, then on to the primary visual cortex of the occipital lobe. Unfortunately, this test has a very spotty history in the operating room environment, with multiple studies reporting poor sensitivity (that is, too many false negatives) and specificity (that is, too many false positives), making the test unreliable.[13,14]

Our own limited experience with VEP monitoring during endovascular procedures is consistent with this conclusion. Using goggles emitting light flashes, we routinely used VEP monitoring in the endovascular suite during provocative testing of the posterior cerebral artery (PCA) in anesthetized patients prior to pedicle embolization of occipital arteriovenous malformations (AVMs). We had several false-negative VEP studies and never saw any changes when testing arteries supplying lesions behind the chiasm. Because of the near-unanimity of opinion regarding the intraoperative experience with VEP monitoring, we do not advocate use of VEP monitoring during cranial or endovascular procedures.

Motor Evoked Potential

MEP—Signal Generators and Pathways

Compared with SEP, motor evoked potential (MEP) is a much more recent test in the IOM field, only being approved by the FDA in 2002. In contrast to the SEP tests described above, MEP monitors an efferent limb (that is, a corticospinal tract) of the central nervous system (CNS). As in SEP, the stimulation in MEP is electrical in nature, but this time stimulation is applied to the region of the cerebral cortex—the primary motor cortex—that gives rise to voluntary movements. Evidence of corticospinal activity can be seen through either field potentials recorded from a spinal epidural electrode,[15] or from an electromyogram (EMG) recorded from limb muscles contralateral to the side being stimulated. MEPs from head and neck muscles innervated by cranial nerves have also been described.[16]

MEP—Vascular Considerations

The motor cortex receives its vascular supply primarily from the anterior cerebral artery (ACA) and middle cerebral artery (MCA). Vascular territories are covered in Chapter 1 and summarized in **Table 11.2**.

MEP—Methods

There are three main methods to stimulate the upper motor neurons of the motor cortex to cause MEPs: (1) electrical stimulation across the skull (transcranial electric), (2) direct electrical stimulation via epidural strip electrodes after a craniotomy, and (3) transcranial magnetic stimulation. Magnetic stimulation in the operating room environment[17] has multiple technical limitations and will not be discussed further.

Assuming the patient's corticospinal tract is normal and anesthesia conditions permit, suitable stimulation for MEP monitoring causes muscles in the patient's contralateral arms and hands to contract. The accompanying compound muscle action potential (CMAP) can be recorded by pairs of subcutaneous needle electrodes in the muscle of interest, without the need for signal averaging. This speed of acquisition represents a substantial advantage of EMG-based MEP monitoring over the SEP. In general, muscles in the hands are easiest to activate with transcranial MEP testing, while those in the legs—especially the large muscles in the thigh—require stronger stimulus intensities for recruitment.

There is considerable debate as to just what properties of the MEP signal are most important to monitor. For SEPs, a common strategy is to apply a stimulus of sufficient intensity so that further increases fail to elicit an increase in response magnitude, indicating that the stimulus is supramaximal. Most publications related to MEP monitoring have adopted a similar approach, whereby warning to the surgical team is not relayed until MEP reductions of from 50% to 100% (that is, complete loss) of the initial (baseline) response amplitude have occurred.[16] This approach requires very high stimulus intensities, leading to strong twitch contractions in muscles of the head, neck, and shoulders.

An alternative approach that we developed is to monitor the stimulus intensity needed to elicit a minimal (that is, threshold) response from a target muscle. Using this 'threshold-level' method, increases in a given muscle's threshold stimulus intensity that cannot be explained by changes in anesthesia or blood pressure have been shown to correspond to a deterioration in corticospinal tract function.[18] By definition, this approach minimizes the amount of charge delivered to the subject for a given MEP trial; therefore, this threshold-level approach minimizes the risks associated with MEP compared with the alternative, supramaximal strategy advocated by others.

We and others have found the threshold-level method to be highly sensitive to changes in corticospinal tract function.[18-20] In a direct comparison of this approach to the "presence-or-absence" method,[21] we recently showed that MEP alarm criteria based on a complete loss of the evoked response lacked sensitivity to the initial stages of corticospinal tract functional change associated with these signal changes. Since one of the goals of intraoperative monitoring is to provide early warning of impending problems, it is clear that alarm criteria based on a signal loss are not consistent with this goal.

This argument takes on even greater significance if MEPs are being used to monitor the functional integrity of corticospinal tract axons within the cranium itself. This is because strong MEP stimulus intensities activate corticospinal tract axons below the cortex (that is, within the internal capsule or brainstem), whereas threshold stimuli activate cells at the level of the cerebral cortex itself.[22] If baseline MEP responses are obtained with very strong stimuli—depolarizing axons caudal to the cerebral cortex or proximal internal capsule—then procedures that place these regions at risk will be running blind with respect to the risk of injury.[23] Only threshold stimuli, causing recruitment of CST axons within the cerebral cortex itself, should therefore be used for these types of cases.

MEP—Indications

Neurosurgical procedures around the spinal cord, ventral brainstem, internal capsule, and posterior portions of the frontal lobe can all lead to paresis. The MEP is intended to provide early warning of impending injury to these regions to lower the risk of these devastating outcomes (see **Table 11.2**).

In the brain, clipping of an aneurysm on the MCA or anterior communicating arteries (ACOM) can lead to inadvertent inclusion of one or more medial lenticulostriate arteries vital to corticospinal tract fibers passing through the internal capsule. Changes in MEPs have been reported in such procedures,[24,25] alerting the surgical team that they need to revise the clip placement. In a manner analogous to that described for EEG use during vascular malformation obliteration, MEPs can be used with sodium amobarbital or methohexital to rule out a shared arterial supply between the motor cortex and the malformation. For this test, it is essential that one avoid use of stimulus intensities beyond threshold-level values, as detailed earlier

MEP—Strengths and Weaknesses

A major strength of the transcranial MEP test is its accuracy for predicting postoperative motor status. In a large series (>800) of spine cases in which MEP findings were compared with postoperative motor function, we found sensitivity and specificity to be 1.000 and 0.997, respectively.[21] Other reports associated with cranial-based procedures show comparably high accuracy of MEPs for predicting postoperative deterioration of motor function. This is not to say that MEP monitoring is not without its drawbacks (**Table 11.2**).

MEP—Risks

The risks associated with transcranial electrical stimulation for causing MEPs are not trivial (**Table 11.2**). If EMG-based responses are being monitored, then train-based stimulation of intensity sufficient to cause evoked responses in limb muscles will typically lead to contraction of head and neck muscles, so the surgeon or proceduralist must exercise caution if an instrument is adjacent to CNS tissue.

MEP—Anesthesia

It is especially important to consider the effects of anesthesia in order to monitor MEPs successfully. Early studies utilizing single-pulse transcranial electric stimulation showed that even very low levels of halogenated agents like isoflurane—levels well below those needed to maintain surgical immobility—caused a loss of MEP responses.[26–28] This anesthetic effect was partially offset by the availability of multi-pulse stimulation, but consistently successful MEP monitoring was still possible only if halogenated agents (iso/des/sevoflurane) were avoided altogether or if their levels were maintained at or below only 50% of the concentration needed to achieve immobility (that is, 0.5 MAC).[29,30] Because even low levels of halogenated agents will cause a gradual elevation in the minimum stimulus energy needed to elicit MEPs,[31] we recommend avoidance of these agents altogether, beyond their use for induction and patient positioning. Finally, for MEP outcome measures based on muscle EMG, total neuromuscular blockade is clearly contraindicated. Partial blockade, provided the level of blockade remains relatively constant (as is possible with infusion pumps), is acceptable with the threshold-level monitoring method, but it will be problematic for outcome criteria based upon the characteristics of the evoked response itself (amplitude, complexity, duration).

Case Study: Carotid Endarterectomy

A 75-year-old male was being treated with an endarterectomy for stenosis of the right common carotid artery (CCA). We were monitoring spontaneous EEG from three sites bilaterally, sampling over the lateral central sulcus (C3/C4), the inferior temporal cortex (T3/T4), and the occipital cortex (O1/O2), with each recording lead being referenced to their respective mastoid processes (M1/M2) on the same side. We also were stimulating median and posterior tibial nerves bilaterally for upper- and lower-limb SEPs.

Fig. 11.1 illustrates multiple 10-second samples of raw (that is, unprocessed) EEG from the six recording electrodes at various times before (**Fig. 11.1A**) and after (**Fig. 11.1B–1F**) clamping the CCA. The top-most traces (**Fig. 11.1A**), sampled approximately 30 seconds before cross-clamping, show a moderately deep level of anesthesia, with near-complete recovery from burst-suppression that was in place a few minutes previously. Roughly 80 to 90 seconds after clamp placement, **Fig. 11.1B** shows a marked reduction in EEG activity across all three of the right-side leads, with the C4-M2 and T4-M2 leads (fourth and fifth from the top of this group) showing the biggest reduction in activity. Note that spontaneous activity in the left-side leads (top three traces of **Fig. 11.1B**) is little changed from pre-clamp (**Fig. 11.1A**) activity levels. Also note that the rhythmic low-frequency spike-like activity move evident in the third through fifth traces of **Fig. 11.1B** is an ECG artifact (roughly 1 per second).

Upon reporting the asymmetric change in EEG evident in **Fig. 11.1B** to the surgical team, the decision was made to deliver a bolus of sodium thiopental for neuroprotection, and this agent was delivered roughly at the time when the EEG in **Fig. 11.1C** was sampled. Note that a marked asymmetry between left-side activity (still substantial) and right-side activity (depressed) is still evident. It was also decided at this time to place a vascular shunt in the CCA to hasten restoration of blood flow, at the cost of a slightly higher risk of thromboembolic stroke.[32] At the next sample shown (**Fig. 11.1D**), there is now almost complete EEG silence, reflecting the global influence of the thiopental in depressing spontaneous activity in cortical neurons. By roughly 10 minutes post-clamping, the total suppression of EEG has diminished, as evidenced by the occasional burst of activity (center region of **Fig. 11.1E**). Shortly after flow is restored (**Fig. 11.1F**), bursts are more frequent and of longer duration, and substantial activity is now evident bilaterally. Eventually the EEG showed full recovery from burst-suppression (not shown) and was judged to be no different than what was seen prior to clamp placement. The patient awoke uneventfully, without evidence of neurologic deficit.

Figure 11.2 summarizes the findings illustrated in **Fig. 11.1** in a graphic manner, by quantifying the EEG power at each recording lead over a 20-minute period (the time axis is vertical), expressing the power at specific signal frequencies (X-axis, ranging from 1 to 20 Hz) via different colors of the visible spectrum (the darker shade being the highest power, and the lighter shade being the lowest power, as indicated by the legend inset into the 'O1-M1' record of **Fig. 11.2**). Shortly after clamp application (top-most horizontal arrows), there is a marked drop-off of EEG power under the frontal and temporal EEG leads on the right side (C4-M2 and C3-M2, respectively), with only a slight change in left-side activity. Even before thiopental is added (middle horizontal arrows), the right-side EEG is very depressed and shows little further depression with drug infusion. In contrast, left-side EEG power declines dramatically after thiopental, as illustrated in **Fig. 11.1D**. Note that the slight recovery of EEG power best seen in the C3-M1 montage around the time the clamp is removed (bottom arrows) reflects the onset of bursting in these leads.

Finally, **Fig. 11.3** shows SEP changes that were seen through this period leading up to (**Fig. 11.3A**) and following CCA clamping (**Figs. 11.3B** and **11.3C**). Both cortical (upper traces) and subcortical (lower traces) responses to median nerve stimulation are visible bilaterally and showed good reproducibility. (Note that the upper trace of each cortical and subcortical pair is the recently acquired record, whereas the lower trace of each pair is the stored baseline record. Thus the lower traces of each cortical and subcortical pair are identical across panels A, B, and C of this figure.) SEPs in response to lower-limb stimulation (not shown) could not be elicited, even at the initiation of the procedure.

Approximately three minutes after the CCA was clamped, the SEP to left median nerve stimulation as recorded over the right cortex was significantly lower in amplitude (arrow in 3B), whereas there was no significant difference in the cortical response to right-side stimulation (reflecting activity in the left cortex) or in the subcortical responses bilaterally. This shows that the effect of CCA clamping was restricted to the right cortex. **Fig. 11.1C**, obtained during the period when power in the right-side EEG was much reduced, shows the ability of SEP signals to withstand the influence of significant depression from higher levels of anesthesia. Shortly after releasing the clamp on the CCA and restoring cerebral blood flow to both hemispheres, the cortical SEP to left-side stimulation (**Fig. 11.3C**) was fully recovered, being essentially indistinguishable from that seen just prior to clamp application (**Fig. 11.3A**). Again, left-side cortical and subcortical responses to right-side median stimulation did not change in any appreciable manner at any time relative to the clamp application.

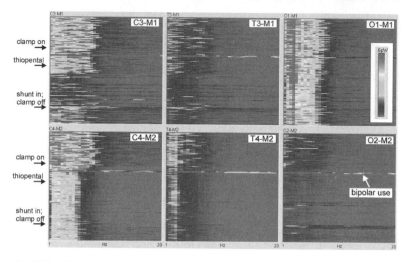

Fig. 11.2 Density spectral array (DSA) depiction of EEG activity spanning a 20-minute period prior to, during, and after removal of clamp on the common carotid artery. Activity from the same six lead pairs listed in the **Fig. 11.1** legend is shown within individual display panels, as labeled. High-power activity is depicted as dark color, whereas low-power activity appears light in color, as summarized by the legend inset in the top-right panel ('O1-M1') of this figure. Shortly after clamping the CCA, there is a marked diminution of EEG power within the right-side leads, best seen in the C4-M2 panel (bottom left; upper (of three) horizontal *arrows*). Shortly thereafter, the bipolar was used for hemostasis, resulting in a brief high-energy artifact that is evident within all six panels (*white arrow* in 'O2-M2' panel). Once sodium thiopental was given to the patient (middle horizontal *arrows*), there was a further reduction in EEG power evident in the left-side leads (since the right-side leads at C4 and T4 were already essentially silent). Once the CCA was released, EEG power showed recovery, but overall power was still diminished within the time period shown compared with pre-clamp levels.

Clinical Pearls

- Intraoperative neuromonitoring (IOM) provides information about functional neurologic status that is not otherwise available in the anesthetized patient.
- Multiple tests are available, designed to interrogate specific CNS systems perfused by nearly all the major cranial and spinal vessels.
- Many tests can be utilized in a provocative manner, so that the results of temporary vascular occlusion can be used to decide whether or not a vessel/malformation/aneurysm can be permanently occluded/obliterated.
- Close cooperation with the anesthesia team is essential for IOM success, due to the non-uniform effect of different anesthetic agents on IOM tests.
- IOM has developed into an essential adjunct for preserving neurologic function during procedures that place the CNS at risk; its use should be considered a standard of care in the modern neurosurgical and cerebro-endovascular suite.

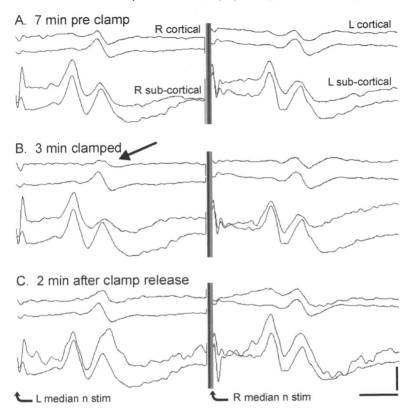

Fig. 11.3 **(A)** SEPs obtained seven minutes before and **(B)** three minutes after clamping the right-side CCA, and then again **(C)** approximately minutes after the clamp was released. Each panel shows responses to stimulation of the left-side and right-side median nerves (left- and right-hand sides of the figure), with cortical potentials (C3 or C4 referenced to Fz) above subcortical potentials (M2 referenced to Fz for both sites). Each record includes the 'active' waveform that was just recorded (that is, corresponding to the comment in the panel heading), and immediately below that waveform is the stored waveform that was collected early in the procedure, after the patient was positioned but before the incision (that is, the baseline). The records show a borderline-significant reduction of the right-side cortical potential (*arrow* in **Fig. 11.3B**) following stimulation of the left median nerve, while the subcortical potential was essentially unchanged. Responses to right-side stimulation (reflecting cortical and subcortical activity in the left brain) were not significantly different from baseline values at any time during the procedure. Horizontal bar = 10 milliseconds; vertical bar = 1.0 µV.

References

1. Penfield W. Mechanisms of voluntary movement. Brain 1954;77(1):1–17
2. Barash PG, Cullen BF, Stoelting RK, et al. *Handbook of Clinical Anesthesia*, 6th ed. Wolters Kluwer Health/Lippincott Williams & Wilkins; 2009
3. Burchiel KJ, Clarke H, Ojemann GA, Dacey RG, Winn HR. Use of stimulation mapping and corticography in the excision of arteriovenous malformations in sensorimotor and language-related neocortex. Neurosurgery 1989;24(3):322–327
4. Pasternak JJ, Lanier WL. Neuroanesthesiology update. J Neurosurg Anesthesiol 2010; 22(2):86–109
5. MacDonald DB, Al Zayed Z, Khoudeir I, Stigsby B. Monitoring scoliosis surgery with combined multiple pulse transcranial electric motor and cortical somatosensory-evoked potentials from the lower and upper extremities. Spine (Phila Pa 1976) 2003;28(2):194–203
6. Isley MR, Edmonds HL Jr, Stecker M; American Society of Neurophysiological Monitoring. Guidelines for intraoperative neuromonitoring using raw (analog or digital waveforms) and quantitative electroencephalography: a position statement by the American Society of Neurophysiological Monitoring. J Clin Monit Comput 2009;23(6):369–390
7. Keyhani K, Miller CC III, Estrera AL, Wegryn T, Sheinbaum R, Safi HJ. Analysis of motor and somatosensory evoked potentials during thoracic and thoracoabdominal aortic aneurysm repair. J Vasc Surg 2009;49(1):36–41
8. Hu Y, Ding Y, Ruan D, Wong YW, Cheung KM, Luk KD. Prognostic value of somatosensory-evoked potentials in the surgical management of cervical spondylotic myelopathy. Spine (Phila Pa 1976) 2008;33(10):E305–E310
9. Møller AR, Jannetta PJ. Preservation of facial function during removal of acoustic neuromas. Use of monopolar constant-voltage stimulation and EMG. J Neurosurg 1984;61(4):757–760
10. Legatt AD. BAEPs in Surgery. In: Nuwer MR, ed. *Intraoperative Monitoring of Neural Function*. Elsevier; 2008:334–349
11. Nakamura M, Roser F, Dormiani M, Samii M, Matthies C. Intraoperative auditory brainstem responses in patients with cerebellopontine angle meningiomas involving the inner auditory canal: analysis of the predictive value of the responses. J Neurosurg 2005;102(4):637–642
12. Glendenning KK, Baker BN. Neuroanatomical distribution of receptors for three potential inhibitory neurotransmitters in the brainstem auditory nuclei of the cat. J Comp Neurol 1988;275(2):288–308
13. Raudzens PA. Intraoperative monitoring of evoked potentials. Ann NY Acad Sci 1982;388:308–326
14. Cedzich C, Schramm J, Fahlbusch R. Are flash-evoked visual potentials useful for intraoperative monitoring of visual pathway function? Neurosurgery 1987;21(5):709–715
15. Burke D, Hicks R, Stephen J, Woodforth I, Crawford M. Assessment of corticospinal and somatosensory conduction simultaneously during scoliosis surgery. Electroencephalogr Clin Neurophysiol 1992;85(6):388–396
16. Dong CC, Macdonald DB, Akagami R, et al. Intraoperative facial motor evoked potential monitoring with transcranial electrical stimulation during skull base surgery. Clin Neurophysiol 2005;116(3):588–596
17. Edmonds HL Jr, Paloheimo MPJ, Backman MH, Johnson JR, Holt RT, Shields CB. Transcranial magnetic motor evoked potentials (tcMMEP) for functional monitoring of motor pathways during scoliosis surgery. Spine (Phila Pa 1976) 1989;14(7):683–686
18. Calancie B, Harris W, Broton JG, Alexeeva N, Green BA. "Threshold-level" multipulse transcranial electrical stimulation of motor cortex for intraoperative monitoring of spinal motor tracts: description of method and comparison to somatosensory evoked potential monitoring. J Neurosurg 1998;88(3):457–470
19. Calancie B, Harris W, Brindle GF, Green BA, Landy HJ. Threshold-level repetitive transcranial electrical stimulation for intraoperative monitoring of central motor conduction. J Neurosurg 2001;95(2, Suppl):161–168

20. Quiñones-Hinojosa A, Alam M, Lyon R, Yingling CD, Lawton MT. Transcranial motor evoked potentials during basilar artery aneurysm surgery: technique application for 30 consecutive patients. Neurosurgery 2004;54(4):916–924, discussion 924

21. Calancie B, Molano MR. Alarm criteria for motor-evoked potentials: what's wrong with the "presence-or-absence" approach? Spine (Phila Pa 1976) 2008;33(4):406–414

22. Rothwell J, Burke D, Hicks R, Stephen J, Woodforth I, Crawford M. Transcranial electrical stimulation of the motor cortex in man: further evidence for the site of activation. J Physiol 1994;481(Pt 1):243–250

23. Szelényi A, Langer D, Kothbauer K, De Camargo AB, Flamm ES, Deletis V. Monitoring of muscle motor evoked potentials during cerebral aneurysm surgery: intraoperative changes and postoperative outcome. J Neurosurg 2006;105(5):675–681

24. Neuloh G, Schramm J. Monitoring of motor evoked potentials compared with somatosensory evoked potentials and microvascular Doppler ultrasonography in cerebral aneurysm surgery. J Neurosurg 2004;100(3):389–399

25. Sasaki T, Kodama N, Matsumoto M, et al. Blood flow disturbance in perforating arteries attributable to aneurysm surgery. J Neurosurg 2007;107(1):60–67

26. Sloan TB, Heyer EJ. Anesthesia for intraoperative neurophysiologic monitoring of the spinal cord. J Clin Neurophysiol 2002;19(5):430–443

27. Calancie B, Klose KJ, Baier S, Green BA. Isoflurane-induced attenuation of motor evoked potentials caused by electrical motor cortex stimulation during surgery. J Neurosurg 1991;74(6):897–904

28. Kalkman CJ, Drummond JC, Ribberink AA. Low concentrations of isoflurane abolish motor evoked responses to transcranial electrical stimulation during nitrous oxide/opioid anesthesia in humans. Anesth Analg 1991;73(4):410–415

29. Quiñones-Hinojosa A, Lyon R, Zada G, et al. Changes in transcranial motor evoked potentials during intramedullary spinal cord tumor resection correlate with postoperative motor function. Neurosurgery 2005;56(5):982–993

30. Ubags LH, Kalkman CJ, Been HD. Influence of isoflurane on myogenic motor evoked potentials to single and multiple transcranial stimuli during nitrous oxide/opioid anesthesia. Neurosurgery 1998;43(1):90–94, discussion 94–95

31. Lyon R, Feiner J, Lieberman JA. Progressive suppression of motor evoked potentials during general anesthesia: the phenomenon of "anesthetic fade." J Neurosurg Anesthesiol 2005;17(1):13–19

32. Salvian AJ, Taylor DC, Hsiang YN, et al. Selective shunting with EEG monitoring is safer than routine shunting for carotid endarterectomy. Cardiovasc Surg 1997;5(5):481–485

Diagnostic Endovenous Procedures

Madhu B. Vijayappa and Dileep R. Yavagal

While endovascular therapies are normally associated with the treatment of vascular disease, there are a myriad of procedures that use endovascular techniques to aid in the diagnosis of various conditions. Some of the more common endovascular diagnostic procedures are discussed below.

Inferior Petrosal Sinus Sampling

Etiology

In the early 1980s, Oldfield and Doppman from the National Institutes of Health introduced bilateral inferior petrosal sinus sampling (IPSS), which is used by both neurosurgeons and endocrinologists to determine whether the potential source of aberrant hormone secretions, such as adrenocorticotropic hormone (ACTH), is the pituitary gland. This diagnostic test is indicated when imaging studies do not demonstrate an obvious pituitary mass that could be considered responsible for hormonal imbalances, such as those seen in Cushing syndrome. When no overt pituitary mass is observed, an ectopic source of ACTH secretion is often suspected, but it is challenging to differentiate between an ectopic source of ACTH and a pituitary source of ACTH clinically or using only biochemical tests. Bilateral IPSS is used to differentiate whether the ACTH causing Cushing syndrome comes from the pituitary or is ectopic in origin. It may also help localize which side of the gland is producing ACTH at abnormally high levels.

Cushing syndrome is a clinical condition that results after prolonged exposure to ACTH. Of the cases in which hypercortisolemia results from an ACTH–dependent process, approximately 80% are due to a pituitary adenoma (Cushing disease), 10% are due to adrenal lesions, and the remaining 10% are secondary to ectopic ACTH secretion. Large pituitary adenomas (>1 cm diameter) are rare and usually present with mild manifestations of Cushing's syndrome. Pituitary microadenomas (<1 cm diameter) are mainly responsible for ACTH-dependent Cushing syndrome. However, precise localization of these microadenomas is often difficult, because of their small size. Surgical removal of tumors secreting ACTH is the treatment of choice in Cushing disease, which makes finding the source of ACTH secretion paramount in the management of Cushing disease.

Diagnosis

When intracranial imaging is either negative or inconclusive for pituitary microadenomas in patients with hormonal imbalances, bilateral IPSS is a very sensitive method for differentiating between pituitary and ectopic ACTH secretion. It must be noted as well that clinically nonfunctional adenomas can occur and that the etiology of hormonal imbalances can and does occur outside the pituitary even with the presence of a pituitary mass. Inferior petrosal sinus sampling is therefore recommended in cases of Cushing syndrome in which clinical, biochemical, or imaging studies have not clearly identified either a pituitary or an ectopic origin of the ACTH production. Several noninvasive tests, such as the 48-hour high-dose dexamethasone suppression test (HDDST), are used to differentiate the sources of ACTH, but these tests have sensitivities of approximately 80%. ACTH levels from IPSS are simultaneously drawn and compared with the levels from both central catheters and the peripheral vein. As ACTH secretion is episodic and sampling can miss hormonal bursts, corticotropin-releasing hormone (CRH) is used as a stimulating agent to increase the sensitivity of the test. In patients without prior CRH use, a basal ratio of central/peripheral ACTH values of 2.0 or greater is strongly indicative of Cushing disease. After CRH administration, a central/peripheral ACTH ratio of 3.0 or greater is strongly indicative of Cushing disease. A unilateral elevation of ACTH (a ratio of interpetrosal ACTH >1.4) suggests laterality and indicates the presence of a microadenoma on the ipsilateral side. Selective venous sampling from the posterior portion of the cavernous sinus is more reliable in lateralizing ACTH-secreting pituitary adenoma. The laterality of increased ACTH can localize the microadenoma and reduce a potential procedure to one side rather than a total hypophysectomy, which would result in complete hormone dependence or panhypopituitarism.

The clinical features of a pituitary adenoma vary depending on the location, size of the tumor, and its secretory function and capability. Pituitary macroadenomas can cause headaches, double vision, loss of peripheral vision leading to blindness, facial pain, or numbness. Hypopituitarism manifests itself by lack of energy, weight loss, nausea, vomiting, constipation, amenorrhea and infertility, dry skin, increased pigmentation of the skin, cold intolerance, and mental status changes. ACTH-secreting adenomas produce Cushing disease, which itself results in moon facies, with acne and flushing, fatty deposits over the back of the neck, stretch marks, easy bruising, posterior subcapsular cataracts, arterial hypertension, aberrant hair growth, diabetes mellitus, muscle loss, fatigue, depression, and psychosis.

Visual acuity can be decreased in one or both eyes. Bitemporal superior quadrantanopsia can be seen in patients with a macroadenoma causing compression of the optic chiasm; larger adenomas can cause bitemporal hemianopsia. Optic atrophy is frequently seen on a fundus exam. Galactorrhea can be seen in patients with prolactinomas. In cases of acromegaly, which is due to excess growth hormone, patients can present with large hands and feet, coarse facial features with frontal bossing, high arched palate, and prognathism. If the disease is left untreated, patients will usually succumb to these chronic conditions.

Conventional imaging studies like CT and MRI have relatively poor sensitivity in identifying pituitary lesions.[1-3] Dynamic MRI, in which the parasellar region is imaged continuously before and after contrast administration, apparently has higher sensitivity with lower specificity for localizing microadenomas. Studies have shown that MRI has a range of sensitivity from 46% to 67% in detecting ACTH-secreting pituitary microadenoma and a range of specificity from 62% to 100%.[1,4,5] However, these imaging studies have inherent diagnostic limitations, given the potential significant incidence of asymptomatic microadenomas and difficulty in locating small ectopic sites.

Evidence-Based Medicine

Sensitivity and Specificity of Inferior Petrosal Sinus Sampling

Inferior petrosal sinus sampling is considered the gold standard for differentiating whether the source of ACTH secretion in patients with Cushing disease is ectopic of from the pututiary.[6-9] The sensitivity of inferior petrosal sampling ranges from 85% to 100% and the specificity ranges from 67% to 100% (**Table 12.1**). A hypoplastic or anomalous inferior petrosal sinus was believed to underlie the false-negative results of inferior petrosal sinus sampling. Other causes of ambiguous results include IPSS performed during a period of normal cortisol levels in patients with intermittent ectopic ACTH secretion and false-positive test results caused by CRH-secreting tumors.[10] During inferior petrosal sinus sampling, diagnostic accuracy can be increased by additional sampling of other anterior pituitary hormones, such as prolactin, for normalization of ACTH ratios. Booth et al. compared the efficacy of IPSS and the results of imaging studies for localization of pituitary tumors and demonstrated a 70% likelihood of accurate localization using inferior petrosal sinus sampling compared with 49% using imaging alone.[11-13] Selective venous sampling from the cavernous sinus is an alternative to inferior petrosal sinus sampling and is highly reliable in lateralizing the tumor location.

Preprocedural Preparation

Inferior petrosal sinus sampling is used for both localization and differential diagnosis in the face of hormonal imbalances and inconclusive imaging studies. Patients selected for IPSS usually have a sustained elevation of free cortisol in their urine (>250 µg/day) and are not on any suppressive drugs. If they are on suppressive medications, the effect of such drugs should be allowed to dissipate completely for some weeks prior to IPSS. Patients who have had a bilateral adrenalectomy are not suitable candidates for IPSS. In these cases, dexamethasone 0.5 mg every 6 hours for 2 to 10 days prior to IPSS suppresses the normal pituitary corticotrophs.

Table 12.1 Sensitivity and Specificity of IPS Sampling

Citation	# of cases	Sensitivity (%)	Specificity (%)
Oldfield et al., 1991	215	100	100
Invitti et al., 1999	85	85	100
Kaltsas et al., 1999	107	97	100
Bonelli et al., 2000	82	92	90
Tsagarakis et al., 2000	30	100	100
Colao et al., 2001	74	90	100
Swearingen et al., 2004	139	90	67
Machado et al., 2007	47	92	100
Tsagarakis et al., 2007	47	98	100

As with other angiographic procedures, NPO status should be enforced the night before, and standard moderate sedation protocols can be used. The patient should also be asked about any history of a deep venous thrombus or IVC filter placement, as this may alter the route of access. Patients should always have routine laboratory tests performed and should be asked about dye allergies and medications that may interfere with the use of contrast materials.

Equipment

Fifteen lavender-top tubes with EDTA should be labeled, numbered, and placed in an ice-water bath prior to beginning IPSS. During the procedure, each sample is drawn into a syringe and transferred into the appropriately labeled lavender-top tube. Samples should be sent to the laboratory immediately for processing, including centrifugation within 1 hour of collection.

Sheath and Catheter

Bilateral femoral venous access is normally obtained. Standard 10 cm long 6 Fr sheaths are used, but in extremely obese patients, a 23 cm long sheath may be necessary. A 5 Fr diagnostic catheter allows for an ample lumen for sampling and drug administration. Ideal catheters are custom steam-shaped Vinuela catheters, but other shapes can be used, such as the JB-1 curve, Berenstein curve, and H-1 curve. Catheters should have gradual curves, resembling a hockey stick, one with a 70 degree curve and a 1 to 2 cm distal straight portion and the other with a 45 degree curve. The 70 degree curve can be achieved using steam. Standard guidewires can be used with these catheters. Standard microcatheters and microwires can be used to access more distal sites, such as the cavernous sinus.

Technique

Both groin areas are prepared, as both femoral veins need to be catheterized. A sheath in the femoral vein provides venous access and a means for administering drugs. Multiple simultaneous inferior petrosal samplings, along with a concurrent peripheral nonselective sample, will yield the best results. Multiple samples are necessary, as the secretory nature of the tumor may be episodic. Systemic anticoagulation is maintained during the procedure with a loading bolus of heparin and a maintainence dose every hour after successful catheterization. Antiplatelets may be administered at least 30 minutes prior to the procedure. The patient's head should be in a neutral position, and fluoroscopic views are done in the AP plane. A catheter with a 70 degree angle can be used to select the innominate vein off the superior vena cava, which will lead to the proximal left subclavian and internal jugular veins. Frequently, a valve is located at the region of thoracic inlet, which may make catheterization of the internal jugular vein challenging. Repetitive prodding during the various phases of respiration with a J-curved hydrophilic-coated guidewire or an angled-tip wire usually results in successful catheterization of the internal jugular vein. In cases of extraordinary difficulty, direct catheterization of the internal jugular vein can be performed. The inferior petrosal sinus enters the jugular vein anteromedially and thus at a relatively acute angle (**Fig. 12.1**). Advancing a 5 Fr catheter into the inferior petrosal sinus can cause ve-

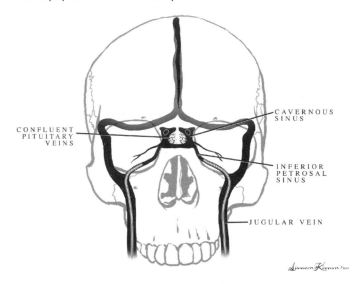

Fig. 12.1 Schematic representation of inferior petrosal sinus. (Reproduced with permission from Lad SP, Patil CG, Laws ER Jr, et al. The role of inferior petrosal sinus sampling in the diagnostic localization of Cushing's disease. Neurosurg Focus 2007;233:E2.)

nous damage or perforation. Thus, catheterization of the inferior petrosal sinus can be difficult, especially if the sinus has type C or type D drainage (**Fig. 12.2**). Warn the patient before catheterizing the sinus about the possibility of hearing strange noises in the ipsilateral ear, a side effect that is usually temporary. The catheter is rotated in the internal jugular vein so that the tip is directed medially and anteriorly. The tip is held several cm below the expected origin of the petrosal sinus, and a glide microwire (guide wire coated with hydrophilic material) is advanced until it enters the medially directed vein. Gentle injection of contrast may be made to outline the anatomy or standard roadmapping technique. A microcatheter can be advanced into the inferior petrosal sinus. If the orifice of the sinus is occluded, venous samples may be inaccurate, but slight withdrawal of the microcatheter while it is kept within the petrosal vein may allow hemodynamically normal flow and more accurate sampling. In some patients, the inferior petrosal sinus may be of small caliber, and this caliber can vary from side to side as a normal anatomical variant. If there is considerable difficulty in catheterizing one side, it is better to stop and consider catheterizing the other side. After successful catheterization of the opposite side, contrast can be used to define the anatomy. In rare cases, like type E (**Fig. 12.2**), an ipsilateral vertebral vein can be used, even though this may yield less selective results, as it is extremely difficult to catheterize the inferior petrosal sinus with this kind of drainage. The tip of the microcatheter can be advanced into the cavernous sinus after catheterizing the inferior petrosal sinus to obtain samples that aid in lateralizing the location of the tumor. Occasionally the venous anatomy can be evaluated by arterial injection.

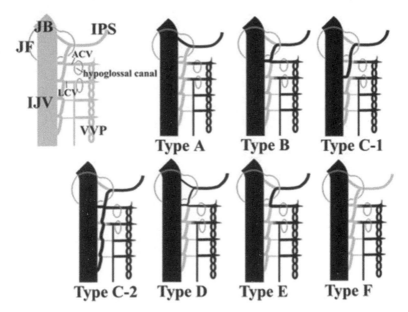

Fig. 12.2 Schematic representation of variations of junction between inferior petrosal sinus and jugular vein. JB, jugular bulb; IJV, internal jugular vein; IPS, inferior petrosal sinus; ACV, anterior condylar vein; LCV, lateral condylar vein; VVP, vertebral venous plexus. Type A, IPS drains JB; Type B, IPS drains to IJV at the level of opening of hypoglossal canal; Type C-1, IPS is a single route communicating to IJV; C-2, another upper venous route exists; Type D, IPS forms a plexus and has multiple junctions to IJV around jugular foramen; Type E, IPS drains directly to VVP with no connection to IJV; Type F, IPS absent. (Reproduced with permission from Mitsuhashi Y, Nishio A, Kawahara S, et al. Morphological evaluation of the caudal end of the inferior petrosal sinus using 3D rotational venography. AJNR 2007;28:1179-1184.)

Two sets of baseline samples are taken, and three sets of samples are obtained after CRH administration. Blood samples for ACTH assay should be obtained simultaneously from both sides of the inferior petrosal sinus and from a peripheral vein before and 3, 5, and 10 minutes after CRH 100 mg is given as a bolus injection. After drawing 2–3 mL of fluid into a waste syringe, 10 mL of blood should be drawn in a 12 mL syringe for baseline samples. Ovine CRH (Bachem, Torrance, CA) is diluted with sterile water and administered slowly at the dose of 1 µg/kg over 1 minute. It usually takes 20–40 seconds to draw a sample; a timer should be used to ensure sampling is done at 3, 5, and 10 min after the CRH administration.

Postprocedural Care

Bilateral inferior petrosal sinus sampling is a safe and reliable procedure. Postprocedural bed rest should last for 6 hours, with flat bed rest in cases closed with direct pressure. Closure devices allow patients to get up sooner. Standard groin observation should follow, including puncture site assessment every 15 minutes for one hour, then every 30 minutes for two hours, then hourly during the ICU stay, as groin hematomas are reported in 3–4% of patients. Patients should be observed for fever, tachycardia, bradycardia, hypertension (with systolic blood pressure more than 170 or less than 90), respiratory distress, acute change in neurological examinations, and urine output of less than 30 mL/hour.

Acute Neurological Change

Acute neurological change is less common in inferior petrosal sinus sampling. The risk of serious complication or death is less than 1%. If the IPS is small, catheter placement can result in ear pain or headache. Contrast injection may also provoke severe but brief headaches; narcotics can be used ease the discomfort or pain. As venous drainage from the pons and brainstem can be directly or indirectly into the inferior petrosal sinus and/or the basilar venous plexus, care should be taken while performing IPSS to avoid any devastating neurological deficits. Patients have been reported to develop jumping vision, unsteadiness, nausea, vomiting, difficulty swallowing, and diplopia.[14,15] Venous subarachnoid hemorrhage has also been reported.[16]

Alternative Therapies

Jugular venous sampling with CRH administration can be used as an alternative to bilateral inferior petrosal sinus sampling in patients with abnormal anatomy. The catheter should be placed at the angle of the mandible, below the petrosal sinus inflow, and blood samples collected before and after administration of CRH.

Technical Pearls

- An adequate dose of heparin should be used to avoid clotting issues.
- The injection of contrast material into the inferior petrosal sinus and surrounding veins should be performed gently.
- Images should be obtained to document the catheter position.
- It is important to demonstrate reflux of contrast material into the ipsilateral cavernous sinus for adequate sampling. If there is no reflux, pituitary effluent will not be adequately reflected in the sample, leading to false lateralization or incorrect diagnosis.

Transvenous Manometry

Recent advances in neuroradiology have demonstrated many causes of venous hypertension resulting in idiopathic intracranial hypertension (IIH). With a number of causes, including paranasal sinus infection, mastoid infection, hypercoaguable states like lupus, leukemia, and postpartum, and obstruction by tumors, venous sinus thrombosis can lead to venous outflow obstruction and reduced CSF absorption.[17] Similarly, a dural arteriovenous fistula draining into the transverse sinus can lead to venous hypertension.[18] Cerebral venography and transvenous manometry are endovascular diagnostic procedures that can objectively measure venous hypertension in patients with idiopathic intracranial hypertension.

Etiology

Idiopathic intracranial hypertension, also known as pseudotumor cerebri, is a syndrome of raised intracranial pressure and normal CSF constituents, without any overt abnormal radiographic findings. It most commonly affects obese women of childbearing age but can also affect all other groups, including men, non-obese females, and children. This condition may be caused by structural or functional obstruction to venous outflow. Intracranial hypertension has been associated with a range of systemic conditions, including hypoparathyroidism, iron deficiency anemia, renal disease, corticosteroid withdrawal, and the use of medications like vitamin A, tetracyclines, lithium, nitrofurantoin, and nalidixic acid.[19]

Diagnosis

The most common clinical presentation of patients with IIH is nausea, vomiting, headaches, visual changes, tinnitus, and occasional abducens nerve palsy.[19] Although IIH is often associated with obesity, many patients may not appear to have any ominous signs on gross physical exam. A physical exam may demonstrate dilated scalp veins. On funduscopic examination, patients will often have papilledema, which can be associated with other ocular abnormalities, including visual field defects and extraocular cranial nerve palsies. These patients often have a normal mental status without neuropsychological or cognitive deficits. However, psychological conditions have been associated with IIH but not in a causal fashion. For some pseudotumor cerebri patients, it has been reported that weight reduction improves their outcome.[20]

While it is frequently negative in finding obvious causes of intracranial hypertension, imaging plays an important role in ruling out any tumor causing obstruction of any of the major sinuses, compressing the optic apparatus, or producing other causes of intracranial hypertension. MR angiography and venography can also be performed to evaluate for any arteriovenous fistulae or sinus thromboses.

Preprocedural Preparation

As with other angiographic procedures, NPO status should be enforced the night before, and standard moderate sedation protocols can be used. The patient should also be asked about any history of a deep venous thrombosis or IVC filter placement, as this may alter the route of access. Patients should always have routine laboratory tests performed and be asked about dye allergies and medications that may interfere with the use of contrast materials.

Equipment

- The femoral vein access is obtained through standard micropuncture access techniques. A 5 Fr sheath is normally used for femoral vein access.
- Venous navigation can be done with standard 0.035 inch J-shaped guidewires and standard diagnostic catheters, for example, a 5 Fr headhunter catheter.
- Standard microcatheters and microwires can be used with fluoroscopically guided roadmapping techniques for access in small-caliber and difficult venous branches.

Technique

Intravenous pressure measurements can be assessed with a transducer connected to a microcatheter. Systemic anticoagulation is maintained during the procedure with an initial heparin bolus followed by a maintainence dose every hour after successful catheterization. The normal central venous pressure ranges measured at the right atrium are usually 0–4 mm Hg in patients in the supine position. Superior sagittal sinus pressures in adults are normally 4–10 mm Hg, depending on the position of the head.[21-23] In patients with idiopathic intracranial hypertension, superior sagittal sinus pressure can range from 13 to 24 mm Hg. If a thrombus is seen in the sinus, the microcatheter can be used to thrombolyse the clot, chemically or mechanically, as necessary. If there is stenosis, a self-expanding intracranial stent can be placed (please refer to the chapter on stenting). Balloon angioplasty is not recommended, due to the elastic recoil of the sinus wall after the procedure.

Technical Pearls

1. An adequate dose of heparin should be used to avoid clotting issues.
2. Venous valves always hinder navigation to the jugular veins. Patience, variable catheter positions, and varying wire tip trajectories are the key to getting past the valves, especially the left side, normally located just to the left of the left pedicles in the anteroposterior (AP) plane.
3. All catheters should be kept ipsilateral to the IPS being sampled so as to not confuse the samples.
4. Two wires with different shapes can be used to access the IPS, one with a wide bend and an up-going tip to catheterize the initial junction of the IPS and then one with a small curve to navigate through the IPS channels.
5. Injection of contrast material into the inferior petrosal sinus and surrounding veins should be performed gently.
6. Images should be obtained to document the catheter position.
7. It is important to demonstrate reflux of contrast material into the ipsilateral cavernous sinus for adequate sampling. If there is no reflux, pituitary effluent will not be adequately reflected in the sample, potentially leading to false lateralization or incorrect diagnosis.

References

1. Graham KESM, Samuels MH, Nesbit GM, et al. Cavernous sinus sampling is highly accurate in distinguishing Cushing's disease from the ectopic adrenocorticotropin syndrome and in predicting intrapituitary tumor location. J Clin Endocrinol Metab 1999;84(5):1602–1610
2. Escourolle H, Abecassis JP, Bertagna X, et al. Comparison of computerized tomography and magnetic resonance imaging for the examination of the pituitary gland in patients with Cushing's disease. Clin Endocrinol (Oxf) 1993;39(3):307–313
3. Kaltsas GA, Giannulis MG, Newell-Price JD, et al. A critical analysis of the value of simultaneous inferior petrosal sinus sampling in Cushing's disease and the occult ectopic adrenocorticotropin syndrome. J Clin Endocrinol Metab 1999;84(2):487–492
4. Tabarin ALF, Laurent F, Catargi B, et al. Comparative evaluation of conventional and dynamic magnetic resonance imaging of the pituitary gland for the diagnosis of Cushing's disease. Clin Endocrinol (Oxf) 1998;49(3):293–300
5. Kaltsas GGM, Giannulis GDC, Newell-Price JDC, et al. A critical analysis of the value of simultaneous inferior petrosal sinus sampling in Cushing's disease and the occult ectopic adrenocorticotropin syndrome. J Clin Endocrinol Metab 1999;84:440–448
6. Findling JWKM, Kehoe ME, Shaker JL, Raff H. Routine inferior petrosal sinus sampling in the differential diagnosis of adrenocorticotropin (ACTH)-dependent Cushing's syndrome: early recognition of the occult ectopic ACTH syndrome. J Clin Endocrinol Metab 1991;73(2):408–413
7. Ilias ITD, Torpy DJ, Pacak K, Mullen N, Wesley RA, Nieman LK. Cushing's syndrome due to ectopic corticotropin secretion: twenty years' experience at the National Institutes of Health. J Clin Endocrinol Metab 2005;90(8):4955–4962
8. Isidori AMKG, Kaltsas GA, Pozza C, et al. The ectopic adrenocorticotropin syndrome: clinical features, diagnosis, management, and long-term follow-up. J Clin Endocrinol Metab 2006;91(2):371–377
9. Oldfield EHDJ, Doppman JL. Petrosal versus cavernous sinus sampling. J Neurosurg 1998;89(5):890–893
10. Young J, Deneux C, Grino M, Oliver C, Chanson P, Schaison G. Pitfall of petrosal sinus sampling in a Cushing's syndrome secondary to ectopic adrenocorticotropin-corticotropin releasing hormone (ACTH-CRH) secretion. J Clin Endocrinol Metab 1998;83(2): 305–308
11. Booth GLRD, Redelmeier DA, Grosman H, Kovacs K, Smyth HS, Ezzat S. Improved diagnostic accuracy of inferior petrosal sinus sampling over imaging for localizing pituitary pathology in patients with Cushing's disease. J Clin Endocrinol Metab 1998;83(7): 2291–2295
12. Doppman JL. There is no simple answer to a rare complication of inferior petrosal sinus sampling. AJNR Am J Neuroradiol 1999;20(2):191–192
13. Oldfield EH, Chrousos GP, Schulte HM, et al. Preoperative lateralization of ACTH-secreting pituitary microadenomas by bilateral and simultaneous inferior petrosal venous sinus sampling. N Engl J Med 1985;312(2):100–103
14. Seyer HHJ, Honegger J, Schott W, et al. Raymond's syndrome following petrosal sinus sampling. Acta Neurochir (Wien) 1994;131(1-2):157–159
15. Lefournier VGB, Gatta B, Martinie M, et al. One transient neurological complication (sixth nerve palsy) in 166 consecutive inferior petrosal sinus samplings for the etiological diagnosis of Cushing's syndrome. J Clin Endocrinol Metab 1999;84(9):3401–3402
16. Bonelli FS, Huston J III, Meyer FB, Carpenter PC. Venous subarachnoid hemorrhage after inferior petrosal sinus sampling for adrenocorticotropic hormone. AJNR Am J Neuroradiol 1999;20(2):306–307
17. Giuseffi V, Wall M, Siegel PZ, Rojas PB. Symptoms and disease associations in idiopathic intracranial hypertension (pseudotumor cerebri): a case-control study. Neurology 1991;41(2 [Pt 1]):239–244

18. Ray BSDH. Thrombosis of the dural venous sinuses as a cause of "pseudotumor cerebri." Ann Surg 1951;134:367–386

19. Wall M. Idiopathic intracranial hypertension. Semin Ophthalmol 1995;10(3):251–259

20. Rowe FJSN, Sarkies NJ. The relationship between obesity and idiopathic intracranial hypertension. Int J Obes Relat Metab Disord 1999;23(1):54–59

21. Iwabuchi TSE, Sobata E, Suzuki M, Suzuki S, Yamashita M. Dural sinus pressure as related to neurosurgical positions. Neurosurgery 1983;12(2):203–207

22. Ross JJ. *Dynamics of the Peripheral Circulation: Determination of the Venous Pressure,* 11th ed. Baltimore: Williams & Wilkins; 1985

23. Ekstedt J. CSF hydrodynamics studies in man: normal hydrodynamic variables related to CSF pressure and flow. J Neurol Neurosurg Psychiatry 1978;41:345–353

III

Treatment of Specific Disease Entities

Management of Cerebral Aneurysms

Eric M. Deshaies

Etiology

Cerebral aneurysms can occur at any age but are most common in the adult population and more common in females. Aneurysmal rupture occurs most commonly in the fifth decade and has an incidence of approximately 10 in 100,000 persons per year (approximately 27,000 individuals per year in the United States). Cerebral aneurysms arise most commonly in the anterior cerebral circulation. The formation, growth, and rupture of cerebral aneurysms are thought to be caused by multiple factors (**Table 13.1**), including environmental factors such as smoking and chemical stimulants (for example, cocaine), genetic predisposition and susceptibility factors, family history of aneurysm, systemic medical comorbidities (such as hypertension or hyperlipidemia), and collagen vascular disease, such as Marfan syndrome, adult polycystic kidney disease, and Loeys-Dietz syndrome.

Diagnosis

Unruptured cerebral aneurysms are frequently identified incidentally during an evaluation for chronic headaches, ill-defined neurological disorders, tumor, and trauma. Ruptured aneurysms often present with an acute onset of headache, meningismus, photophobia, and in severe cases, coma and death (**Fig. 13.1**, **Table 13.2**). Up to 30% of ruptured aneurysm patients are found to have complained of a headache days before, which may have been from a "sentinel" hemorrhage.

Evidence-Based Medicine

There has been a paucity of well-designed clinical studies that have examined cerebral aneurysms, both from a natural history and a treatment perspective. The following reports are the best currently available studies from the literature that examine both the natural history of unruptured aneurysms as well as some differences between microsurgical and endovascular management of cerebral aneurysms.

Table 13.1   Risk Factors for Aneurysm Formation

Smoking
Hypertension
Atherosclerosis
Connective tissue disorders
Alcohol
Hemodynamic stresses
Illicit drugs
Genetics/family history

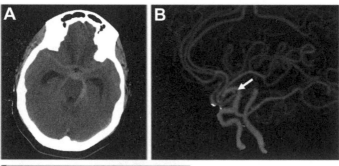

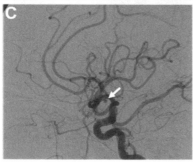

Fig. 13.1 Aneurysmal subarachnoid hemorrhage. **(A)** Admission head CT of a patient with sudden-onset headache, nausea, and vomiting demonstrating diffuse, thick subarachnoid hemorrhage, most prominent on the left, with hydrocephalus. **(B)** CT angiogram and **(C)** catheter angiogram demonstrating a small MCA aneurysm (*arrows*).

The International Study of Unruptured Intracranial Aneurysms-1 (ISUIA-1)[1]

Purpose

The International Study of Unruptured Intracranial Aneurysms-1 (ISUIA-1) was designed to establish the natural history of unruptured intracranial aneurysms (retrospective arm) and the risk of surgical clip ligation (prospective arm). There were two groups within each study arm: one (Group 1) had no history of previous subarachnoid hemorrhage (SAH) and the other (Group 2) did have a history of previous SAH from another aneurysm.

Table 13.2 Grading Scales for Patients with SAH: WFNS and Hunt & Hess

WFNS*	H&H*	GCS score	Motor deficit	Clinical description
I	I	15	Absent	Asymptomatic, mild headache or slight nuchal rigidity
II	II	13–14	Absent	Moderate to severe headache, nuhcal rigidity and no other neurological deficit except cranial nerve palsy
II	III	13–14	Present	Drowsiness, confusion, or mild focal deficit
III	IV	7–12	Present or absent	Stupor, moderate to severe hemiparesis, and possibly early decerebrate rigidity and vegetative disturbances
IV	V	3–6	Present or absent	Deep coma, decerebrate rigidity, and moribund appearance

*The World Federation of Neurosurgical Societies (WFNS) grade utilizes the combination of GCS score and motor deficit, while the Hunt and Hess (H&H) grade utilizes only the clinical description.

Eligibility

The inclusion criteria selected patients from the United States, Europe, and Canada with unruptured aneurysms and those with a history of SAH from another aneurysm, who presented with headache (HA), central nervous (CN) palsy, stroke, ill-defined spells, mass effect, seizure, brain tumor, or degenerative central nervous system (CNS) disease. Exclusion criteria included fusiform, mycotic, or traumatic aneurysms, aneurysms less than or equal to 2 mm, SAH or intracranial hemorrhage (ICH), no consent to follow-up, or malignant brain tumor.

Results

The average aneurysm size was 10.9 mm (Group 1) and 5.7 mm (Group 2). The rupture risk was predicted by location (for both Group 1 and Group 2) and size (Group 1). A higher rupture risk was observed for larger (**Table 13.3**), posterior circulation (**Table 13.4**) aneurysms and for older age (RR = 1.31).

Criticisms

(1) Posterior communicating artery (PCOM) aneurysms were categorized as "posterior circulation" despite originating from the internal carotid artery (ICA), (2) surgical morbidity and mortality were greater than that previously reported (**Table 13.5**), and (3) the average size of aneurysms in Group 1 was almost twice that of Group 2.

Table 13.3 ISUIA-1: Aneurysm Size and Annual Rupture Risk

	Annual rupture risk	
Aneurysm size (mm)	Group 1	Group 2
2–10	0.05	0.5
10–24	<1	<1
25	6	—

Table 13.4 ISUIA-1: Relative Risk of Aneurysm Rupture, Based on Location

| | Annual rupture risk | |
Location	Group 1	Group 2
Basilar tip	13.8	5.1
Vertebrobasilar artery	13.6	—
Posterior communicating artery	8	—

Table 13.5 ISUIA-1: Surgical Morbidity and Mortality

| | Annual rupture risk | |
Time after surgery	Group 1	Group 2
30 days	17.5%	13.6%
1 year	15.7%	13.1%

The International Study of Unruptured Intracranial Aneurysms-2 (ISUIA-2)[2]

Purpose

The International Study of Unruptured Intracranial Aneurysms-2 (ISUIA-2) was a prospectively randomized trial designed to assess further the natural history of unruptured intracranial aneurysms and to compare outcomes of surgical and endovascular repair. Enrolled patients were randomized to one of three study arms: (1) prospective observational, (2) surgical clip ligation, and (3) endovascular repair.

Eligibility

The criteria for ISUIA-2 were the same as those for ISUIA-1.

Results

There was increased rupture risk for larger and posterior circulation aneurysms (including PCOM) (**Table 13.6**), and those less than 7 mm with a previous SAH from another aneurysm (**Table 13.7**). Patient age greater than or equal to 50 years, posterior circulation, and aneurysm size greater than or equal to 12 mm were predictors of poor surgical outcome. Complete aneurysm obliteration rates were 55% for the endovascular arm (**Table 13.8**) and 264 aneurysms required additional treatments.

Criticisms

(1) Aneurysms less than 7 mm are reported as having a 0% rupture risk, which is misleading given that most ruptured aneurysms are between 6 and 9 mm; (2) morbidity and mortality were higher for surgical treatment, but the cumulative risk of subsequent procedures for failed initial treatment is not discussed.

Table 13.6 ISUIA-2: 5-year Aneurysm Rupture Risk

	Annual rupture risk	
Size (mm)	Anterior circulation	Posterior circulation
2–7	0	2.6
7–12	2.6	14.5
13–24	14.5	18.4
³25	40	50

Table 13.7 ISUIA-2: 5-year Aneurysm Rupture Risk for Aneurysms <7 mm with History of SAH from Another Aneurysm

	Annual rupture risk	
	No SAH history	SAH history
Anterior	0	1.5
Posterior	2.6	3.4

Table 13.8 ISUIA-2: Endovascular Aneurysm Obliteration Rates

Obliteration type	Percent
Complete	55
Incomplete	24
No obliteration	18

The International Subarachnoid Aneurysm Trial (ISAT)[2]

Purpose

The International Subarachnoid Aneurysm Trial (ISAT) was a prospectively randomized multicenter clinical trial designed to evaluate the safety and efficacy of coil embolization versus surgical clip ligation for ruptured aneurysms.

Eligibility

Patients with ruptured intracranial aneurysms eligible for either treatment modality were randomized to the surgical or endovascular arm. Those deemed better treated with surgery or coiling were not randomized in this study.

Results

There was a 22.6% RRR (6.8% ARR) at one year in dependency and death after endovascular treatment. A second treatment was required for 136 endovascular and 34 surgical patients; a majority underwent a second treatment using the other modality (**Table 13.9**). There was statistically no difference in rebleed rates between the two groups, using an intent-to-treat analysis (**Table 13.10A**).

Table 13.9   ISAT: Retreatment after Initial Allocated Treatment

Initial allocation	Number of retreatments	Retreatment allocation	
		Endovascular	Neurosurgery
Endovascular	136	53	83
Neurosurgery	34	30	4

Table 13.10   ISAT: Number of Rebleeds Using (A) an Intent-to-Treat Analysis and (B) Excluding Those Who Rebled While Waiting for Treatment

A		
Timing of rehemorrhage	**Endovascular**	**Neurosurgery**
Before first procedure	14	23
<30 days after procedure	20	6
30 days–1 year	6	4
>1 year	2	0
TOTAL	42	33

B		
Before first procedure	Excluded	Excluded
<30 days after procedure	20	6
30 days–1 year	6	4
>1 year	2	0
TOTAL	28	10

Criticisms

(1) Only 25% of the patients met inclusion criteria for randomization; (2) 93% of aneurysms were less than or equal to 10 mm; (3) 89% were WFNS 1 (63%) or 2 (26%); (4) location was heavily weighted toward the anterior communicating artery (ACOM) and PCOM, limiting generalization of the results to other aneurysm locations (**Table 13.11**); (5) the number of basilar bifurcation aneurysms was small, suggesting that they were likely better treated with endovascular therapy; and (6) when the number of patients who bled again while waiting for treatment are removed, rebleed rates were actually higher for the endovascular group (**Table 13.10B**).

Table 13.11 ISAT Distribution of Aneurysm Location

ACOM	973
PCOM	536
MCA	257
BA	17

Abbreviations: ACOM, anterior communicating artery; BA, basilar artery; MCA, middle cerebral artery; PCOM, posterior communicating artery.

Preprocedural Preparation

Unruptured Aneurysms

During preparations for endovascular treatment of an unruptured aneurysm, conditions that predispose the patient to procedural risks must be elicited from the patient (Chapter 6). Pretreatment with antiplatelet agents, required when using vascular reconstruction devices (stents), must also be considered.

Ruptured Aneurysms

In addition to those preparations defined for unruptured aneurysms, aneurysmal SAH patients require additional preparation prior to endovascular treatment. The SAH patient is generally ill and neurologically impaired. Rerupture rates are typically 4% over the first 24 hours, 20% over two weeks, 50% over six months, and then 3% annually. Rerupture is generally lethal. Initial assessment of SAH patients should be done expeditiously (**Table 13.12**).

Equipment Check List

The nuances of the equipment and techniques can be found elsewhere in this handbook (Chapters 7 and 8). Here we will describe only those details pertinent to aneurysm coiling.

Table 13.12 ABCVs of SAH: Recommendations for Preprocedural Preparation

Assessment	Result	Action
Airway	Unable to protect airway, GCS£8	Intubation
Breathing	Required intubation	Mechanical ventilation (pCO$_2$ 35–45)
Circulation	Hypertension, cardiac ischemia, arrhythmia	Normotensive (SBP 90–130), cardiac enzymes
Ventricles	Hydrocephalus	EVD at 15 cm, ICP <20 cm H$_2$O

Sheath and Guide Catheter

A 6 Fr sheath is standard because it will allow for a 6 Fr guide catheter, which is the smallest diameter that can accommodate the multiple microcatheters needed for balloon-assisted coiling or stent-assisted coiling and still allow for continuous flush and contrast injections during the procedure.

Glide Wire

Generally, angled glide wires will allow catheterization of the internal carotid artery (ICA) and vertebral arteries (VAs). Shapeable or stiff glide wires may be preferred depending on the anatomy (Chapter 7).

Microcatheter

Selection of the microcatheter depends on the size of the aneurysm neck and dome, coil choice, proximal vessel tortuosity, and user preference. (See Chapters 7 and 8 for detailed information.)

Microwire

A softer microwire is safer for accessing smaller aneurysms but less stable. (See Chapters 7 and 8.)

Coils

Different coil shapes, sizes, and coatings have been developed to reduce aneurysm recurrence rates. Coils shapes are divided into complex 3D (framing coils) and 2D helical (filling coils). Coil properties can be divided into bare platinum and bioactive coils, and liquid embolic agents (Onyx-500, see Chapters 7 and 8). Choice depends on size of the aneurysm and the preference of the physician.

Stents

Intracranial stents, also known as vascular reconstruction devices, are available in different diameters, lengths, and stent cell design, that is, open-cell or closed-cell design. Stents can be used either to hold the coils in place or to be stand-alone devices for flow diversion techniques.

Technique

Anesthesia

Aneurysm coil embolization can be performed under either conscious sedation or general anesthesia.

Conscious Sedation

An advantage of sedation is that in patients with comorbidities that preclude general endotracheal intubation, neurological exams can be followed during the procedure. The disadvantages include motion artifacts; in addition, sedation is not well tolerated by confused or uncooperative patients.

General Anesthesia

Advantages of general anesthesia include better control of patient blood pressure and oxygenation, along with less motion artifact. The disadvantages include the patient's inability to follow a neurological exam and systemic hypotension.

Coil Embolization Procedure

Vessel Engagement

After sterilization of the puncture site and the attainment of vascular access (Chapter 6), the vessel of interest is engaged with a guide catheter attached to a continuous heparinized saline flush (1 unit heparin/cc). For unruptured aneurysms, an intravenous heparin (70–100 U/kg) bolus can be given after the sheath is inserted and activated coagulation time (ACTs) checked every 20 min (goal ACT = 200–250) to reduce the risk of thromboembolic complications. In ruptured aneurysm cases, heparinization can be held until after the first coil is placed to prevent rebleeding. A baseline CBA of the cervical and intracranial circulation can be evaluated for stenosis, spasm, dissection, and emboli, as well as be used to obtain aneurysm measurements. Hemodynamically significant stenosis or spasm may need to be treated before advancing a guide catheter past the lesion.

Stent-Assisted and Balloon-Assisted Coiling

Both stent-assisted and balloon-assisted coiling can prevent the coil mass from herniating into the parent artery.

- Stent-Assisted Coiling: There are two techniques: (1) A stent is deployed across the aneurysm neck, then the dome is accessed with a microcatheter through the stent tines or (2) the two-microcatheter technique, or "jailing technique," is performed, in which a stent is deployed across the aneurysm neck after the first microcatheter has been placed in the aneurysm; this effectively jails the first microcatheter between the stent and the arterial wall so that access to the aneurysm is not lost after stent placement (**Fig. 13.2A**). "Y" stenting for wide-necked bifurcation aneurysms (middle cerebral artery, MCA, and basilar artery, BA) requires two stents placed in the proximal parent artery extending into each distal arterial branch (**Fig. 13.3**). An advantage of this stent placement is that the stent serves as a permanent buttress for the coil mass. Disadvantages include long-term use of antiplatelet agents and delayed in-stent stenosis.
- Balloon-Assisted: Here, the "jailing technique" is performed by inflating a balloon across the aneurysm neck rather than placing a stent. The tech-

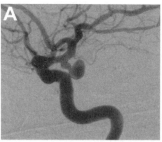
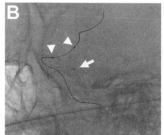

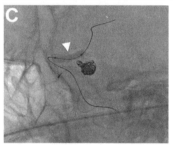

Fig. 13.2   Microcatheter "jailing" technique. **(A)** Lateral injection of a left internal carotid artery demonstrating a complex posterior carotid wall aneurysm. **(B)** Radiopaque markers on balloon catheter (*arrowheads*) placed over the neck of the aneurysm, within which is another microcatheter (*arrow*). **(C)** Inflation of the balloon (*arrowhead*) and subsequent coiling of the aneurysm. Given the difficulty of catheterization, the balloon is used in this case to keep the microcatheter from kicking back into the parent artery.

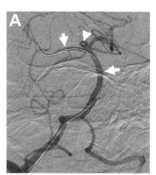
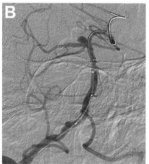

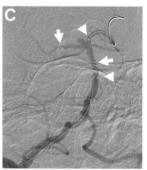

Fig. 13.3   Y-stenting technique for aneurysms located at branching or bifurcating segments. **(A)** A microcatheter has been placed in the basilar apex aneurysm (*arrowhead*). A microwire was placed in the distal right PCA where a stent was deployed; tines are marked by the *arrows*. **(B)** Another microwire is carefully navigated into the distal left PCA through the stent. **(C)** The second stent is deployed, tines marked by the *arrowheads*, while the original stent remains in place, tines marked by *arrows*.

nique is similar to that described above (**Fig. 13.2B**). Advantages of balloon assistance are that this technique avoids the long-term use of antiplatelet agents and in-stent stenosis. The disadvantages are serial balloon deflations to minimize ischemia time and risk of vessel rupture during each inflation.

Aneurysm Microcatheterization

Microcatheter and microwire choices are based on parent vessel tortuosity, aneurysm dome and neck size, and the physician's preference (Chapter 6). There are two approaches to catheterizing an aneurysm: direct and indirect.

- Direct: The microwire is advanced directly into the aneurysm, and the microcatheter is advanced over it. This technique is riskier for smaller aneurysms, because the microcatheter can jump forward if there is significant forward tension and rupture the aneurysm dome. This forward tension is more commonly encountered in tortuous vessels.
- Indirect: The microwire and microcatheter are advanced into the distal parent artery, past the aneurysm, then pulled back toward the neck so any excess forward tension can be removed from the system before direct entry into the aneurysm. This approach is safer for smaller aneurysms and those arising from proximal tortuous parent arteries.

Aneurysm Coiling

- Three-D framing coils are generally used to frame the aneurysm. Typically the diameter of the first coil matches that of the aneurysm dome or is slightly undersized for ruptured aneurysms to lower the risk of the aneurysm rebleeding when the coil is deployed. If the aneurysm is oval, then the average of the length and width can be a good starting coil diameter. Once the aneurysm is framed, 2D filling coils can be used to complete the coil nest to occlude the aneurysm.
- "Onion-skinning" is a technique in which the framing coil loop is the largest, with subsequent filling coils being serially down-sized in loop size and coil length.
- Angiography before detaching each coil assesses its position, the residual size of the aneurysm, herniation into the parent artery, contrast extravasation suggestive of rupture, and thromboembolic events.
- The goal is to insert coils until either no contrast fills the aneurysm or the microcatheter is pushed out by the coils and cannot be re-accessed.
- A completion angiogram can evaluate aneurysm filling, distal emboli, vessel occlusions, and coil herniation.

Onyx HD-500 Embolization

Onyx HD-500 (ev3, Plymouth, MN) embolization is used for wide-necked very large and giant aneurysms. Balloon-assisted injection of Onyx 500 is used to form a "kernel" initially on the microcatheter tip, then by a slow injection of the glue, the "kernel" expands and the glue fills the aneurysm. Special training in the use of Onyx 500 must be obtained, because it acts differently than the Onyx 18 and 34 used for arteriovenous malformation (AVM) embolization.

Flow-Diverting Stents

Flow-diverting stents, such as the Pipeline (Chestnut Medical Technologies, CA), are among the newest technologies for aneurysm embolization. There have been mixed results with their use, ranging from successful embolization of wide-necked and giant aneurysms to post-stenting aneurysm rupture from increased intra-aneurysmal luminal pressures. Additionally, there have been reports of perforator thrombosis after treatment. Further investigations are needed to determine the safety and efficacy of flow-diverting stents.

Grading Angiographic Embolization Results

Raymond Roy Occlusion Classification System

The Raymond Roy Occlusion Classification system (RROC) angiographically grades aneurysm occlusion after embolization.[3] See **Table 13.13** for information on this system.

Aneurysm Embolization Grade (AEG)

The aneurysm embolization grade (AEG) is an angiographic grading scale that predicts the rate of recurrence, based on aneurysm filling characteristics.[4] See **Table 13.14** for further information.

Removing the Catheter Systems

Once the microcatheter (MC) has been removed and the guide catheter has been pulled back into the proximal ICA or VA, a CBA through the guide catheter can evaluate the vessels for dissection and spasm.

Table 13.13   Raymond-Roy Occlusion Classification

RROC	Occlusion type
1	No filling of neck or dome
2	No filling of neck, dome fills
3	Filling of neck and dome

Table 13.14   Aneurysm Embolization Grade (AEG)

AEG	Angiographic results	Predicted angiographic stability
A	No filling of aneurysm neck or dome	Stable
B	Contrast stasis in neck, no filling of dome	Stable or improve
C	Contrast stasis in neck and dome	Stable or improve
D	Contrast flow in neck, no filling of dome	Worsen
E	Contrast flow in neck and dome	Worsen

Postprocedural Care

Unruptured Aneurysms

In circumstances where there were no technical complications or adverse anesthesia events during coil embolization of an unruptured aneurysm, postprocedural care is typically straightforward, characterized by an overnight hospital stay and basic postprocedural care (**Table 13.15**).

Acute Neurological Change

In cases of acute neurological change, consider the possibility of a thromboembolic event, acute hemorrhage, or arterial dissection; consider emergent cerebral angiography and intervention if a head CT does not show acute hemorrhage.

Post-Coiling Headaches

In the absence of SAH or hydrocephalus, post-coiling headaches can be due to coil mass effect, cerebral edema, or chemical meningitis. Anecdotally, we have found that Decadron 4 mg by mouth or intravenously every six hours effectively alleviates these headaches.

Arteriotomy Site Complications

Arteriotomy site complications are discussed in Chapters 6 and 10.

Laboratory Studies

Laboratory studies are discussed in Chapter 9.

Antiplatelet Agents

Antiplatelet agents are discussed in Chapter 4.

Table 13.15 Postprocedural Recommendations for Unruptured Aneurysms

1. Admission to a neuroscience observation unit.
2. Hourly neurological exams, vital signs, and arteriotomy site checks.
3. Keep access site immobilized.
4. Monitor fluid balance (I's/O's).
5. Resume diet.
6. Adequate hydration to improve renal clearance of the dye load.
7. Check hematocrit and creatinine level next day.
8. Medication recommendations: Consider aspirin 325 mg and Plavix 75 mg orally daily, depending on the use of a stent and the degree of coil-to-artery interface.

Table 13.16 Suggested Schedule for Follow-Up Imaging

Time from coiling (months)	3	9	15	24	36	48	60

Outpatient Follow-Up Imaging

Consider cerebral angiography or nagnetic resonance angiography (MRA) as more useful imaging studies for following coiled aneurysms for recurrence because of less metal artifact than computed tomography angiography (CTA). Suspicion for recurrence on MRA should be further evaluated with CBA. The risk of rupture with residual aneurysm filling after coil embolization is unclear, but based on post-clipping data, it is approximately 0.4% annually. Guidelines have not been established for follow-up imaging schedules, but suggestions are listed in **Table 13.16**. During this 5-year follow-up evaluation with MRA or cerebral angiography, recurrences should be considered for retreatment, either with coil re-embolization, combined stent-coil, or surgical clip ligation.

Ruptured Aneurysms

A detailed discussion of ICU management for SAH is beyond the scope of this handbook, and the reader is referred to other well-written neurocritical care texts and the American Stroke Association Guidelines (see citation 3 in the Recommended Reading section below). A brief overview, however, is provided here.

After a ruptured aneurysm is secured, measures are taken to protect against vasospasm; some physicians will employ prophylactic vasospasm treatment and others will wait until there is radiographic or clinical evidence of cerebral vasospasm before initiating therapy (**Table 13.17**).

Fisher Grading Scale

The Fisher grading scale predicts the risk of developing vasospasm, based on the amount of SAH on CT (**Table 13.18**).

"Triple-H Therapy"

Hypertensive-Hypervolemic-Hemodilution (HHH) therapy is used to maximize blood flow through the spastic cerebral arteries after the aneurysm has been secured. Side effects include pulmonary edema, myocardial infarction (MI), pneumonia, hypercapnia, hyponatremia, reversible leukoencephalopathy from a disrupted blood-brain barrier, and nosocomial infections from indwelling arterial and venous catheters, all of which can impair oxygen delivery and result in poor long-term neurological outcomes.

- *Hypertension*: This must be used only after the aneurysm is secured! It is recommended to maintain a systolic blood pressure (SBP) of 160–200 mm Hg with vasopressors when necessary. This is the only component of HHH demonstrated to be effective.
- *Hypervolemia*: It is recommended that a central venous pressure (CVP) greater than or equal to 8 mm Hg be maintained with colloid (5% albumin

Table 13.17 Postprocedural Recommendations for Ruptured Aneurysms

1. Admission to a unit where vasopressors can be administered.
2. Hourly neurological, vital signs, and arterial line monitoring.
3. EVD when hydrocephalus is present or ICP/Licox monitoring when needed.
4. Strict monitoring of fluid balance, keeping the patient hypervolemic with NS. Monitor for SIADH, CSW, or occasionally DI, which can be an early sign of vasospasm. Watch for fluid overload, i.e., CHF, pulmonary edema.
5. If vasopressors fail to resolve vasospasm, intra-arterial vasodilators (verapamil, cardene, or nitroglycerin) or balloon angioplasty should be considered.
6. CBC, metabolic panel to check hematocrit and creatinine levels.
7. Daily transcranial Doppler to assess vasospasm. CTA and CTP as an adjunct to monitoring vasospasm by directly evaluating arterial diameter and blood flow.
8. Echocardiogram and EKG to assess cardiac function before using vasopressors, and HHH therapy to minimize risk of CHF and pulmonary edema.
9. CXR to evaluate pulmonary edema (from HHH) or ARDS (from SAH).
10. Brain CT when indicated to evaluate for HC.
11. Medications to consider for vasospasm prevention/protection: a. Nimotop 60 mg PO Q4 x 21 days; Level 1 evidence shows it is a neuroprotectant and may reduce risk of vasospasm. b. Statins: Lipitor 80 mg PO daily; Level 2 evidence demonstrates both a neuroprotective effect and a reduction in vasospasm. c. Magnesium sulfate (12 g/1 L NS) iv at 50 mL/hr; Level 2 evidence demonstrates neuroprotective effects.[6,7] d. Enoxaparin Lovenox 20 mg SC BID; Level 2 evidence indicates that it reduces vasospasm.[8]

Abbreviations: BID, twice daily; CBC, complete blood count; CHF, congestive heart failure; CTA, computed tomography angiogram; CTP, CT perfusion; CSW, cerebral salt wasting; EKG, electrocardiogram; EVD, extracranial ventricular drain; HCT, head CT; NS, normal saline; SIADH, syndrome of inappropriate ADH secretion; SAH, subarachnoid hemorrhage.

Table 13.18 Fisher Grade with Modification

Grade	Description
1	No blood
2	Diffuse deposition or thin layer, no clots >3 mm thick or vertical layers >1 mm thick
3	Dense collection of blood >1 mm thick in the vertical plane (interhemispheric fissure, insular cistern, or ambient cistern), or >5×3 mm in longitudinal and transverse dimension in the horizontal plane (stem of sylvian fissure, sylvian fissure, and interpeduncular cistern)
4	Intracerebral or intraventricular clots, but with only diffuse or no blood in basal cisterns

250 mL intravenously every 6 hours as necessary for CVPs less than 8) or crystalloid (NS 75 mL/hour qtt or 3% HS 50 mL/hour intravenous drip; the goal is a Na^+ level of 140–150).

- *Hemodilution*: Although hemodilution is never intentionally achieved, it can result from a dilutional anemia. A hemocrit (HCT) of 30 provides optimal rheolytic properties of blood to improve oxygenation; HCT greater than 30 has poor rheolytic properties; HCT less than 30 impairs oxygenation.

Cerebral Blood Flow

- Cerebrovascular tone is regulated predominantly by the CO_2 and O_2 content in the blood. Vascular tone directly influences cerebral blood flow by regulating the luminal diameter in response to changes in blood flow proximally. Increasing CO_2 and decreasing O_2 contents cause vasodilation (reduced vascular tone), resulting in increased cerebral blood flow and oxygen delivery. Under normal circumstances (mean arterial blood pressure [MAP] 60–150 mm Hg), cerebral blood flow is relatively constant due to a protective mechanism called autoregulation. Outside of these limits, cerebral autoregulation is lost, and cerebral perfusion pressure (CPP) becomes dependent upon the MAP and intracranial pressure (ICP). These parameters are related by the following equation: $CPP = MAP - ICP$.
- The CPP is usually maintained between 70 and 90 mm Hg in adults (60–70 mm Hg in children) when the autoregulatory mechanism is functioning properly. When the CPP is below 70 mm Hg for a sustained period of time, the brain is at risk for ischemic damage. Below the range of autoregulation, the blood vessels cannot effectively constrict further to maintain normal perfusion pressures; above this range, the arteries are maximally dilated, allowing for blood flow to be dependent upon MAP and ICP. Radiologic perfusion studies, such as CT perfusion and MR perfusion, can help determine the tissue at risk, meaning the area that can potentially be salvaged in cases of acute stroke and/or cerebrovascular insufficiency or that is at an increased risk for reperfusion injury (edema/hemorrhage) once blood flow is re-established.[4]
- Ischemic stroke occurs secondary to either arterial occlusion from a thrombus or atherosclerotic plaque, or from inadequate blood flow or acute flow failure. Chronic flow failure is often compensated by the development of pial collateralization via extracranial to intracranial anastomoses. The pial collateralization associated with moyamoya disease is an excellent example of this concept. The development of arterial collaterals occurs when the cerebral perfusion remains above the ischemic threshold (greater than 20 cc/g/min). Permissive hypertension, or induced hypertension, can temporarily improve blood flow distal to an arterial stenosis either directly or through collateral flow via a complete circle of Willis. An acute hypertensive episode that significantly increases blood flow to an area with newly developing collaterals or to an area that has been ischemic can lead to reperfusion injury, characterized by hemispheric edema and intracranial hemorrhage. Therefore, rigid blood pressure control in those circumstances is critical to decrease the risk of complications potentially associated with revascularization.

Cerebral Vasospasm

- Cerebral vasospasm, or involuntary smooth muscle contraction within the intracranial arterial wall, can occur in response to intra- or extraluminal injury. For example, local intraluminal injury from catheter trauma or (more frequently) diffuse extraluminal injury from aneurysmal subarachnoid hemorrhage can both result in cerebral vasospasm. The precise etiology of cerebral vasospasm from aneurysmal SAH is unclear. However, the most popular theory is that the by-products of the hemoglobin degradation pathway that circulate in the subarachnoid space induce cerebral vasospasm. A detailed description of the proposed mechanisms of cerebral vasospasm is beyond the scope of this textbook. However, the main theories have included alterations in the nictric oxide, endothelin, and calcium channel pathways. After aneurysmal subarachnoid hemorrhage, 30–70% of patients will develop angiographic cerebral vasospasm. In approximately 30–40% of these patients, vasospasm will become symptomatic and require endovascular therapy using vasodilators, such as nitroglycerin, calcium channel blockers, and balloon angioplasty in severe cases.
- Noninvasive techniques that are useful for monitoring cerebral vasospasm have been developed, including transcranial Doppler studies (TCDs), CT/MR angiography and perfusion, xenon CT analysis, positron emission tomography (PET) scanning, and transcranial cerebral oximetry (TCCO); TCD and CT/MR angiography and perfusion are the most common.[5-8] These studies are all limited by the fact that they are "snapshots" in time and do not allow for continuous monitoring. More invasive techniques, such as the Licox cerebral oximetry monitoring system, indirectly monitor for cerebral vasospasm by continuously monitoring cerebral oxygenation. The limitations of Licox are twofold: it is invasive and it measures a small localized volume. Less-invasive continuous cerebral oxygen monitoring techniques are needed.
- Since the identification of clinical and angiographic cerebral vasospasm in the 1970s and 1980s, multiple pharmaceutical agents have been introduced for its treatment. The calcium channel blocker nimodipine (Nimotop) was the first agent to be used for the treatment of cerebral vasospasm in the mid to late 1980s.[5] Though it is commonly thought to reduce the incidence of cerebral vasospasm, it actually was shown to be an effective neuroprotectant and not a spasmolytic for intracranial cerebral vasospasm. Since that time, other calcium channel blockers, such as verapamil and papaverine, have been also been introduced to the clinical arena.
- Treatment strategies for reducing the untoward effects of cerebral vasospasm can be divided into two main categories: (1) those that reduce vasospasm or improve blood flow and (2) those that act as neuroprotectant agents (which are described in more detail in Chapter 5 but will be briefly mentioned below).
- Triple-H therapy (Hypertension, Hypervolemia, Hemodilution) aims to improve blood flow through the spastic arteries. The most commonly used therapies that reduce vasospasm include the use of pharmaceutical agents, such as nitro-containing compounds or calcium channel blockers, and balloon angioplasty. Neuroprotectants include magnesium sulfate, statin therapy, and calcium channel blockers. These pharmaceutical agents can have harmful side effects, in particular in the elderly population, who frequently

have underlying cardiac, peripheral vascular, and pulmonary co-morbidities that can complicate the treatment phase of the post-SAH period. In these patients, early endovascular intervention with intra-arterial administration of spasmolytic agents and balloon angioplasty may reduce these risks.

Imaging Studies for Vasospasm

TCDs, CTA, CTP, MRA or MRP, and DSA are all imaging modalities that are used to detect vasospasm, evaluate cerebral blood flow, and monitor response to HHH; TCDs are the least sensitive. Careful monitoring of cardiac and pulmonary status is necessary to avoid MI, congestive heart failure (CHF), and pulmonary edema, which can ultimately result in poor cerebral perfusion and oxygenation.

Medications

- *Nimodipine (Nimotop 60 mg by mouth every 4 hours × 21 days):* Nimodipine is a calcium channel blocker that functions as a neuroprotectant against secondary ischemia and may reduce the risk of vasospasm. Side effects include peripheral vasodilatation, which can reduce the MAP during HHH. In such a situation, we recommend changing to Nimotop 30 mg q2 degrees to reduce fluctuation in systolic blood pressure (SBP).
- *Magnesium sulfate (magnesium sulfate 12 g/1 L NS intravenously at 50 mL/hour):* There is level 2 evidence that demonstrates neuroprotective effects of magnesium sulfate.[6,7] Larger randomized clinical trials are currently in progress to better determine its efficacy as a neuroprotectant.
- *Enoxaparin (Lovenox 20 mg subcutaneously twice a day):* There is evidence that enoxaparin reduces vasospasm and is not associated with a higher incidence of deep vein thrombosis compared with controls.[8]
- *Statins (Pravastatin 40 mg by mouth daily):* Though recently controversial, statins may work through the endothelial nitric oxide synthase (eNOS) pathway to relax smooth muscle cells in the arterial walls, thereby reducing cerebral vasospasm.

Electrolyte Abnormalities

H_2O and Na^+ imbalances, frequently seen after SAH, can lead to cerebral edema; the two most common imbalances being SIADH and CSW.

- SIADH is a hyponatremic *hypervolemia*. Correct with fluid restriction, sodium chloride tablets for mild cases, and hypertonic saline solution for more severe cases. Hyponatremia should be corrected slowly to avoid pontine myelinolysis.
- CSW occurs from excess renal Na^+ excretion causing a hyponatremic hypovolemia. Correct with normal saline or 3% HS.
- Diabetes insipidus occurs from excess water reabsorption by the kidneys secondary to increased release of ADH. This syndrome can be seen in poor-grade SAH patients and those with early anterior cerebral artery vasospasm secondary to hypothalamic-pituitary-axis dysfunction.

Hydrocephalus

Post-SAH hydrocephalus can result in a poor neurological exam. An EVD can be life-saving by decompressing the ventricular space and reducing ICPs.

- Non-communicating or obstructive hydrocephalus develops from intraventricular hemorrhage impeding normal CSF flow, usually by blocking the foramen of Monro or the sylvian aqueduct.
- Communicating or non-obstructive hydrocephalus develops from blood breakdown products generally thought to be from an interruption of CSF reabsorption by the arachnoid granulations.

Seizures

Generalized tonic-clonic seizures can increase brain oxygen consumption in the setting of a brain that is poorly perfused from vasospasm. Though the benefits of anticonvulsants are disputed, we use anticonvulsants in all ruptured aneurysm patients until the aneurysm is secured and in comatose patients throughout the vasospasm period to avoid undetected subclinical seizures, which have been identified in up to 25% of SAH patients.

Outpatient Follow-up Imaging

Outpatient follow-up imaging is the same as for unruptured aneurysms (**Table 13.16**).

Potential Complications and Adverse Events

Aneurysm Rupture

Aneurysm rupture is uncommon (less than 1%) during embolization but usually occurs at the time of accessing the aneurysm and placing the first coil. A cerebral angiogram can confirm a suspected rupture, in which case rapid coiling of the aneurysm should be performed to stop the bleeding. A CT scan evaluates the extent of hemorrhage and determines if surgical clot evacuation is necessary.

Aneurysm Recurrence

Aneurysm recurrence is reported to be as high as 20% two years after coiling with bare platinum coils. This recurrence rate may be lower in small narrow-necked aneurysms and those treated with biologically active coils.

Thromboembolic Complications

Thromboembolic complications are reported to be as high as 9% without an antiplatelet preload, which reduces this risk to less than 2%. Heparinization (ACT of 200–250) during the procedure reduces this complication rate, but heparin should not be administered until at least the first coil has been deployed in the aneurysm to reduce the risk of bleeding. Preloading with antiplatelet agents in the setting of a ruptured aneurysm is not safe, nor is it necessary unless a stent is required for wide-necked aneurysms. In such a case, intravenous Rheopro can be used after the aneurysm is secured and the clinical assessment concludes that there is a low risk for needing any further invasive devices, such as an external ventricular drain. Once this has been decided against, aspirin and Plavix can be started for patients with secured ruptured aneurysms that required a stent.

Cranial Neuropathies

Large cavernous, PCOM, and SCA aneurysms can exert mass effect and cause CN III palsy. Large PICA aneurysms can cause lower cranial neuropathies. Neuropathies may worsen after embolization from further compression of the CN by the coil mass. However, there are reports of neuropathies improving after coiling; this improvement is attributed to a reduction in pulsatile injury to the CN.

Alternative Treatments

Surgical clip ligation is the traditional treatment for aneurysms and should still be considered a good alternative to coil embolization for young patients with few comorbidities, for anterior circulation or wide-necked aneurysms, and those that fail endovascular treatment.

Anterior Circulation Aneurysms (PCOM, SHy, ACh, ICAt, ACOM, MCA)

Ipsilateral pterional craniotomy is the workhorse approach for these aneurysms (**Fig. 13.4**). Sylvian fissure dissection and identification of the ICA, M1, A1, and optic nerves, followed by peri-aneurysmal dissection, are mandatory before clipping the aneurysm (**Fig. 13.5**). Aneurysm clips come in a large variety of shapes and sizes for optimal aneurysm occlusion. A bifrontal craniotomy and interhemispheric approach are required for peri-calossal and calossal-marginal aneurysms.

Posterior Circulation Aneurysms

(1) BA and PCA aneurysms can be approached via pterional, combined pterional-anterior temporal, or subtemporal routes, depending on the height of the basilar apex relative to the posterior clinoids. (2) A transpetrosal approach allows access to SCA and AICA aneurysms but carries a risk of loss of hearing, facial nerve injury, and CSF leak. (3) A far-lateral suboccipital craniotomy is used for VBJ and PICA aneurysms (**Figs. 13.6** and **13.7**).

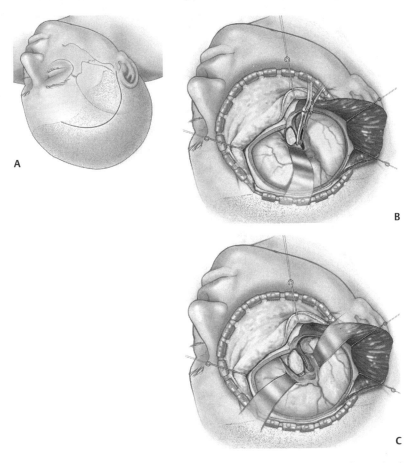

Fig. 13.4 Anterior circulation aneurysms. Positioning, skin incision, and extradural bone removal. **(A)** Scalp incision is from midline to zygoma. **(B)** The sphenoid ridge is flattened and the posterior orbital roof and lateral orbital wall are removed. **(C)** Extradural bone removal can be extended to include the anterior clionid process. (With permission from Macdonald RL. *Neurosurgical Operative Atlas*, 2nd ed. Thieme; 2008, figure 2.4a-c.)

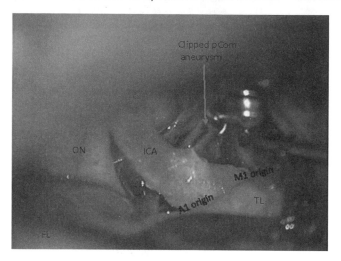

Fig. 13.5 After the sylvian fissure is dissected, the ICA, A1, M1, and optic nerves are identified prior to dissecting around the aneurysm in preparation for clip ligation.

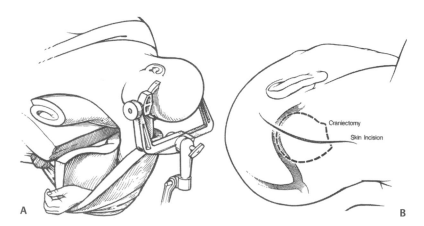

Fig. 13.6 Posterior circulation aneurysms. **(A)** The lateral position for a lateral suboccipital craniotomy and the position of the skin incision and bone flap and **(B)** the exposed dura after the bone has been removed. (With permission from Samson DS, Batjer HH. *Intracranial Aneurysm Surgery: Techniques.* Futura Publishing; 1990.)

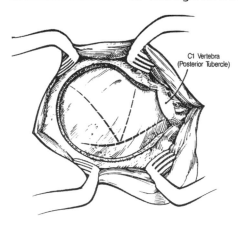

C1 Vertebra
(Posterior Tubercle)

Fig. 13.7 Far-lateral suboccipital craniotomy depicted here shows removal of the occipital bone from the level of the transverse sigmoid sinus superolaterally to the foramen magnum inferiorly and includes a C1 hemilaminectomy. The dotted lines represent the dural opening such that the dural flaps allow the most visualization.

Technical Pearls

1. If hydrocephalus is present in a SAH patient with a wide-necked aneurysm that may require placement of a stent, surgical clip ligation should be considered, because ASA and Plavix will increase the risk of bleeding complications from EVD insertion and potential ventriculoperitoneal shunt placement.

2. Empirically, we have found a cocktail that temporarily reverses antiplatelet effects when it is administered immediately before placement of an EVD or the performance of a short bedside procedure on a patient taking clopidrogel (Plavix): 10 packs of platelets, 0.1 mcg of DDAVP, 10 mg of Decadron, and 2 units of FFP. We find this cocktail to be so effective that it should at least be mentioned here, although the reader is cautioned that this cocktail has not yet been reported nor the individual components tested. In our experience with almost 30 patients over the past few years, no significant hemorrhages have occurred with EVD placement using this cocktail, and the series is currently being prepared for publication.

3. Coiling only the part of the aneurysm that bled (usually the dome) is called "band-aid coiling," and it may temporarily reduce the risk of re-bleeding. Subsequent endovascular or surgical intervention should be performed at a later date once the patient is more stable.

4. Before each coil is detached, angiography should be performed to confirm that there is no coil herniation out of the aneurysm or stenosis of the parent artery by the coil mass, to detect contrast extravasation consistent with rupture, and to quantify residual aneurysm filling.

5. Leaving the coil pusher at the tip of the microcatheter (MC) when removing the system after placement of the last coil can prevent the coil tail from catching in the MC tip and pulling the coil into the parent artery.

Recommended Reading

Bederson JB, Connolly ES, Batjer HH, et al. Guidelines for the management of aneurysmal subarachnoid hemorrhage. AHA/ASA guidelines. Stroke 2009;40:1–32

International Study of Unruptured Intracranial Aneurysms Investigators. Unruptured intracranial aneurysms—risk of rupture and risks of surgical intervention. N Engl J Med 1998;339(24):1725–1733

Molyneux A, Kerr R, Stratton I, et al.; International Subarachnoid Aneurysm Trial (ISAT) Collaborative Group. International Subarachnoid Aneurysm Trial (ISAT) of neurosurgical clipping versus endovascular coiling in 2143 patients with ruptured intracranial aneurysms: a randomised trial. Lancet 2002;360(9342):1267–1274

Wiebers DO, Whisnant JP, Huston J III, et al.; International Study of Unruptured Intracranial Aneurysms Investigators. Unruptured intracranial aneurysms: natural history, clinical outcome, and risks of surgical and endovascular treatment. Lancet 2003;362(9378):103–110

Yamada NK, Cross DT III, Pilgram TK, Moran CJ, Derdeyn CP, Dacey RG Jr. Effect of antiplatelet therapy on thromboembolic complications of elective coil embolization of cerebral aneurysms. AJNR Am J Neuroradiol 2007;28(9):1778–1782

References

1. International Study of Unruptured Intracranial Aneurysms Investigators. Unruptured intracranial aneurysms—risk of rupture and risks of surgical intervention. N Engl J Med 1998;339(24):1725–1733

2. Molyneux A, Kerr R, Stratton I, et al.; International Subarachnoid Aneurysm Trial (ISAT) Collaborative Group. International Subarachnoid Aneurysm Trial (ISAT) of neurosurgical clipping versus endovascular coiling in 2143 patients with ruptured intracranial aneurysms: a randomised trial. Lancet 2002;360(9342):1267–1274

3. Raymond J, Guilbert F, Weill A, et al. Long-term angiographic recurrences after selective endovascular treatment of aneurysms with detachable coils. Stroke 2003; 34(6):1398–1403

4. Deshaies EM, Adamo MA, Boulos AS. A prospective single-center analysis of the safety and efficacy of the hydrocoil embolization system for the treatment of intracranial aneurysms. J Neurosurg 2007;106(2):226–233

5. Tseng MY, Czosnyka M, Richards H, Pickard JD, Kirkpatrick PJ. Effects of acute treatment with pravastatin on cerebral vasospasm, autoregulation, and delayed ischemic deficits after aneurysmal subarachnoid hemorrhage: a phase II randomized placebo-controlled trial. Stroke 2005;36(8):1627–1632

6. Muroi C, Terzic A, Fortunati M, Yonekawa Y, Keller E. Magnesium sulfate in the management of patients with aneurysmal subarachnoid hemorrhage: a randomized, placebo-controlled, dose-adapted trial. Surg Neurol 2008;69(1):33–39, discussion 39

7. Collignon FP, Friedman JA, Piepgras DG, et al. Serum magnesium levels as related to symptomatic vasospasm and outcome following aneurysmal subarachnoid hemorrhage. Neurocrit Care 2004;1(4):441–448

8. Wurm G, Tomancok B, Nussbaumer K, Adelwöhrer C, Holl K. Reduction of ischemic sequelae following spontaneous subarachnoid hemorrhage: a double-blind, randomized comparison of enoxaparin versus placebo. Clin Neurol Neurosurg 2004;106(2):97–103

9. Wiebers DO, Whisnant JP, Huston J III, et al.; International Study of Unruptured Intracranial Aneurysms Investigators. Unruptured intracranial aneurysms: natural history, clinical outcome, and risks of surgical and endovascular treatment. Lancet 2003; 362(9378):103–110

Cranial Vascular Malformations

Junichi Yamamoto

Etiology

The prevalence of cranial vascular malformations is between 15 and 18 per 100,000 adults.[1] The detection rate ranges between 1.12 and 1.34 per 100,000 person years.[2,3] Autopsy data suggest that there is an overall frequency of detection of arteriovenous malformations (AVMs) in approximately 4.3% of the population.[4,5] Autopsy data suggest that as few as 12% of arteriovenous malformations are symptomatic during life.[6] Cerebral arteriovenous malformations are thought to be congenital vascular lesions consisting of abnormal direct connections between the arterial and venous systems (**Fig. 14.1**).[7,8] The exact embryological origin is still unknown, but both persistence of a primitive arteriovenous connection and development of such a connection before or after birth have been suggested.[2]

Genetic Factors

AVMs are traditionally thought to be sporadic, congenital vascular lesions. It has been suggested that cerebral AVMs originate at or before the 40 mm to 80 mm embryo length stage and may be related to a primary abnormality of primordial

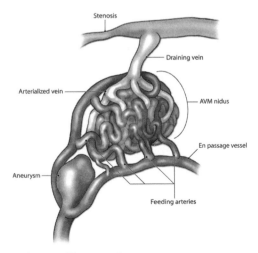

Fig. 14.1 Angioarchitectural features of AVMs.

capillary or venous formation.[7] Familial occurrences have been reported.[8] However, genetic factors for brain AVMs are still largely unexplored because of the low incidence of familial cases, but genetic data for these congenital malformations are being pursued. Cerebral AVMs are diagnosed much more in adults than in children.[8,9] Some AVMs, however, are associated with congenital or hereditary syndromes (**Table 14.1**).[10]

Environmental Factors

Triggering environmental factors for AVM hemorrhage have yet to be well defined. The trigger could be mechanical, hormonal, thrombotic, hemodynamic, thermal, ischemic/hypoxemic, or inflammatory in nature.[11,12]

Diagnosis

Presentation

Intracranial AVMs are occasionally seen in the elderly but are typically diagnosed before the patient has reached the age of 40 years. The most common presentations of AVMs are hemorrhage (>50%) and seizure (20%–25%); less common are headaches (15%), focal neurological deficits from steal phenomenon (5%), and tinnitus.[13-16]

AVM rupture most commonly causes intracerebral hemorrhage followed by subarachnoid and intraventricular hemorrhages, although isolated cases of subdural hematomas have been reported. Severe vasospasm from AVM-related hemorrhage is uncommon.[14] Seizures can be either focal or generalized and may be an indicator of the location of the lesion. In children younger than two years of age, presentation can include congestive heart failure, a large head due to hydrocephalus, and seizures.

Occasionally, an AVM-related steal phenomenon can cause focal neurological deficits by altering perfusion in the tissue near the AVM.[15,17] The steal phenomenon can result from cerebral artery hypotension, leading to ischemia in brain tissue adjacent to the lesion.[18,19] Venous hypertension and any mass effect of the malformation are alternative explanations for the progression of focal neurological deficits.[20]

Table 14.1   AVM-Associated Syndromes

Rendu-Osler-Weber
Klippel-Trenaunay
Parks-Weber
Wyburn-Mason
Sturge-Weber

Clinical Examination

Thorough physical and neurological examinations are needed. Specific findings are related to the location of the lesion in question. When the lesion is associated with other congenital or systemic conditions, other physical exam findings can be found.

Diagnostic Imaging Studies

CT and CT angiography are the first and best imaging studies in hemorrhagic AVM cases, especially in an emergent setting. MRI may not be the first choice for imaging, due to the time required for acquisition of images. However, MRI can provide superior visualization of surrounding brain structures. Further, MR fluid attenuation inversion recovery (FLAIR) imaging can be helpful for detecting small AVM hemorrhages, focal parenchymal changes and mass effect. On MRI, AVMs are detected by inhomogeneous signal voids on T1- and T2-weighted sequences. Gradient-echo sequences can detect hemosiderin, which suggests prior hemorrhage. MR angiography provides information on the vascular anatomy of the AVM but frequently has a lower spatial resolution than CT angiography or cerebral angiography. However, time-resolved MR angiography continues to improve and has been used for general follow-up after treatment as well as radiosurgery treatment planning. A functional MRI can be used to determine the eloquence of the surrounding brain parenchyma, potentially altering management strategies.

Cerebral angiography is an invasive study but remains the gold standard for defining the angioarchitecture of AVMs. Most institutions advocate cerebral angiography at some point in the management phase of AVMs. Cerebral angiography not only can provide highly detailed information on anatomic features in all phases, including points of fistulous connections, associated aneurysms, nidal size, and arterial and venous flow patterns necessary for utilizing the Spetzler-Martin grading scale, but also can provide important hemodynamic information regarding dominant arterial filling and pedicle arrangements. A meta-analysis demonstrated that the risk of conducting diagnostic angiography is significantly lower in patients with AVMs (0.3–0.8%) than in those evaluated for transient ischemic attack or stroke (3.0–3.7%).[21]

Spetzler-Martin Grading Scale

The Spetzler-Martin grading scale predicts the neurological outcome in case of surgical resection, and it has become the scale most often used by treating physicians to describe anatomic details for a specific AVM[22] (**Table 14.2**). In the endovascular era, the Spetzler-Martin scale has generated much debate regarding its utility in assessing endovascular outcomes. Thus, alternative grading scales have been postulated but not frequently accepted. Therefore, the Spetzler-Martin grading scale has remained the dominant classification scale. In this classifica-

Table 14.2   Spetzler-Martin Grading Scale

Graded feature	Points assigned
Size	
Small (<3 cm)	1
Medium (3–6 cm)	2
Large (>6 cm)	3
Eloquence of Adjacent Brain	
Non-eloquent	0
Eloquent	1
Pattern of Venous Drainage	
Superficial	0
Deep	1

tion scale, AVMs are defined by three variables: size, location, and the pattern of venous drainage.

- Sizes are graded as small (0 to 3 cm, 1 point), medium (3 to 6 cm, 2 points), or large (greater than 6 cm, 3 points).
- AVM location is divided into eloquent (1 point) and non-eloquent (0) regions. Eloquent areas include sensorimotor, language, and visual areas, as well as the thalamus, hypothalamus, internal capsule, brainstem, cerebellar peduncles, and deep cerebellar nuclei.
- The pattern of venous drainage can affect surgical accessibility and is divided into superficial (0) and deep (1 point). Only cortical venous drainage and cerebellar venous drainage into the straight or transverse sinus are considered to be superficial. However, the importance of drainage patterns has been challenged in recent years, as superficial venous drainage can often obstruct surgical resection whereas deep drainage does not obstruct resection.

The scale does not include characteristics like associated aneurysms, venous stasis or stenosis, or venous aneurysms or varicies that have been associated with increased hemorrhagic risk. It has been established that several morphologic factors, such as small AVMs, impaired venous drainage, deep draining vein, single draining vein, feeding artery or nidal aneurysm, venous varix, and high intranidal pressure, are all associated with AVM hemorrhage, but their absolute relevance remains unclear. Clinical outcomes after surgical resection of intracranial AVMs can be predicted with this scale.[23] The predicted lifetime risk of hemorrhage is:

$$1 - (1 - \text{annual hemorrhage risk})^n$$

where n = the remaining years of life expected. This risk should be weighed against the risk of surgery as predicted by the Spetzler-Martin grading scale (**Table 14.3**), the experience of the neurosurgeon, and prior clinical status after presentation.

Table 14.3 Surgical Outcome Predicted by the S-M Grading Scale[22]

S-M grade	No deficits	Minor deficits	Major deficits
1	100%	0%	0%
2	95%	5%	0%
3	84%	12%	4%
4	73%	20%	7%
5	69%	19%	12%

Evidence-Based Medicine

The main goal of AVM treatment is to eliminate the risk of hemorrhage and all related symptoms, such as seizures and neurologic deficits, without any or with only minimal morbidity or mortality to the patient. The available methods of treatment are microsurgery, radiosurgery, endovascular treatment with embolization, or a combination of these techniques.

Several factors are considered in the decision to treat an AVM, such as symptoms, age of the patient, medical condition, the size and location of the AVM, the type of venous drainage, the history of hemorrhage, and the natural history of AVMs in general.

Existing data indicate that only complete eradication of the lesion provides the most complete protection from future hemorrhage; partial treatment may not be helpful and may, in fact, increase the rate of future hemorrhage.

A current attempt to unravel the mysteries of unruptured AVMs has been undertaken by several prospective databases across the world. In the United States, the ARUBA trial encompasses a prospective database involving multiple academic centers where AVMs are randomized to either observation or treatment when the treating physician feels the AVM does not pose any immediate risk. While this trial is still undergoing enrollment, it will hopefully shed some light regarding what the natural history of AVMs dictates as true hemorrhagic risk. Although promising, this trial has met with much criticism.

Bleeding and Rebleeding Rates

- The AVM hemorrhage rate has been classically reported to be approximately 2%–4% per year,[24–30] but the actual rupture risk may differ between distinct patient subgroups.
- The first episode of bleeding is associated with a mean mortality rate of 10%, which increases to 15% with the second hemorrhage and to 20% with the third one. An additional 20% mean rate of neurological morbidity accompanies each hemorrhage.[31] After a hemorrhagic episode, the rate of rehemorrhage increases to 6% in the first year and then returns to 2%–4% per year thereafter.[31] Grade IV and V AVMs appear to have a lower rate of hemorrhage, which is estimated at 1.5% per year.[31]

- Data from the New York Islands AVM Hemorrhage Study suggest that the AVM detection rate is 1.21/100,000 person-years, and the incidence of AVM hemorrhage is 0.42/100,000 person-years.[32]
- Data from the prospective, longitudinal, population-based Northern Manhattan Stroke Study suggest that the crude incidence for first-ever AVM-related hemorrhage is 0.55/100,000 person-years.[33]

Surgery

- The Spetzler-Martin grading scale has also been applied prospectively. Grade I, II, or III AVMs were found to have low treatment-associated morbidity.[34] However, grade IV lesions conferred 31.2% treatment-associated morbidity, and grade V lesions had 50% new treatment-associated morbidity. In addition, the rate of permanent deficit was 29.9% for grade IV lesions and 16.7% for grade V lesions.[34] The authors recommend surgery for all grade I and II lesions. Grade III lesions should be treated on a case-by-case basis. Grade IV and V lesions require a multidisciplinary approach with individual analysis.[34] However, these figures were developed at a time when there were no other adjunctive therapies, such as endovascular embolization. Current multimodality therapy may alter these results, but the data have yet to be determined.
- In one study, 67 patients underwent resection of AVMs less than 3 cm in their largest diameter, regardless of location. Complete angiographic obliteration of the AVM by microsurgical technique was accomplished in 63 patients (94%) with a surgical morbidity of 1.5% and no operative mortality. Patients with hemispheric AVMs had a cure rate of 100% and no neurological morbidity.[35]
- Accumulating data suggest that partial AVM resection does not reduce, but rather increases, the risk of future hemorrhage.[36] Partially treated grade IV and V AVMs carry a 10.4% risk of hemorrhage, compared with a 1% risk in patients with no previous treatment.[31]

Embolization

- The rate of complete obliteration of brain AVMs by using embolization as the sole method of treatment is thought to be between 5% and 40%.[37] These AVMs are usually smaller than 3 cm in diameter and have only one or two feeding arteries. The chance of complete obliteration was inversely proportional to AVM volume and the number of feeding pedicles. To achieve permanent obliteration, a nonbiodegradable agent should be used to occlude the AVM nidus. Complete obliteration of the brain AVM should be demonstrated by the immediate postprocedure angiogram and confirmed by follow-up angiography.[37]
- Valavanis and Yasargil reported complete AVM obliteration with embolization alone in 39% of 387 patients. In the subgroup analysis of 182 AVMs that were treated with intent-to-cure, they reported a cure rate of 75%.[38] Yu et al. reported achieving complete obliteration rates of 60% in patients treated with embolization alone.[39] An initially high degree of obliteration of the AVM nidus may be followed by its recurrence shortly after embolization. The ex-

tent to which the collateral supply develops and the time required for its development may depend on the degree of nidus obliteration and the material used for the obliteration.[40]

- Although the reported rates of complete endovascular obliteration vary, most estimates are in the range of 10%. However, it is important to note that these estimates are based on series that predate the introduction and widespread application of the liquid embolic Onyx (MicroTherapeutics, Inc., Irvine, CA) and, therefore, may be expected to increase with Onyx.[36]

Radiosurgery

Radiotherapy is recommended for small (<3 cm in diameter), deep malformations for which a surgical approach involves passing through functionally important brain tissue, for malformations in an eloquent area, and for ones in which the large number of feeding arteries or the presence of endovascularly inaccessible feeders makes embolization impractical. In general, the success of radiotherapy is inversely proportional to the size of the AVM nidus to be treated.[41] AVMs with nidal volumes less than 10 mL (diameter <3 cm) are frequently curable by radiosurgery, with rates of obliteration at 2 years estimated at between 80% and 88%.[39,42] However, it takes two to three years before the efficacy of the treatment can be determined, and the hemorrhage risk either remains or can increase up to 11–16% during the first six months after treatment. Furthermore, secondary complications from the effects of radiation on the surrounding parenchyma or cranial nerves may confer unacceptable morbidity.

Combination Therapy

The goal of combination therapy is to maximize the benefits of each option and decrease the overall morbidity and mortality of AVM treatment. Embolization of AVMs can be beneficial prior to microsurgical resection or radiosurgery (**Table 14.4**) to reduce the treatment volume or potential blood loss during resection.[45,46,47]

Gobin et al. reported their experience with 125 patients undergoing embolization (predominantly with n-BCA) prior to radiosurgery. They achieved total occlusion in 11.2% of AVMs after embolization alone, with an additional 76% of lesions reduced sufficiently in size to undergo radiotherapy. A 65% rate of total occlusion was observed after radiotherapy in patients undergoing combined treatment.[43] Despite the straightforward rationale for pre-radiosurgical embolization, very little data currently exist to support this approach. From the existing data, no compelling evidence exists to justify or refute the usefulness of pre-radiosurgical embolization.[36]

Preprocedural Preparation for AVMs

Unruptured AVMs

- Similar to other endovascular interventions.
- Check blood level of antiseizure medications if the patient takes them.
- Review all CT, MRI, and angiography imagery thoroughly prior to the procedure.
- Often done on an elective basis.

Table 14.4   Benefits of AVM Embolization before Microsurgery and Radiosurgery

Microsurgery	Radiosurgery
Occludes the deep and surgically inaccessible feeding pedicles.	Decreases the size of large AVM (>3 cm) so radiosurgery can be performed.
Decreases blood flow and nidal size, resulting in less blood loss during the surgery.	Treat AVM-associated aneurysms prior to radiosurgery (radiosurgery may not be effective for the aneurysms).
Onyx or n-BCA in the feeding arteries or nidus provides a good road map during resection.	Smaller residual AVMs have higher radiosurgical cure rate.[69,80,81]
Treat AVM-associated aneurysms prior to the surgical resection.	

Ruptured AVMs

- Same for unruptured AVMs.
- Head CT or MRI to assess intracranial hemorrhage, hydrocephalus, or other acute intracranial lesions.
- Often done on a more emergent basis. Surgical evacuation of a significant hematoma may precede the actual treatment of the AVM by several weeks.

AVM-Associated Aneurysms

- Same for unruptured AVMs.
- In case of ruptured AVM aneurysms, treatment of the aneurysm should be done before or during definitive treatment of AVM. Although rare, if the aneurysm rupture confers a significant amount of hemorrhage into the subarachnoid space, vasospasm should be anticipated, which may change the timing or strategy of definitive AVM therapy.
- Despite its inherent difficulty, determination of the source of hemorrhage should be considered, that is, whether the AVM or aneurysm is the source.

Equipment

Sheath

Selection of a sheath is often based on preference and the experience of the operators. A 4 Fr or 5 Fr sheath 11 cm long is most commonly used for diagnostic angiography. A 6 Fr or 7 Fr sheath 11 cm long or longer (up to 35 cm) for tortuous proximal access or a 6 Fr Shuttle Select Tuohy-Borst introducer (Cook, Inc.) (90 cm in length) can be used for embolization.

Catheters

Angled glidecaths are useful for uncomplicated or Type I arches. The Simmons II catheter is useful for tortuous great vessels or a complicated aortic arch. For more stability, co-axial guiding systems like the 6 Fr Envoy (MPC or Sim 2) (Cordis Neurovascular, Inc., Miami Lakes, FL), 6 Fr Neuron (ID 0.070 or 0.051) (Penumbra, Inc., Alameda, CA) catheter, or 6 Fr Chaperon MP2 (Microvention, Inc., Aliso Viejo, CA) guide catheters can be used through a 6 Fr or 7 Fr shuttle sheath. Two techniques to place guiding catheters or long or shuttle sheaths in the common and internal carotids and vertebral arteries of difficult aortic arches are described in **Table 14.5**. In addition, distal access catheters can be used in conjunction with standard guide catheters to stabilize the catheter system further and allow for more stable distal access.

Glide Wires

Most commonly, a 0.035 or 0.038 guide wire is used in 150 cm or 260 cm lengths. Stiff wires are normally used for tortuous access. Exchange length 0.035 or 0.038 glide wires can be used as well, especially in anticipation of exchanging a diagnostic catheter for a guide catheter. The Amplatz J-wire can be useful, especially in cases where the external carotid artery is used as an anchor while delivering a guiding catheter or shuttle sheath.

Microcatheter

As mentioned above, selection of the microcatheter is most frequently based on the preference and experience of the operator, as well as the microcatheter's trackability or support. Tips are shapeable with hot steam. Several pre-shaped microcatheters are available, among them 45 degree, 90 degree, J, C, or S-shaped tips. Microcatheters are divided into flow-guided and microwire-directed types (**Table 14.6**).

Microwire

Selection is based on preference and experience. Larger and stiffer wires have more stability and trackability, but they also have more risk of perforation of the vessels (**Table 14.7**).

Table 14.5 Techniques for Catheterizing the Carotid and Vertebral Arteries in Difficult Aortic Arches

1. Exchange technique using a diagnostic catheter and exchanging length (260 cm) of stiff or regular glide wire.
2. Co-axial technique by using 6 Fr 125 cm 0.038 Sim2 Sidewinder II Supertorque (Cordis Neurovascular, Inc., Miami Lakes, FL). First, the target vessel is catheterized with this catheter. Then a stiff 0.035 glide wire or 0.038 glide wire is advanced distally, and a 6 Fr or 7 Fr shuttle sheath is advanced over the catheter and wire.

Table 14.6 Microcatheters Used for AVM Embolization

Flow-guided	Microwire-directed
*Marathon Flow Directed Micro Catheter (1.5 Fr/2.7 Fr) (Micro Therapeutics, Inc, d/b/a ev3 Neurovascular, Irvine, CA)	• *Echelon-14 Micro Catheter (1.9 Fr/2.4 Fr) • *Echelon-10 Micro Catheter (1.7 Fr/2.1 Fr) (Micro Therapeutics, Inc, d/b/a ev3 Neurovascular, Irvine, CA)
Balt Magic (1.2 Fr, 1.5 Fr, 1.8 Fr, 2.5 Fr/3 Fr) (Balt/Boston Scientific, Fremont, CA)	• Prowler 10 Micro Catheter (2.3 Fr/1.7 Fr) • Prowler 14 Micro Catheter (2.3 Fr/1.9 Fr) • Prowler Select Plus Micro Catheter (2.8 Fr/2.3 Fr) (Cordis Neurovascular, Inc., Miami Lakes, FL)
	• Excelsior SL-10 Micro Catheter (1.7 Fr/2.4 Fr) • Excelsior 1018 Micro Catheter (2.6 Fr/2.0 Fr) (Boston Scientific Corporation, Natick, MA)

*Important Note: Only the Marathon and Echelon microcatheters from ev3 are DMSO/Onyx compatible.

Table 14.7 Microwires

Mirage 0.008 hydrophilic guide wire X-pedion-14 hydrophilic guide wire X-pedion-10 hydrophilic guide wire (Micro Therapeutics, Inc, d/b/a ev3 Neurovascular, Irvine, CA)
Synchro2 soft micro guide wire Synchro2 standard micro guide wire (Boston Scientific Corporation, Natick, MA)
Silver Speed 10 micro guide wire Silver Speed 14 micro guide wire (Micro Therapeutics, Inc, d/b/a ev3 Neurovascular, Irvine, CA)
Agility 14 standard Agility 10 soft Agility 14 soft (Cordis Neurovascular, Inc., Miami Lakes, FL)

Technique

Anesthesia

The choice of anesthetic technique is controversial and depends largely on local practice and training. The patient's tolerance for lying supine for long periods should be assessed, and in women, the possibility of pregnancy should be ascertained.[37]

General Anesthesia

Factors such as age (for example, infants and young children), an uncooperative or very nervous patient, and acutely ruptured AVMs favor the use of general anesthesia. There are many benefits to using general anesthesia for AVM embolization

(**Table 14.8**). A disadvantage of general anesthesia is the inability to perform a neurological examination during the procedure. Neurophysiological monitoring, such as EEGs, SSEPs and MEPs, is useful to monitor the patient's neurological status under general anesthesia. However, visual and language areas cannot be reliably monitored with current electrophysiological techniques. Additionally, gaseous anesthesia cannot be used with neuromonitoring; total intravenous anesthetic (TIVA) is required, and this must be discussed with the anesthesiologist beforehand. There is no evidence that either general endotracheal anesthesia or intravenous sedation is associated with a lower rate of complications.[44]

Conscious Sedation and Local Anesthesia

The primary goals of anesthetic choice for intravenous sedation include alleviation of pain or discomfort and anxiety and patient immobility. The anesthetic must allow for a rapid decrease in the level of sedation when neurological testing is required.[20] Versed and fentanyl are commonly used or low-dose propofol infusion if required. Postoperatively, most patients are monitored in the intensive care unit for signs of hemodynamic instability or neurological changes.

Benefits of conscious sedation over general anesthesia include the ability to monitor a neurological exam throughout the entire procedure (including visual and language areas) and the ability to test the feeding arteries to the AVM with barbiturate and lidocaine to verify whether any of them are supplying an eloquent region of the brain before embolization.

Embolization

Two FDA-approved liquid embolic materials are: TruFill n-butyl cyanoacrylate (n-BCA) (Cordis Neurovascular, Inc., Miami Lakes, FL); and Onyx (ethylene-vinyl alcohol copolymer EVOH) (Micro Therapeutics, Inc., Irvine, CA). n-BCA used to be the most

Table 14.8 Advantages/Disadvantages of General Anesthesia during AVM Embolization

Advantages	Disadvantages
Airway control	Unable to follow a neurological exam
Blood pressure control during embolization	
ICP management	
Less motion artifact, allowing for better visualization of vascular structures	
Patient comfort	
Control of unexpected complications	
Controlled elevation of the arterial pressure when ischemic complications occur	
Option to use adenosine for temporary cardiac arrest to decrease the flow through the AVM during the glue placement in high-flow AVMs	

frequently used embolic agent. However, Onyx, a more recent non-adhesive liquid embolic material that theoretically permits slower filling, better penetration, and better obliteration of the nidus, provides a solid nidus cast due to its longer precipitation time and lack of adherence.

n-Butyl Cyanoacrylate

An adhesive liquid monomeric agent, n-butyl cyanoacrylate (n-BCA) quickly polymerizes and becomes solid when in contact with a solution containing anions, such as the hydroxyl groups in blood.[45] Such a process causes occlusion, marked inflammatory endothelial response, and ultimately fibrosis.[46] Although recanalization can occur, it is rare after an adequate embolization.

The safety of n-BCA in AVM embolization has been tested in a prospective, randomized, multicenter trial on 114 patients.[47] The rate of polymerization and the rate of injection determine how far the agent will travel within the cerebral vasculature before solidifying. The n-BCA itself is radiolucent and must be mixed with a radiopaque agent, typically ethiodol oil mixture (Lipiodol) for most applications. In addition to imparting radiopacity to the n-BCA, the oil acts as a retardant, slowing the rate of polymerization and thus allows the n-BCA to penetrate farther in the feeding vessel before solidifying. Micronized tantalum powder can also be added to improve radiopacity and visualization.

n-BCA should be prepared with clean gloves free of ionic solutions (such as blood, contrast, or saline). The microcatheter should be flushed with 5% dextrose in water prior to the injection. n-BCA should be injected under fluoroscopy or subtracted fluoroscopy.

The physical characteristics of n-BCA offer unique working properties (**Table 14.9**). The viscosity of n-BCA can be adjusted by changing the amount of ethiodol added to the mixture. Decreasing the amount of ethiodol in the mixture can increase viscosity, which can be useful for high-flow AVMs. For deeper and more

Table 14.9   n-BCA Working Properties

Advantages[36]	Disadvantages
Potential for penetration deep into the AVM nidus.	Proper delivery of the agent into the nidus requires accurate polymerization time.
Durable occlusion of the embolized vessel or pedicle.	Prolonged injections are difficult, so that only a limited amount of nidal vessels can usually be occluded with a single injection.
Ability to be delivered through small, flexible, flow-directed catheters that can be manipulated safely and atraumatically into the most distal locations within the cerebrovasculature.	Catheter retention is a possible risk if the adhesive properties of n-BCA make withdrawal traumatic or impossible.[36,48–50]
Delivered into the pedicle easily and quickly; infusions generally require <1 minute.	Rapid removal of the catheter is required when reflux is seen at the tip of the catheter.
Ethiodol dosing can adjust the viscosity to adjust nidal penetration (more ethiodol, increased penetration).[48]	Diagnostic angiography cannot be done during the injection.

homogeneous nidal penetration, a lower viscous mixture is recommended.[48] Commonly a solution containing 30–35% n-BCA is used, and a thicker one can be used for high-flow AVMs. To maintain delayed polymerization, adjustments to the pH of the solution can also be performed.[49,50]

Onyx

The application of the ethylene-vinyl alcohol copolymer (EVOH) in the endovascular treatment of intracranial AVMs was first described by Taki et al.[51] and Terada et al.[52] in the early 1990s. EVOH is now commercially available as the nonadhesive liquid embolic system under the names Onyx-18 and Onyx-34 (ev3 Micro Therapeutics, Inc., Irvine, CA). Since July 2005, Onyx-18 and Onyx-34 have been approved in the United States by the Food and Drug Administration. The numbers 18 and 34 quantify the viscosity of Onyx in centipoises (cp). Onyx-18 contains 6% EVOH and 94% dimethyl sulfoxide (DMSO), and Onyx-34, 8% EVOH and 92% DMSO. Micronized tantalum powder (35% weight/volume) is added for radiopacity (**Fig. 14.2**). Onyx must therefore be shaken for at least 20 minutes before injection to achieve homogeneous radiopacity of the mixture.

DMSO is potentially angiotoxic, but this effect is negligible if it used with the recommended infusion rates (**Table 14.10**).[45,53] The Onyx precipitation process begins on the surface while the core is still liquid, resulting in a soft, nonadherent mass. Therefore, Onyx has a lava-like flow pattern within blood vessels without any fragmentation during the injection. Due to these properties and because Onyx is not absorbable, it is capable of producing permanent vascular occlusion (**Table 14.11**).[53,54] Although long-term data are currently lacking, Onyx is, like n-BCA, a permanent agent.[48,55,56] Natarajan et al. showed histopathological evidence of foreign body giant cell and angionecrosis in 39% and 43% of their surgically resected AVMs treated with Onyx and suggested that Onyx is not inert. No long-term studies have been performed with regard to the toxicity or carcinogenicity of Onyx.[57]

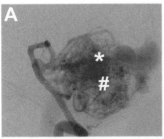
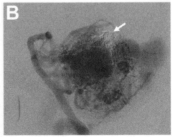
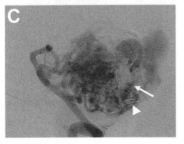

Fig. 14.2 Embolization of a posterior fossa AVM. **(A)** Large posterior fossa AVM with prominent arterial supply from both the SCA (*asterisk*) and AICA (*pound sign*) branches. **(B)** The initial Onyx cast (*arrow*) can be seen in the area of reduced nidal filling. **(C)** Second embolization with Onyx can be seen (*arrow*) as well as with coils (*arrowhead*). Coils can sometimes be used to give the Onyx cast something to attach itself to.

Table 14.10   Procedure for Onyx Injection

1. Aqueous solutions will precipitate Onyx polymer, so make sure no blood or aqueous solutions are on the table or gloves; recommend setting up a separate clean table.
2. Flush the microcatheter with DMSO prior to injecting Onyx.
3. Injection rate should be ≤0.1 cc per minute to avoid angiotoxicity.
4. Avoid significant Onyx reflux around the microcatheter tip to lower the risk of microcatheter entrapment.
5. Depending on the size of the vessel and flow into the AVM, Onyx can be injected slowly and steadily or puffed into the vessel; the first is the traditional technique.

Table 14.11   Onyx Working Properties

Advantages	Disadvantages
Nonadhesive, reducing the possibility of the catheter adherence.	The diluent, DMSO, can be potentially angiotoxic, particularly with rapid injections.
Allows the operator a much greater degree of flexibility with respect to the volume and rate of the injection.	DMSO volume and injection time (0.1 cc/minute) need to be monitored closely to achieve a safe embolization.
The operator may temporarily halt infusion periodically to perform angiography and assess the status of the AVM nidus and draining veins before continuing the infusion.[36]	Limited to ev3 microcatheters because of their demonstrated DMSO compatibility.
Can halt infusion for up to 2 minutes before risking solidification of the Onyx at the catheter tip and catheter occlusion.	Visibility can be limited in smaller feeding pedicles due to the separation of Onyx and the added opacifying agent tantalum.
Onyx is a soft, sponge-like mass that is easy to handle during microsurgery.	Although Onyx is nonadhesive, only partial reflux can be allowed around the catheter tip or the microcatheter may adhere to the Onyx cast.
The embolized vessels are completely filled by the embolic agent and are less fragile because of the lower inflammatory reaction and the absence of polymerization heat compared with n-BCA-embolized AVMs.	
Less intraoperative blood loss and a shorter duration of surgical procedures for Onyx compared with n-BCA in an animal model; ONYX seemed to provide benefits for surgeons.[47]	

Removing the Microcatheter Systems

The difficulty in removing the catheter depends on the tortuosity of the catheterized vessels, the duration of the precipitation, the distance of the reflux, and the experience of the investigator who is pulling on the catheter.[53]

n-Butyl Cyanoacrylate

When proximal reflux occurs, injection should be terminated. Then the microcatheter is aspirated and briskly removed. Working with two experienced physicians, one to aspirate and the other to pull, is highly recommended. Retained microcatheters have been widely reported without significant clinical morbidity.

Onyx

Stretching or fracturing of the microcatheter may occur with Onyx, even though the risk is lower than with n-BCA. Nevertheless, when the catheter is trapped, it is better to leave it in place than to risk a potential rupture of a vessel. Waiting a few seconds following completion of injection before attempting catheter retrieval is recommended to avoid fragmentation of Onyx into non-target vessels. Difficulty in retrieval may be caused by: (1) a distal, long, tortuous pedicle; (2) vasospasm; or (3) Onyx reflux. In cases of resistance when the catheter is pulled out, specific maneuvers are recommended for retrieval (**Table 14.12**). More than 20 cm of traction to the microcatheter is not recommended to minimize the risk of catheter separation. Transient focal neurological deficits or changes in SSEP or/and MEP could happen while pulling the microcatheter out, most likely secondary to exces-

Table 14.12   Microcatheter Removal after Embolization

Onyx	n-BCA
Pull carefully to assess the severity of resistance.	When proximal reflux occurs, terminate the injection.
Remove any "slack" (redundant loops) in the catheter.	Aspirate through the microcatheter.
Gently apply steady traction to the catheter (cm by cm, ~3–4 cm of stretch to the catheter), then hold this traction for a few seconds and release; this process can be repeated intermittently until the catheter is retrieved.	Rapidly pull the microcatheter out; two experienced interventionists are preferred for this maneuver—one aspirates while the other rapidly pulls the microcatheter out.
OR	
Remove all slack from the catheter and create slight tension by putting a few cm of traction on the catheter.	
Firmly hold the microcatheter and then pull it, using a quick wrist snap motion, 10–15 cm (from left to right).	

sive stretch of the vessel (based on personal experiences). We recommend gentle and intermittent (or continuous) traction instead of rapid pulling out in cases of resistance or an adherent tip. A monorail snare recovery technique to remove an adherent microcatheter in the external carotid artery has recently been reported.[58]

Entrapped Microcatheters

In some circumstances, it may be safer to leave the microcatheter in place rather than risk causing hemorrhagic or other complications. This is accomplished by stretching the catheter and cutting the shaft at the groin sheath, allowing the catheter to remain in the artery; antiplatelet therapy may be required, typically with aspirin.

Postprocedural Care

Acute Neurological Change

The mortality rate associated with brain AVM embolization varies from 0.9% to 1.6%. The overall morbidity rate ranges from 5% to 12.8%. The most common complications associated with brain AVM embolization are infarct and hemorrhage. Vessel dissection or vasospasm from the guide catheter can also cause an acute neurological change.

Normal perfusion pressure breakthrough can also occur following aggressive treatment of large AVMs and can cause focal neurological deficits or hemorrhagic complications. This entails normal brain becoming edematous from the hemodynamic changes within the brain parenchyma surrounding the AVM.[37]

Stroke

Infarct results from occlusion of normal arterial branches to vital parenchyma, redistribution of blood flow after embolization, occlusion of an AVM feeder that is also supplying the normal parenchyma ("en passage" feeder), and/or unintentional embolization of an artery from glue reflux.

Systemic heparinization may help to reduce the risk of ischemic complications. Intra-arterial thrombolysis (using t-PA, platelet glycoprotein IIb/IIIa antagonists) or mechnical thrombectomy may be needed in the event of a thromboembolic complication.

Intracranial Hemorrhage

Overall, the rate of periprocedural bleeding complications reported in the literature ranged between 2% and 16.7% after endovascular use of Onyx.[53,59-67] Causes of acute post-embolization hemorrhage include: (1) inappropriate venous outflow occlusion of a partially embolized AVM, (2) increased pressure in feeding arteries as a result of embolization, (3) normal perfusion pressure breakthrough, (4) hyperemia of normal brain circulation or redistribution of cerebral blood flow into adjacent regions, (5) venous thrombosis secondary to stasis caused by substantial obliteration of the AVM, (6) inflammatory reaction or mural necrosis induced by the embolic material (DMSO, etc.), (7) ischemic tissue around an abnormal blood vessel that bled under pressure, and (8) rupture of an intranidal or pedicle aneurysm.[68] The development of unexplained bradycardia and hypertension (the Cushing response) should raise the suspicion of intracranial hemorrhage. In such a case, the procedure should be aborted, and a CT scan obtained. Many modern angio suites have the ability to perform CT-like scans in the angio suite. If the CT scan is positive for hemorrhage and the patient is not under general anesthesia, he or she should be intubated and an external ventricular drain inserted to monitor and control intracranial pressure if the hemorrhage is severe.

Hydrocephalus

Hydrocephalus may occur as a result of intraventricular hemorrhage secondary to a ruptured AVM, requiring a ventricular drain. As the ventricular blood is cleared, patients may develop a chronic communicating hydrocephalus warranting a ventriculoperitoneal shunt. In rare instances, a noncommunicating hydrocephalus can result from compression of the aqueduct by large AVMs.

Seizures

Patients with a history of seizures should be adequately medicated preoperatively with anti-epileptic agents. Those without a history of seizures should also be premedicated with anti-epileptic agents if they had an intracranial hemorrhage or are considered to have a high risk for seizures due to the anatomical location of the AVM. If status epilepticus develops, the patient should be intubated and either administered medications to break the status or put into a barbiturate or propofol coma until burst suppression is acquired on continuous EEG monitoring.

Follow-Up Imaging Studies

Postembolization cerebral angiography remains the gold standard for evaluating residual AVM anatomy and flow. CT is useful for evaluating acute hemorrhagic lesions, but CTA provides limited information about residual AVM because of embolic artifact. MRI can demonstrate details of ischemic or hemorrhagic lesions and can be useful in localizing any residual nidus of the AVM due to limited glue artifact.

Alternative Therapies

At present, there are five major treatment paradigms available for patients with cerebral AVM: (1) observation, (2) surgical resection, (3) endovascular embolization, (4) radiosurgery, and (5) combination therapy. The AVM can be observed expectantly, with the understanding that there is a continued risk of hemorrhage and possible resultant neurological deficits, depending on the location. Alternatively, intervention can be undertaken with the goal of complete AVM obliteration, because subtotal therapy does not seem to provide protection from hemorrhage.[69-71]

Observation

According to the study by Ondra et al., observation alone carries an average hemorrhage risk of 3% to 4%.[28] The surgical resection of Grade IV and V AVMs is generally associated with a risk of operative morbidity and mortality that exceeds the risks associated with the natural history of the lesion. Han et al. analyzed outcomes in a series of 73 consecutive patients with Grade IV and V AVMs. They recommended no treatment for most patients in this group (55 out of 73) and reported a relatively low risk of hemorrhage in these patients (1% per yr). In addition, in this series as well as in several additional reports, partial AVM treatment substantially increased the yearly risk for hemorrhage.[31] In the current age of multimodality therapy, the clinical outcomes have not been completely determined. Furthermore, although the literature is not conclusive, treatment of AVM-related aneurysms may at least reduce the rupture risk from that lesion. Thus, a standard set of guidelines to treat AVMs is far from complete, due to the multitude of possible AVM configurations.

Surgical Resection

Despite advances in radiosurgery and endovascular techniques, surgical resection continues to play an important role in the management of brain AVMs and is still touted to be the only cure. Cure is thought to be immediate and permanent after complete resection by microsurgery. However, several case reports have noted purported recurrences after total surgical resection. Surgical treatment is favored in patients in good medical condition with a good life expectancy who harbor small to medium-sized AVMs in anatomically accessible locations. The risk of major complications from surgical excision is very low for AVM lesions smaller than 3 cm.[34] Most cerebral AVMs of Spetzler-Martin Grades I and II can be surgically removed by experienced neurosurgeons with acceptably low morbidity and mortality.[31]

Radiosurgery

Radiosurgery, performed either alone or in combination with endovascular embolization, has made possible the safe and effective treatment of some brain AVMs without the need for surgical resection.[72–74] However, radiosurgery does carry the risk of radiation injury to adjacent normal parenchyma and cranial nerves and a delayed onset of obliteration (15–30 months), with a possible increased risk of hemorrhage during the first 6 months (11–16%). Radiosurgery can produce an angiographic and clinical cure for many different types of lesions. Optimally, the lesion should be small (<10 cc total volume). The efficacy of radiosurgical obliteration of lesions <2.5 cm in diameter ranges from 74% to 80% and decreases to 50% for lesions between 2.5 and 3 cm in diameter.[75,76] The full effect of radiosurgery usually does not become apparent for at least 2 years.

After endovascular embolization, microsurgery, or the combination has reduced the size of a difficult AVM nidus as much as possible, radiosurgery can often treat the remnant definitively. The risk of major complications in AVMs <2 cm is very low[74]; for lesions <3 cm in diameter it is <5%.[39,75,76] Until the lesion is completely obliterated by radiosurgery, it is believed and reported to still offer a hemorrhagic risk.[77–79]

Combination Therapy

More so than any other vascular lesion of the central nervous system, the treatment of brain AVMs requires a multimodality and multidisciplinary approach. All patients should be evaluated by physicians with expertise in endovascular embolization, microneurosurgical resection, and radiosurgery. After careful consideration of the clinical data and AVM architecture, a risk-to-benefit ratio for treatment can be estimated. As soon as a treatment plan is agreed on, all parties must have a clear understanding of their individual roles to facilitate successful treatment.[36]

Clinical Pearls

1. Diagnostic angiography remains the gold standard for assessing AVM anatomy, including the feeding arteries, en passage vessels, pedicle or/and intranidal aneurysms, nidus, and draining veins.
2. Obtaining several angiographic angles for the injection of embolic materials reduces the risk of accidental occlusion of normal artery or large draining veins.
3. Rotational angiography or DSA with three-dimensional reconstruction is useful to better understand the anatomy of AVMs.
4. Systolic blood pressure during the procedure should be controlled at normal or less than normal, depending on the size, location, and flow of the AVMs; after the embolization, blood pressure is usually kept lower than the baseline systolic pressure for 24 to 72 hours.
5. Microcatheter runs with 1 cc syringe and gentle hand injection are useful to see more detailed anatomy, including en passage vessels, and normal arteries close to the catheter tip which could be occluded by reflux.
6. Provocative testing involves the use of Amytal (30–50 mg), Brevital (2–4 mg), or lidocaine (30–40 mg), usually injected through the microcatheter before definitive embolization in patients who are awake.
7. Under general anesthesia, both MEP and SSEP can be monitored to avoid false-negative results; vision and language cannot be monitored under general anesthesia.
8. A pre-treatment functional MRI can also be very helpful when determining the safety of each potential therapy.

Recommended Reading

Hurst RW, Rosenwasser RH. Eds. *Interventional Neuroradiology*. Informa Healthcare USA, Inc; 2008

Morris P. *Interventional and Endovascular Therapy of the Nervous System*. Springer; 2001

Stieg PE, Batjer HH, Samson D. *Intracranial Arteriovenous Malformations*. Informa Health-Care; 2006

Morris P. *Practical Neuroangiography*, 2nd ed. Lippincott Williams & Wilkins; 2006

Stieg PE, Batjer HH, Samson D. *Surgical Neuroangiography: Vol. 1 Clinical Vascular Anatomy and Variations*, 2nd ed. Springer; 2001

References

1. Kaplan HA, Aronson SM, Browder EJ. Vascular malformatons of the brain. An anatomical study. J Neurosurg 1961;18:630–635
2. Fleetwood IG, Steinberg GK. Arteriovenous malformations. Lancet 2002;359(9309): 863–873
3. Al-Shahi R, Fang JS, Lewis SC, Warlow CP. Prevalence of adults with brain arteriovenous malformations: a community based study in Scotland using capture-recapture analysis. J Neurol Neurosurg Psychiatry 2002;73(5):547–551
4. Michelson WJ. Natural history and pathophysiology of arteriovenous malformations. Clin Neurosurg 1979;26:307–313
5. McCormick WF, Schochet SS Jr. *Atlas of Cerebrovascular Disease.* Philadelphia: WB Saunders Co; 1976:422
6. McCormick WF. Classification, pathology, and natural history of angiomas of the central nervous system. Wkly Update Neurol Neurosurg 1978;14:2–7
7. Mullan S, Mojtahedi S, Johnson DL, Macdonald RL. Embryological basis of some aspects of cerebral vascular fistulas and malformations. J Neurosurg 1996;85(1):1–8
8. van Beijnum J, van der Worp HB, Schippers HM, et al. Familial occurrence of brain arteriovenous malformations: a systematic review. J Neurol Neurosurg Psychiatry 2007;78(11):1213–1217
9. Ezura M, Kagawa S. Spontaneous disappearance of a huge cerebral arteriovenous malformation: case report. Neurosurgery 1992;30(4):595–599
10. Chaloupka JC, Huddle DC. Classification of vascular malformations of the central nervous system. Neuroimaging Clin N Am 1998;8(2):295–321
11. Lasjaunias PL. *Vascular Diseases in Neonates, Infants, and Children: Interventional Neuroradiology Management.* Springer-Verlag; 1997:51–65
12. Yasargil MG. Pathological considerations. In: Yasargil MG, ed. *Microneurosurgery: AVM of the Brain, History, Embryology, Pathological Considerations, Hemodynamics, Diagnostic Studies.* Thieme Verlag; 1987:49–211
13. Brown RD Jr, Wiebers DO, Torner JC, O'Fallon WM. Frequency of intracranial hemorrhage as a presenting symptom and subtype analysis: a population-based study of intracranial vascular malformations in Olmsted County, Minnesota. J Neurosurg 1996;85(1):29–32
14. Maeda K, Kurita H, Nakamura T, et al. Occurrence of severe vasospasm following intraventricular hemorrhage from an arteriovenous malformation. Report of two cases. J Neurosurg 1997;87(3):436–439
15. Brown RD Jr, Wiebers DO, Forbes G, et al. The natural history of unruptured intracranial arteriovenous malformations. J Neurosurg 1988;68(3):352–357
16. Wilkins RH. Natural history of intracranial vascular malformations: a review. Neurosurgery 1985;16(3):421–430
17. Mast H, Mohr JP, Osipov A, et al. 'Steal' is an unestablished mechanism for the clinical presentation of cerebral arteriovenous malformations. Stroke 1995;26(7):1215–1220
18. Carter LP, Gumerlock MK. Steal and cerebral arteriovenous malformations. Stroke 1995;26(12):2371–2372
19. Nornes H, Grip A. Hemodynamic aspects of cerebral arteriovenous malformations. J Neurosurg 1980;53(4):456–464
20. Miyasaka Y, Kurata A, Tanaka R, et al. Mass effect caused by clinically unruptured cerebral arteriovenous malformations. Neurosurgery 1997;41(5):1060–1063, discussion 1063–1064
21. Cloft HJ, Joseph GJ, Dion JE. Risk of cerebral angiography in patients with subarachnoid hemorrhage, cerebral aneurysm, and arteriovenous malformation: a meta-analysis. Stroke 1999;30(2):317–320
22. Spetzler RF, Martin NA. A proposed grading system for arteriovenous malformations. J Neurosurg 1986;65(4):476–483
23. Schaller C, Schramm J, Haun D. Significance of factors contributing to surgical complications and to late outcome after elective surgery of cerebral arteriovenous malformations. J Neurol Neurosurg Psychiatry 1998;65(4):547–554

24. ApSimon HT, Reef H, Phadke RV, Popovic EA. A population-based study of brain arteriovenous malformation: long-term treatment outcomes. Stroke 2002;33(12):2794–2800
25. Fults D, Kelly DL Jr. Natural history of arteriovenous malformations of the brain: a clinical study. Neurosurgery 1984;15(5):658–662
26. Graf CJ, Perret GE, Torner JC. Bleeding from cerebral arteriovenous malformations as part of their natural history. J Neurosurg 1983;58(3):331–337
27. Brown RD Jr, Wiebers DO, Forbes GS. Unruptured intracranial aneurysms and arteriovenous malformations: frequency of intracranial hemorrhage and relationship of lesions. J Neurosurg 1990;73(6):859–863
28. Ondra SL, Troupp H, George ED, Schwab K. The natural history of symptomatic arteriovenous malformations of the brain: a 24-year follow-up assessment. J Neurosurg 1990;73(3):387–391
29. Kondziolka D, McLaughlin MR, Kestle JRW. Simple risk predictions for arteriovenous malformation hemorrhage. Neurosurgery 1995;37(5):851–855
30. Brown RD Jr. Simple risk predictions for arteriovenous malformation hemorrhage. Neurosurgery 2000;46(4):1024 Letter
31. Han PP, Ponce FA, Spetzler RF. Intention-to-treat analysis of Spetzler-Martin grades IV and V arteriovenous malformations: natural history and treatment paradigm. J Neurosurg 2003;98(1):3–7
32. Stapf C, Mohr JP, Pile-Spellman J, Solomon RA, Sacco RL, Connolly ES Jr. Epidemiology and natural history of arteriovenous malformations. Neurosurg Focus 2001;11(5):e1
33. Sekhon LHS, Morgan MK, Spence I, Weber NC. Chronic cerebral hypoperfusion: pathological and behavioral consequences. Neurosurgery 1997;40(3):548–556
34. Hamilton MG, Spetzler RF. The prospective application of a grading system for arteriovenous malformations. Neurosurgery 1994;34(1):2–6, discussion 6–7
35. Sisti MB, Kader A, Stein BM. Microsurgery for 67 intracranial arteriovenous malformations less than 3 cm in diameter. J Neurosurg 1993;79(5):653–660
36. Fiorella D, Albuquerque FC, Woo HH, McDougall CG, Rasmussen PA. The role of neuroendovascular therapy for the treatment of brain arteriovenous malformations. Neurosurgery 2006 Nov;59(5 Suppl 3):S163–177, discussion S3–13.
37. Dabus G, Adel JG, Miller JW, Parkinson RJ, Shaibani A, Bendok BR. Brain arteriovenous malformations: current endovascular strategies. Contemporary Neurosurgery 2006;28:22
38. Valavanis A, Yaşargil MG. The endovascular treatment of brain arteriovenous malformations. Adv Tech Stand Neurosurg 1998;24:131–214
39. Yu SCH, Chan MSY, Lam JMK, Tam PHT, Poon WS. Complete obliteration of intracranial arteriovenous malformation with endovascular cyanoacrylate embolization: initial success and rate of permanent cure. AJNR Am J Neuroradiol 2004;25(7):1139–1143
40. Yu SC, Chan MS, Lam JM, Tam PH, Poon WS. Complete obliteration of intracranial arteriovenous malformation with endovascular cyanoacrylate embolization: initial success and rate of permanent cure. AJNR Am J Neuroradiol 2004;25(7):1139–1143
41. Kwon Y, Jeon SR, Kim JH, et al. Analysis of the causes of treatment failure in gamma knife radiosurgery for intracranial arteriovenous malformations. J Neurosurg 2000;93(Suppl 3):104–106
42. Lunsford LD, Kondziolka D, Flickinger JC, et al. Stereotactic radiosurgery for arteriovenous malformations of the brain. J Neurosurg 1991;75(4):512–524
43. Gobin YP, Laurent A, Merienne L, et al. Treatment of brain arteriovenous malformations by embolization and radiosurgery. J Neurosurg 1996;85(1):19–28
44. Manninen PH, Gignac EM, Gelb AW, Lownie SP. Anesthesia for interventional neuroradiology. J Clin Anesth 1995;7(6):448–452
45. Debrun GM, Aletich V, Ausman JI, Charbel F, Dujovny M. Embolization of the nidus of brain arteriovenous malformations with n-butyl cyanoacrylate. Neurosurgery 1997;40(1):112–120, discussion 120–121
46. Wikholm G, Lundqvist C, Svendsen P. The Göteborg cohort of embolized cerebral arteriovenous malformations: a 6-year follow-up. Neurosurgery 2001;49(4):799–805, discussion 805–806

47. The n-BCA Trial Investigators. N-Butyl cyanoacrylate emblization of cerebral arteriovenous malformation: results of a prospective, randomized, multi-center trial. AJNR Am J Neuroradiol 2002;23:748–755

48. Linfante I, Wakhloo AK. Brain aneurysms and arteriovenous malformations: advancements and emerging treatments in endovascular embolization. Stroke 2007;38(4): 1411–1417

49. Wakhloo AK, Perlow A, Linfante I, et al. Transvenous n-butyl-cyanoacrylate infusion for complex dural carotid cavernous fistulas: technical considerations and clinical outcome. AJNR Am J Neuroradiol 2005;26(8):1888–1897

50. Lieber BB, Wakhloo AK, Siekmann R, Gounis MJ. Acute and chronic swine rete arteriovenous malformation models: effect of ethiodal and glacial acetic acid on penetration, dispersion, and injection force of N-butyl 2-cyanoacrylate. AJNR Am J Neuroradiol 2005;26(7):1707–1714

51. Taki W, Yonekawa Y, Iwata H, Uno A, Yamashita K, Amemiya H. A new liquid material for embolization of arteriovenous malformations. AJNR Am J Neuroradiol 1990; 11(1):163–168

52. Terada T, Nakamura Y, Nakai K, et al. Embolization of arteriovenous malformations with peripheral aneurysms using ethylene vinyl alcohol copolymer. Report of three cases. J Neurosurg 1991;75(4):655–660

53. Weber W, Kis B, Siekmann R, Kuehne D. Endovascular treatment of intracranial arteriovenous malformations with Onyx: technical aspects. AJNR Am J Neuroradiol 2007;28(2):371–377

54. Murayama Y, Viñuela F, Ulhoa A, et al. Nonadhesive liquid embolic agent for cerebral arteriovenous malformations: preliminary histopathological studies in swine rete mirabile. Neurosurgery 1998;43(5):1164–1175

55. Akin ED, Perkins E, Ross IB. Surgical handling characteristics of an ethylene vinyl alcohol copolymer compared with N-butyl cyanoacrylate used for embolization of vessels in an arteriovenous malformation resection model in swine. J Neurosurg 2003;98(2):366–370

56. Jahan R, Murayama Y, Gobin YP, Duckwiler GR, Vinters HV, Viñuela F. Embolization of arteriovenous malformations with Onyx: clinicopathological experience in 23 patients. Neurosurgery 2001;48(5):984–995, discussion 995–997

57. Natarajan SK, Ghodke B, Britz GW, Born DE, Sekhar LN. Multimodality treatment of brain arteriovenous malformations with microsurgery after embolization with Onyx: single-center experience and technical nuances. Neurosurgery 2008;62(6):1213–1225, discussion 1225–1226

58. Kelly ME, Turner R, Gonugunta V, Rasmussen PA, Woo HH, Fiorella D. Monoral snare technique for the retrieval of an adherent microcatheter from an Onyx cast: technical case report. Neurosurgery 2008;63[ONS Suppl 1]:ONSE91

59. Fournier D, ter Brugge KG, Willinsky R, Lasjaunias P, Montanera W. Endovascular treatment of intracerebral arteriovenous malformations: experience in 49 cases. J Neurosurg 1991;75(2):228–233

60. Pe'rez-Higueras A, Rossi Lopez R, Quinones Taria D. Endovascular treatment of cerebral AVM: our experience with Onyx. Interv Neuroradiol 2005;11:141–157

61. Pierot L, Januel AC, Herbreteau D, et al. Endovascular treatment of brain arteriovenous malformations using Onyx: preliminary results of a prospective multicenter study. Interv Neuroradiol 2005;11:159–164

62. Tevah J, Huete I. Endovascular treatment of cerebral AVMs with a new material: Onyx. Interv Neuroradiol 2005;11(Suppl 1):165–170

63. van Rooij WJ, Sluzewski M, Beute GN. Brain AVM embolization with Onyx. AJNR Am J Neuroradiol 2007;28(1):172–177, discussion 178

64. Song DL, Leng B, Xu B, Wang QH, Chen XC, Zhou LF. Clinical experience of 70 cases of cerebral arteriovenous malformation embolization with Onyx, a novel liquid embolic agent. [in Chinese] Zhonghua Wai Ke Za Zhi 2007;45(4):223–225

65. Mounayer C, Hammami N, Piotin M, et al. Nidal embolization of brain arteriovenous malformations using Onyx in 94 patients. AJNR Am J Neuroradiol 2007;28(3):518–523

66. Weber W, Kis B, Siekmann R, Jans P, Laumer R, Kühne D. Preoperative embolization of intracranial arteriovenous malformations with Onyx. Neurosurgery 2007;61(2):244–252, discussion 252–254

67. Panagiotopoulos V, Gizewski E, Asgari S, Regel J, Forsting M, Wanke I. Embolization of intracranial arteriovenous malformations with ethylene-vinyl alcohol copolymer (Onyx). AJNR Am J Neuroradiol 2009;30:99–106

68. Picard L, Da Costa E, Anxionnat R, et al. Acute spontaneous hemorrhage after embolization of brain arteriovenous malformation with N-butyl cyanoacrylate. J Neuroradiol 2001;28(3):147–165

69. Friedman WA, Bova FJ, Mendenhall WM. Linear accelerator radiosurgery for arteriovenous malformations: the relationship of size to outcome. J Neurosurg 1995;82(2):180–189

70. The Arteriovenous Malformation Study Group. Arteriovenous malformations of the brain in adults. N Engl J Med 1999;340(23):1812–1818

71. Jafar JJ, Davis AJ, Berenstein A, Choi IS, Kupersmith MJ. The effect of embolization with N-butyl cyanoacrylate prior to surgical resection of cerebral arteriovenous malformations. J Neurosurg 1993;78(1):60–69

72. Sasaki T, Kurita H, Saito I, et al. Arteriovenous malformations in the basal ganglia and thalamus: management and results in 101 cases. J Neurosurg 1998;88:285–292

73. Pollock BE, Gorman DA, Schomberg PJ, Kline RW. The Mayo Clinic gamma knife experience: indications and initial results. Mayo Clin Proc 1999;74(1):5–13

74. Pollock BE, Flickinger JC. A proposed radiosurgery-based grading system for arteriovenous malformations. J Neurosurg 2002;96(1):79–85

75. Colombo F, Pozza F, Chierego G, Casentini L, De Luca G, Francescon P. Linear accelerator radiosurgery of cerebral arteriovenous malformations: an update. Neurosurgery 1994;34(1):14–20, discussion 20–21

76. Karlsson B, Lax I, Söderman M. Factors influencing the risk for complications following gamma knife radiosurgery of cerebral arteriovenous malformations. Radiother Oncol 1997;43(3):275–280

77. Friedman WA, Blatt DL, Bova FJ, Buatti JM, Mendenhall WM, Kubilis PS. The risk of hemorrhage after radiosurgery for arteriovenous malformations. J Neurosurg 1996;84(6):912–919

78. Maruyama K, Kawahara N, Shin M, et al. The risk of hemorrhage after radiosurgery for cerebral arteriovenous malformations. N Engl J Med 2005;352(2):146–153

79. Nataf F, Ghossoub M, Schlienger M, Moussa R, Meder JF, Roux FX. Bleeding after radiosurgery for cerebral arteriovenous malformations. Neurosurgery 2004;55(2):298–305, discussion 305–306

80. Pollock BE, Flickinger JC, Lunsford LD, Maitz A, Kondziolka D. Factors associated with successful arteriovenous malformation radiosurgery. Neurosurgery 1998;42(6):1239–1244, discussion 1244–1247

81. Karlsson B, Lindquist C, Steiner L. Prediction of obliteration after gamma knife surgery for cerebral arteriovenous malformations. Neurosurgery 1997;40(3):425–430, discussion 430–431

82. Al-Shahi R, Bhattacharya JJ, Currie DG, et al.; Scottish Intracranial Vascular Malformation Study Collaborators. Prospective, population-based detection of intracranial vascular malformations in adults: the Scottish Intracranial Vascular Malformation Study (SIVMS). Stroke 2003;34(5):1163–1169

83. Stapf C, Mast H, Sciacca RR, et al.; New York Islands AVM Study Collaborators. The New York Islands AVM Study: design, study progress, and initial results. Stroke 2003;34(5):e29–e33

Intracranial Arteriovenous Fistulae

Stacey Quintero Wolfe and Mohammad Ali Aziz-Sultan

Etiology

Intracranial arteriovenous fistulae are of two main types: carotid-cavernous fistulae and dural arteriovenous fistulae. Carotid-cavernous fistulae (CCF) are abnormal vascular connections between the internal and/or external carotid artery and the cavernous sinus. Dural arteriovenous fistulae (DAVF) are direct connections between the arterial and venous systems within the dura, which bypass the capillary bed. Dural arterial feeders can be from the internal carotid artery, external carotid artery, or vertebral system; they most commonly connect into one of the dural sinuses.

Classification

CCFs can be classified according to various criteria: pathogenetically (traumatic versus spontaneous fistulae), hemodynamically (high- versus low-flow fistulae) or angiographically (direct versus dural fistulae), but they are most commonly described according to the Barrow classification (**Table 15.1**).[1] Type A CCFs are by far the most common (72%); Type D is the most common low-flow CCF (21%).[2] Direct CCFs usually occur secondary to trauma causing carotid laceration or rupture of a cavernous carotid artery aneurysm. Indirect CCFs are acquired lesions, thought to originate from an insult to a dural venous sinus that stimulates an inflammatory response, with subsequent neovascularization, angiogenesis, and the development

Table 15.1 Barrow Classification of Carotid-Cavernous Fistulae

Type	Fistulous vessels	Comments
A	Carotid artery to cavernous sinus (CS)	Direct, high flow, most common
B	Dural ICA branches to CS: Meningohypophyseal trunk (66%), inferolateral trunk (30%)	Indirect, low flow
C	ECA branches to CS: internal max (67%), middle mening (59%), accessory mening (31%), ascending pharyn (24%)	Indirect, low flow
D	Both ICA and ECA branches	Indirect, most common low flow

of pathological shunts at the arteriolar level. Alternatively, the fistula may be the initial event, with turbulent arterialized blood flow in the dural venous sinus inciting a process of thrombosis. Another theory supposes the existence of small dural channels between arteries and a venous sinus that may enlarge, should that sinus thrombose. A third theory suggests that spontaneous low-flow CCFs form after the rupture of a dural artery traversing the cavernous sinus. Indirect dural CCFs most commonly occur in perimenopausal women, implying a hormonal influence. In the largest series of studies on indirect CCFs to date (n = 135), Meyers reports that 73% occurred in women with a mean age of 60 years.[3]

DAVFs may be classified according to their pattern of flow (**Fig. 15.1**). Djindjian first classified DAVF according to angioarchitecture in 1978 (**Table 15.2**).[4] In 1995, Cognard (**Table 15.3**) further classified both cranial and spinal arteriovenous fistulae with prognostic and treatment implications.[5] Borden simplified the classification, emphasizing that the major factor in predicting a clinical course centers on the presence of cortical venous drainage and direction of flow (**Table 15.4**).[6] Unlike drainage into the sinuses, cortical veins are not protected by the dura and cannot withstand arterial pressures. Therefore, DAVFs with cortical drainage are at a higher risk for rupture and hemorrhage.

Dural arteriovenous fistulae can occur from direct trauma, sinus occlusion, tumor invasion, vascular collagen diseases, or infections involving the sinus. Inflammatory changes from these conditions can cause angiogenesis, demonstrated by high concentrations of vascular endothelial growth factor (VEGF) found near fistulae. There are also embryological theories, which state that there are primitive direct connections between the arteries and veins that can reopen in the setting of an inflammatory response or a sinus occlusion. Dural fistulae can present anywhere the dura is in proximity to venous drainage (**Fig. 15.1**), but they are usually classified by several common locations: transverse/sigmoid sinuses (**Fig. 15.2**), cavernous sinus (**Fig. 15.3**), superior sagittal sinus (SSS) (**Fig. 15.4**), anterior fossa (ethmoidal) (**Fig. 15.5**), petrosal (**Fig. 15.6**) and sylvian fissure/middle fossa.

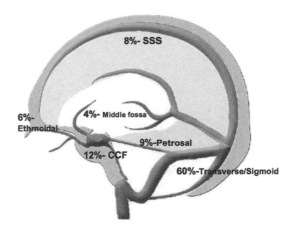

Fig. 15.1 This figure shows the relative distribution of intracranial DAVFs. Most are located in the transverse and sigmoid sinuses and carry a low risk of intracranial hemorrhage, whereas DAVFs found in the ethmoidal, middle fossa, and petrosal regions often present with hemorrhage.

Table 15.2 Djindjian DAVF Classification

Type I: Drainage into a venous sinus
Type II: Drainage into a venous sinus with reflux into cortical veins
Type III: Drainage into cortical veins
Type IV: Presence of venous lakes

Djindjian R, Merland JJ, Theron J. *Super-Selective Arteriography of the External Carotid Artery.* Springer-Verlag; 1978:606–628

Table 15.3 Cognard DAVF Classification

Type I: Anterograde drainage into a venous sinus
Type IIa: Retrograde drainage into a venous sinus
Type IIb: Anterograde drainage into a venous sinus and cortical veins
Type III: Drainage into cortical veins only
Type IV: Drainage into cortical veins only with venous ectasias

Cognard C, Gobin Y, Pierot L, et al. Cerebral dural arteriovenous fistulas: clinical and angiographic correlation with a revised classification of venous drainage. Radiology 1995;194:671–680

Table 15.4 Borden DAVF Classification

Type I: Antegrade flow into a venous sinus
Type II: Retrograde flow into a venous sinus
Type III: Retrograde into cortical veins

Borden JA, Wu JK, Shucart WA. A proposed classification for spinal and cranial dural arteriovenous fistulous malformations and implications for treatment. J Neurosurg 1995;82:166–179

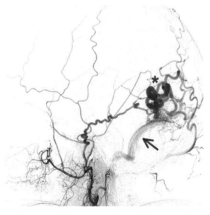

Fig. 15.2 A lateral angiogram of the external carotid artery showing a DAVF fed by the posterior limb of the middle meningeal artery draining into the transverse sinus (*arrow*) with cortical venous drainage (*asterisk*).

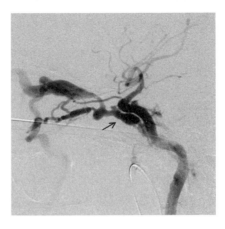

Fig. 15.3 Lateral angiogram of a direct CCF showing immediate filling of the cavernous sinus (*arrow*) with drainage into the superior and inferior orbital veins through a tear in the carotid artery.

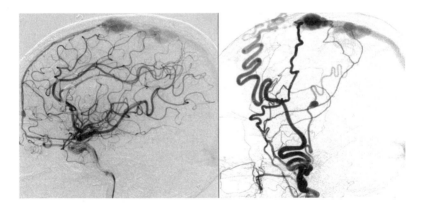

Fig. 15.4 Lateral angiogram of the internal (left) and external carotid artery (right) showing a DAVF fed by the anterior meningeal artery (left) and the superior temporal and middle meningeal arteries (right) draining into the superior sagittal sinus. Note the common fistulous point into a venous varix.

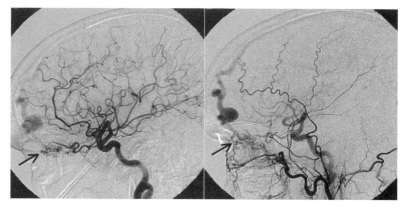

Fig. 15.5 Lateral angiograms of the right internal (left) and external (right) carotid arteries showing an ethmoidal fistula filling from the ophthalmic (left) and internal maxillary artery (right), with the common venous drainage to a frontal cortical vein and into the anterior SSS. Note the common fistulous point on both injections (*arrow*).

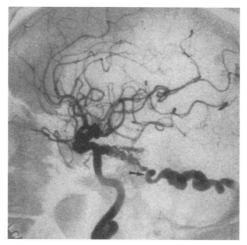

Fig. 15.6 A lateral angiogram showing a petrosal fistula filling from the tentorial artery through the tentorium into the petrosal vein (*arrow* shows the fistulous point).

Presentation

CCFs commonly present with ophthalmological symptoms, such as proptosis, chemosis, conjunctival injection, diplopia, secondary glaucoma, and loss of vision (**Table 15.5**). These symptoms are related to the degree of shunting and the route of venous drainage. They occur as a result of venous hypertension, due to high-pressure arterial flow invading a low-pressure venous system. Headache may occur due to engorgement or partial thrombosis of the cavernous sinus, with stretching of the dura, or due to cortical venous drainage, with cerebral venous hypertension. Subarachnoid or intracerebral hemorrhage from rupture of arterialized cortical

Table 15.5   Presenting Symptoms of CCFs

Proptosis
Chemosis
Conjunctival injection
Diplopia
Secondary glaucoma
Loss of visual acuity or perception

veins may also occur as the presenting symptom. Although retrograde cerebral venous drainage is more common in direct, high-flow fistulae, Meyers et al. report that 31% of patients with indirect CCFs presented with this symptom,[3] a significant risk factor for hemorrhage

Patients with dural fistulae can present with several different clinical scenarios, ranging from asymptomatic presentation to fatal intracerebral hemorrhages. The most common presentation is pulsatile tinnitus, which the physician may auscultate as a bruit. Other presentations can include headaches or deteriorating mentation from the effects of venous congestion. Hydrocephalus may occur as a result of obstructive outflow from a large venous varix, or impaired CSF drainage due to high venous pressures. The most ominous sign is the presence of cortical venous drainage. DAVFs that drain into cortical veins are at high risk of presenting with intracerebral or subarachnoid hemorrhage.

Anatomy

The cavernous sinus is a contiguous network of multiple venous sinusoids sur rounded by a double leaflet of dura. A fibrous diaphragm divides the cavernous sinus into inferoanterior and superoposterior chambers, but most connect either anteriorly or posteriorly through the intercavernous sinus.

The venous drainage of the cavernous sinus includes the inferior petrosal sinus (IPS), basilar plexus, and, less commonly, the superior petrosal sinus posteriorly (**Fig. 15.7**). The IPS drains directly into the internal jugular vein in only 45% of cases and into the cervical plexus via intermediate veins in the remainder.[7] Due to the proximity of Dorello's canal to the IPS, wire navigation, especially in an unopacified or thrombosed IPS, can lead to damage of the abducens nerve. Anterior venous drainage is composed of the superior ophthalmic vein (SOV) and inferior ophthalmic vein (IOV) as they flow toward the angular and facial vein. In a minority of cases, lateral connections may occur, with inflow from the superficial middle cerebral vein.

Diagnosis

Dural fistulae can be imaged using MRA/MRV or CTA, looking for either enlarged feeding arteries or thrombosed or engorged draining veins. The definitive method for diagnosis, however, is angiography, which is also necessary for grading and treatment planning. Fistula location, flow pattern, angioarchitecture and drainage can be visualized and used to predict the clinical course.

Evidence-Based Medicine

Carotid-Cavernous Fistulae

To date, no randomized clinical trials have evaluated the treatment and outcome of CCFs. Clinical studies regarding the treatment of these lesions will be discussed in the "Technique" section.

Dural Arteriovenous Fistulae

1. Davies et al. of the Toronto group followed 102 patients for an average of 33 months and found that 81% of patients treated conservatively had symptom resolution or improvement, compared with 86% of treated patients.[8]
2. Sarma et al. of the Toronto group found that less than 1% of patients develop transformation of benign dural venous drainage to cortical venous drainage.[9] It appears safe to treat benign DAVFs conservatively, with periodic clinical and angiographic follow-up. Assessment should occur if there are any changes in symptoms, including disappearance of a bruit, which may signal a change in the venous drainage and potential cortical venous drainage.
3. Van Dijk et al. from the Toronto group describe the natural history of DAVFs with cortical venous drainage.[10] Twenty of 118 patients with aggressive DAVFs refused treatment or underwent only partial treatment and were followed for an average of 4.3 years. Of these patients, 35% suffered an intracranial hemorrhage, an additional 30% experienced nonhemorrhagic neurologic decline, and there was a 45% mortality rate. This resulted in an annual event rate of 15% (hemorrhagic 8.1% and nonhemorrhagic 6.9%) and an annual mortality rate of 10.4%. Although this is a small cohort of patients, the aggressive nature of DAVFs with cortical venous drainage is clear, and treatment should be strongly encouraged.
4. Duffau et al. from the Salpetriere Hospital in France report a high rate of early rebleeding in DAVFs with cortical venous drainage.[11] Twenty patients presented with hemorrhage and, within the first two weeks following the hemorrhage, 35% experienced a second intracranial hemorrhage.
5. Davies et al. of the Toronto group report their series of 23 patients with aggressive DAVFs (cortical venous drainage) undergoing surgical resection or disconnection to have a complication rate of 13%,[8] while 29% of patients undergoing conservative treatment died due to intracranial hemorrhage during the study period.
6. Cognard et al. report their results of 30 DAVFs treated with Onyx embolization.[5] Ten patients had type II, 8 had type III, and 12 had type IV Cognard fistulae. Sixteen presented with hemorrhage. Complete angiographic cure was obtained in 24 cases. Two (6.7%) clinical complications occurred: rebleeding in one patient due to draining vein thrombosis and a transient cranial nerve palsy in a second patient.

Preprocedural Preparation

If arterial access will be through the internal carotid or vertebral arteries, patients should be heparinized during the procedure. Navigation of the external carotid circulation or the venous system does not require anticoagulation. Some embolic materials, such as Onyx or bioactive coils, can lead to an inflammatory response and a course of perioperative steroids may be helpful.

Equipment

Sheath and Guide Catheter

Regardless of the route, it is important to provide proximal catheter support, typically with a 6 Fr sheath (65 cm) and an Envoy (DePuy Orthopaedics, Warsaw, IN) guide catheter (5 or 6 Fr) tri-axial system. The venous anatomy is often tortuous, and catheterization may involve traversing thrombosed vessels. In a transvenous approach, using a 4 Fr Terumo catheter (Terumo Cardiovascular Systems, Ann Arbor, MI) to access distal veins or smaller sinuses, such as the inferior petrosal sinus, may be helpful. We use a similar setup for arterial approaches.

Wire

An angled 0.038 hydrophilic glide wire can be used to navigate the guide catheter. The stiffer version can be used to "drill" through areas of stenosis. The "buddy wire" technique may be used to help prevent kick-back of the guide catheter by placing a second wire (0.018–0.035) within the guide catheter alongside the microcatheter.

Microcatheter

The method of treatment dictates the microcatheter selection. The use of coils requires a microcatheter capable of accepting 10 to 18 system coils. If the procedure uses liquid embolics, a DMSO-compatible microcatheter (for Onyx) and microcatheters built to withstand the pressure of embolization (Onyx and n-BCA), must be used. For compartmentalized, stenotic venous access, a larger, stiffer microcatheter may be helpful. If the vessel is small or tortuous, a smaller, more navigable microcatheter (0.010) may be helpful.

Microwires

Unlike access for most intracranial lesions, in the transvenous approach, stiff microwires may be more helpful, especially in cases of venous stenosis or occluded varices. In the scenario of dura-encased arteries and venous sinuses, these stiffer wires are relatively safe.

Embolic Material

The treatment objective, rate of flow, and location of the microcatheter dictate which devices can be used. Distal embolization into small branching arterial feeders can be better achieved with a liquid embolic such as n-BCA (mixed 1:2 to 1:4) or Onyx (18 rather than 34). Local occlusion can be best achieved with coils or a combination of coils with a liquid embolic (n-BCA 1:1 or 1:2 or Onyx 34). PVA is no longer favored as it is associated with higher rates of recanalization.

Anesthesia

General anesthesia is preferred in most cases of DAVF treatment because their complexity requires a prolonged procedure time. Manipulation and embolization within dural vessels, as well as use of DMSO, can be extremely painful. Visualization and accuracy are also better maintained under general anesthesia.

Technique

Carotid-Cavernous Fistulae

Endovascular embolization is the preferred treatment for CCFs. Direct CCFs were treated primarily transarterially when detachable balloons were available. Currently, transarterial or transvenous embolization with balloon reconstruction may allow coil obliteration of the cavernous sinus, but this rarely reconstructs the arterial wall. Liquid embolics may be used for remodeling of the fistulous points, but these products have the potential for distal embolization due to high flow. Onyx 500 is a highly viscous liquid embolic that, with balloon remodeling, allows for precise, controlled embolization. As opposed to other liquid embolics, its viscous properties allow for focal embolization with less embolic material to accomplish remodeling of the carotid artery and fistulous point. Covered stents are another excellent alternative, if there is minimal tortuosity that allows navigation of these stiff devices.

The transarterial route for indirect CCF is often unsuccessful, as embolization of meningeal branches is difficult and dangerous because of their small caliber and vast anastomoses. The transvenous approach for embolization was pioneered by Debrun in the 1980s and quickly became the treatment of choice.[2] The IPS is the simplest and shortest venous route to the cavernous sinus possible in approximately 60% of cases.[7] When the IPS cannot be visualized angiographically, a channel can usually be found by probing with a steerable guidewire, but the success rate is only 37.5%.[7] When the IPS is not accessible, the basilar plexus or the facial and angular veins are other endovenous options (**Fig. 15.7**). Since the removal of balloons from the market, coil embolization has been the standard method of cavernous sinus occlusion. Liquid adhesives, such as n-BCA and Onyx, may be used through the arterial or venous side and have the ability to permeate the cavernous sinus, although they carry the risk of embolic complications and stroke. More recently, the use of Onyx is proving extremely promising, due to its ability to permeate deeply into channels.

If none of these transvenous routes can be successfully cannulated, direct surgical cannulation of the SOV is an excellent alternative (refer to Chapter 7). Briefly, a 2 cm incision is made medially in the skin crease above the upper eyelid. An operating microscope is used to incise the orbicularis oculi muscle and open the orbital septum, under which the arterialized SOV is found. A 4 Fr vascular sheath is placed, and embolization of the cavernous sinus may then be performed through the SOV. Although percutaneous treatment of a dural CCF via deep orbital puncture of the SOV was described, we do not recommend this technique, with its unnecessarily high risk of damage to orbital structures.

Complications specific to transvenous embolization include over-packing the cavernous sinus (with resultant cranial nerve palsies), dissection, vessel perforation, and embolic complications. The abducens nerve is especially sensitive to pressure from over-packing, as it is fixed within the trabeculae of the sinus. Meyers et al. reported their permanent procedure-related morbidity to be 2.3%.[3]

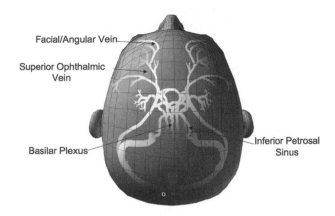

Fig. 15.7 Endovenous routes to the cavernous sinus include the inferior petrosal sinus, basilar plexus, facial vein, and superior ophthalmic vein.

Dural Arteriovenous Fistulae

Unlike arteriovenous malformations, which rupture if the venous outflow is occluded early, dural fistulae thrombose and occlude when the venous drainage is obliterated by surgical or endovascular means. Due to the ease of localizing the venous drainage and the difficulty in catheterizing small arterial feeders, fistula locations such as ethmoidal and petrosal are best treated surgically. Most other DAVFs are best treated by transvenous, or occasionally transarterial, endovascular techniques.

Treatment of benign dural fistulae, such as those in the transverse sinus that rarely transform into malignant lesions, is usually palliative, performed through a transarterial route. In addition, transarterial embolization should be used in the scenario of direct arteriovenous shunts and may be helpful to better elucidate a DAVF by slowing down the flow. Other than palliation, the most common fistula requiring transarterial embolization is the CCF. Transarterial embolization is only rarely indicated through the intracerebral circulation and carries the risk of stroke from distal embolus or reflux.

Transarterial embolization involves cannulating various branches of the external carotid artery with a microcatheter. The microcatheter should be navigated under roadmap guidance as close to the fistulous point as possible. Once proper position has been reached, a microinjection should be performed to assess the rate and pattern of flow. Depending on the rate of flow and size of the fistula, an embolic agent of proper viscosity can be selected. At times the flow may be rapid, requiring the use of a proximal balloon or coil to slow flow. An alternative method to prevent liquid embolics from traveling distally in the venous circulation may be to place a balloon within the sinus during transarterial embolic injection.

The transvenous route can be used for more definitive therapy of DAVFs, as the durability of treatment lies in occluding the venous side of the fistula. The guide catheter is navigated from the IVC through the atrium into the SVC, then into the innominate and jugular veins through which the sinuses and/or facial vein can be accessed. Navigating the venous system extracranially can be complicated by valves. To navigate past these valves requires some diligence in "probing" with your glide wire or using Valsalva maneuvers to open them. Once within the jugular vein, the microcatheter can be navigated to the fistulous point. The fistulous point is often secluded in the walls of the sinus and can be best visualized by changing the mask of the arterial phase to render the arteries white and the venous phase black. Patience and persistence are often required to catheterize this parallel channel by probing with the micro guide wire, as the microcatheter tends to stay in the main lumen of the sinus. Occasionally, using a microcatheter to travel from the arterial side through the fistula is helpful in defining it. Once the fistulous point is cannulated, several different embolic materials may be used, depending on the rate and pattern of flow seen on the microinjection. If the flow is rapid, a balloon or coil may be used proximally to slow flow. A coil may be used within the sinus to act as a basket and prevent distal flow of the liquid embolic. Liquid embolics offer the best penetration but may be hazardous if they flow into the main sinus.

Complex fistulae may require a combined arterial and venous approach. With the newer liquid embolic agents, transarterial embolization can be done with a balloon in the venous side to prevent embolizing material into the main venous system. Also, if unable to cure the fistula, it can be slowed down dramatically by embolizing from both the arterial and venous side. This may be especially helpful in cases of severe venous hypertension and global cerebral dysfunction from high-flow fistulae.

After completion of embolization, it is important to restudy the remaining vessels. By nature, fistulae create a very strong sump effect and may stay open by recruiting other vessels, even though the initial feeders of the fistula have been obliterated. In addition, the DAVF may open channels that had not been visualized at the start of the case. For this reason, follow-up angiography is imperative, and it is usually performed at three months if only arterial obliteration is achieved or at six months if there is confidence in complete venous obliteration.

Postprocedural Care

Patients are sent to an intensive care setting post-embolization. Dramatic changes in hemodynamics from aggressive embolization can lead to intracerebral hemorrhage, requiring the avoidance of hypertension. Embolic material in the venous system may lead to venous infarction. Also, fluid balance should be carefully monitored to prevent potential fluid overload, as these cases may take a long time and involve multiple catheter flushes. A short course of steroids or NSAIDs may aid in pain management since embolic agents may evoke an inflammatory reaction in the surrounding dura, especially when occluding the cavernous sinus for CCFs, in which case this may also offer protection to traversing cranial nerves.

Alternative Therapies

Surgery

Although endovascular therapy is now the primary modality for the treatment of most DAVFs, surgical occlusion, specifically of ethmoidal and petrosal fistulae, is still considered to be the gold standard.

Radiosurgery

Recently, several reports of DAVFs treated with the gamma knife have shown encouraging, albeit incomplete, results. Improvement is seen in most cases, but obliteration is seen in around 60–65%.[12] Radiosurgery may prove to be an excellent adjunctive therapy for inaccessible or incompletely treated DAVFs.

Technical Pearls

1. There is usually a single fistulous point upon which all feeding arteries converge and from which the venous drainage is the same, regardless of which artery is injected. To identify the fistula, look for the point where all venous drainage looks the same on different arterial angiograms.
2. When diagnostic angiography is performed for a direct CCF, an Allcock test (manual compression of the carotid artery in question while injecting the vertebral artery) may help to find the exact fistulous point by removing the overlap of the supraclinoid ICA and allowing the fistula to fill retrograde, through the posterior communicating artery.
3. Standard angiography of DAVFs may lead to a confusing picture of overlapping arteries and veins, making it difficult to pinpoint the fistulous point. The anatomy of a fistula can best be visualized by increasing the frame rate (6/second) to better assess fast-flowing fistulae and then shifting the mask to start at the end of the arterial phase. This renders the arteries white and the veins black. The interface between arteries and venous drainage can then be clearly seen.
4. Many fistulae are found in the wall of the sinus and have multiple septations with compartmentalization. The actual fistulous point may not drain directly into the sinus, but rather exist parallel to the sinus within the dural leaves, which can mislead you into thinking that it is in the same lumen. In cases of transvenous embolization, probing for the fistula from within the lumen of the sinus to find this compartment may be the key to endovascular cure.
5. In a high-flow fistula, use of a balloon within the venous sinus may slow blood flow enough to deliver liquid embolic into the fistulous point without embolization into the sinus or distal venous system. Similarly, a balloon inflated on the arterial side may also slow rapid flow and prevent significant arterial reflux of the liquid embolic agent.
6. To minimize sensitivity of cranial nerves to direct pressure, we give Decadron 10 mg IV before embolization and continue this for 24–48 hours postoperatively. Additionally, NSAIDs may be used for headache associated with sinus thrombosis.

Recommended Reading

Awad IA, Little JR, Akarawi WP, Ahl J. Intracranial dural arteriovenous malformations: factors predisposing to an aggressive neurological course. J Neurosurg 1990;72(6):839–850

Barrow DL, Spector RH, Braun IF, Landman JA, Tindall SC, Tindall GT. Classification and treatment of spontaneous carotid-cavernous sinus fistulas. J Neurosurg 1985;62(2):248–256

Davies MA, Saleh J, ter Brugge K, Willinsky R, Wallace MC. The natural history and management of intracranial dural arteriovenous fistulae: Parts 1 and 2. Benign and aggressive lesions. Interv Neuroradiol 1997;3:295–311

Debrun GM, Viñuela F, Fox AJ, Davis KR, Ahn HS. Indications for treatment and classification of 132 carotid-cavernous fistulas. Neurosurgery 1988;22(2):285–289

Sarma D, ter Brugge K. Management of intracranial dural arteriovenous shunts in adults. Eur J Radiol 2003;46(3):206–220

References

1. Barrow DL, Spector RH, Braun IF, Landman JA, Tindall SC, Tindall GT. Classification and treatment of spontaneous carotid-cavernous sinus fistulas. J Neurosurg 1985;62(2):248–256

2. Debrun GM, Viñuela F, Fox AJ, Davis KR, Ahn HS. Indications for treatment and classification of 132 carotid-cavernous fistulas. Neurosurgery 1988;22(2):285–289

3. Meyers PM, Halbach VV, Dowd CF, et al. Dural carotid cavernous fistula: definitive endovascular management and long-term follow-up. Am J Ophthalmol 2002;134(1):85–92

4. Djindjian R, Merland JJ, Theron J. *Super-Selective Arteriography of the External Carotid Artery.* Springer-Verlag; 1978:606–628

5. Cognard C, Januel AC, Silva NA Jr, Tall P. Endovascular treatment of intracranial dural arteriovenous fistulas with cortical venous drainage: new management using Onyx. AJNR Am J Neuroradiol 2008;29(2):235–241

6. Borden JA, Wu JK, Shucart WA. A proposed classification for spinal and cranial dural arteriovenous fistulous malformations and implications for treatment. J Neurosurg 1995;82(2):166–179

7. Klisch J, Huppertz HJ, Spetzger U, Hetzel A, Seeger W, Schumacher M. Transvenous treatment of carotid cavernous and dural arteriovenous fistulae: results for 31 patients and review of the literature. Neurosurgery 2003;53(4):836–856, discussion 856–857

8. Davies MA, Saleh J, ter Brugge K, Willinsky R, Wallace MC. The natural history and management of intracranial dural arteriovenous fistulae: Parts 1 and 2. Benign and aggressive lesions. Interv Neuroradiol 1997;3:295–311

9. Sarma D, ter Brugge K. Management of intracranial dural arteriovenous shunts in adults. Eur J Radiol 2003;46(3):206–220

10. van Dijk JMC, terBrugge KG, Willinsky RA, Wallace MC. Clinical course of cranial dural arteriovenous fistulas with long-term persistent cortical venous reflux. Stroke 2002;33(5):1233–1236

11. Duffau H, Lopes M, Janosevic V, et al. Early rebleeding from intracranial dural arteriovenous fistulas: report of 20 cases and review of the literature. J Neurosurg 1999;90(1):78–84

12. Friedman JA, Pollock BE, Nichols DA, Gorman DA, Foote RL, Stafford SL. Results of combined stereotactic radiosurgery and transarterial embolization for dural arteriovenous fistulas of the transverse and sigmoid sinuses. J Neurosurg 2001;94(6):886–891

Ischemic Stroke Intervention

Abu Yahia Lodi, Randall C. Edgell, Jason A. Felton, and Michael S. Park

Etiology

Ischemic stroke affects 500,000 to 700,000 patients annually in the United States.[1] The most common etiologies of ischemic stroke are large-artery atherosclerosis (20–30%) cardiac (20–30%), small-vessel or lacunar stroke (20–30%), and cryptogenic stroke. Risk factors associated with atherosclerotic stenoses include hypertension, diabetes, hyperlipidemia, and family history. Stroke risk can be stratified through the presence of symptomatology and degree of stenosis (**Table 16.1**). It is generally thought that atherosclerotic lesions cause stroke through plaque rupture, local platelet aggregation, and finally artery-to-artery embolism. Critical stenoses can lead to cerebral hypoperfusion, resulting in watershed area strokes. Other abnormalities caused by vasculopathies, disorders of coagulation, and systemic conditions can also lead to stroke (**Table 16.2**).

Large-artery atherosclerotic stenosis of the intracranial vessels (ICAD), most commonly through hypoperfusion, is thought to cause 8–10% of ischemic strokes in the United States, an even higher risk for stroke than cervical stenosis, most often in Asian and African Americans. Symptomatic patients with >50% ICAD have approximately a 10% annual risk of ischemic stroke, even when treated with an appropriate antiplatelet agent. This risk increases to 22% in the first year in patients with >70% stenosis and stroke.[2] Atrial fibrillation is the most common cause of cardioembolic stroke, which varies significantly depending on the presence of other comorbid conditions (hypertension, age) and ranges from 2–10%. Other important causes of cardiac embolism are valvular disease, heart failure, and congenital cardiac anomalies. Lacunar infarctions most often occur in the distribution of the perforator arteries of the circle of Willis, commonly as a result of lipohyalinosis, and they are commonly associated with chronic, poorly controlled hypertension. Lacunar infarctions cause dense neurological deficits, due to high density of white matter in small volumes of tissue (<1 cm, brainstem, basal ganglia, and thalamus).[3]

Table 16.1 Stroke Risks

Symptomatology	Stenosis severity	Stroke risk
Asymptomatic	>60%[3]	2% annual[4]
Symptomatic*	50–69%	4% annual
Symptomatic*	>70%[3]	13% in the first year after first stroke/TIA[5]

*Symptomatic usually involves neurological changes or transient ischemic attacks (TIAs).

Table 16.2   Etiology of Stroke

Major etiology of stroke	Specific mechanisms
Embolism	Atherosclerosis, vasculitis, moyamoya, FMD, connective tissue disease, dissection, infection, cardiac tumor/thrombus, arrhythmia, paradoxical cardiac embolism
Hypoperfusion	Cardiac failure, congestive heart failure, cardiac arrhythmia, medication overdose, infection, shock, extra/intracranial vascular disease/stenosis
Focal occlusion	Atherosclerosis of small vessels, vasculitis, vasospasm, angiopathies, arteritis, coagulopathies or hypercoagulable states of multiple causes, platelet dysfunction

Abbreviation: FMD, fibromuscular dysplasia.

Other, less common causes of ischemic stroke include arterial dissection, hypercoagulable states, genetic mutations of the mitochondria and enzymes of glycolysis, and fibromuscular dysplasia. A more extensive review of these and other etiologies is beyond the scope of this text.

Diagnosis

History

The medical history and physical examination taken in the setting of acute stroke, possibly requiring intravenous or intra-arterial thrombolysis, are very different from those taken when evaluating other types of neurological disease. Time is of the essence! The history obtained must be brief and highly focused. The confirmation of an event compatible with an acute vascular event and the time of symptomatic onset are the most crucial pieces of information, as they determine not only the possibility but also the kind of therapy, such as intravenous or intra-arterial thrombolytics or mechanical thrombolysis (see below).

Physical Examination

The physical examination of an acute stroke patient being evaluated for possible endovascular treatment is based on the National Institutes of Health Stroke Scale (NIHSS),[6] a quick, fifteen-item scoring system that includes criteria regarding level of consciousness, attention, cranial nerves, and motor, sensory, cerebellar, and language functioning (**Table 16.3**). If patients have an NIHSS score greater than 10, it is suggestive of large-artery occlusions, with an 80–90% sensitivity and specificity (**Fig. 16.1**).[4,5]

In the subacute or chronic phase of ischemic stroke, the modified Rankin scale (MRS) can be used to measure the degree of global disability or dependence in patients (**Table 16.4**).[4,5] In addition to a thorough neurologic assessment, auscultation of the carotid arteries for bruits and an examination of the heart for murmurs (e.g., valve abnormalities) and arrhythmias are also necessary.

Table 16.3   National Institutes of Health Stroke Scales (NIHSS)

Level of consciousness	0–3 points
Orientation	0–2 points
Responses to commands	0–2 points
Eye movements	0–2 points
Visual fields	0–3 points
Facial motor activity	0–3 points
RUE motor activity	0–4 points
LUE motor activity	0–4 points
RLE motor activity	0–4 points
LLE motor activity	0–4 points
Sensory function	0–2 points
Limb ataxia	0–2 points
Articulation	0–2 points
Language	0–3 points
Neglect	0–2 points

Abbreviations: LLE, left lower extremity; LUE, left uppper extremity; RLE, right lower extremity; RUE, right upper extremity.

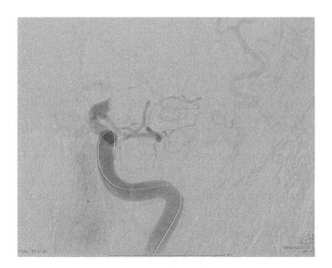

Fig. 16.1   Carotid terminus occlusion.

Table 16.4 Modified Rankin Scale

0	No symptoms.
1	No significant disability. Able to carry out all usual activities, despite some symptoms.
2	Slight disability. Able to look after own affairs without assistance, but unable to carry out all previous activities.
3	Moderate disability. Requires some help, but able to walk unassisted.
4	Moderately severe disability. Unable to attend to own bodily needs without assistance and unable to walk unassisted.
5	Severe disability. Requires constant nursing care and attention, bedridden, incontinent.
6	Dead.

Laboratory Studies

Basic laboratory studies, including serum creatinine, glucose, platelet count, and coagulation studies, should be sent immediately (**Table 16.5**). Because waiting for the results of these tests can delay possible intervention more often than neuroimaging will, they should therefore be prioritized.

Imaging

Computed tomographic (CT) imaging is usually the most readily available and economical mode of acute stroke imaging. Non-contrast imaging allows rapid differentiation between ischemic and hemorrhagic stroke. It is able to detect ischemia with a sensitivity of 65% and specificity of 90% after 6 hours of stroke onset but appears normal in over one third of patients with acute ischemia.[7-9] Early ischemic changes are also weakly correlated with poor outcome after IA chemical thrombolysis. These changes include blurring of the gray-white junction in the cortex or basal ganglia and/or subtle sulcal effacement in the ischemic territory. In large-artery occlusive stroke, it is sometimes possible to identify a linear or circular hyperdensity corresponding to the thrombosed artery (hyperdense to middle cerebral artery [MCA]/ basilar artery [BA] sign or hyperdense dot sign). When a large (>1/3 MCA territory or complete brain stem) area of hypodensity is noted, thrombolysis should not be attempted (**Fig. 16.2**). A CT angiogram (CTA), which should span from the aortic arch to the vertex, can also confirm the presence and location of large-artery occlusions (**Fig. 16.2A**). This imaging adds little time to the study when it is performed on a modern multi-detector scanner, but it can save significant time in the angiography suite by focusing the angiographer on the vessel in question. CTA has up to a 98% sensitivity and specificity for large-artery occlusion.[10] One concern over the routine use of contrast CT scans in acute stroke patients is dye-induced nephropathy. However, Josephson et al. found only a 0.37% incidence of dye-related renal failure among 1075 patients with acute stroke.[11] Further, newer generation contrast agents with higher relaxivities allow lower contrast loads and are associated with lower incidences of nephrotoxicity.

Table 16.5 Laboratory and Alternative Imaging Orders Under Consideration for Patients with New Onset Ischemia

Laboratory or diagnostic test	Reason for investigation; alternatives
Laboratory	
Basic metabolic panel, including glucose and A1C	Metabolic abnormalities, uncontrolled diabetes
Lipid profile and hepatic function profile, including ammonia	Dyslipidemias, hepatologies causing coagulopathies, encephalopathies
Complete blood count with differential; platelet function	Hematologic abnormalities, platelet dysfunction, infection, systemic conditions
Coagulation profile	Coagulopathies, medication effects or therapeutic levels
Arterial blood gas	Pulmonary/renal exchange pathology
Cardiac enzyme profile	Cardiac injuries or dysfunction
Erythrocyte sedimentation rate (ESR) and C-reactive protein levels	Infection, inflammatory states
Antinuclear antibody (ANA)	Connective tissue disorders
Homocysteine	Systemic vascular disease
Diagnostic	
Electrocardiogram	Cardiac arrythmias
Transthoracic echocardiogram	Valvular dysfunction, PFO; may need transesophageal echo to identify arch abnormalities if unable to visualize
Carotid duplex ultrasound	Extracranial stenosis
Lower extremity Dopplers	Deep venous thromboses

Perfusion imaging, an emerging area of acute stroke imaging, allows differentiation between normal tissues, those at risk for progression to infarct (the ischemic penumbra), and infarcted tissues (the ischemic core). CT perfusion (**Fig. 16.3**) has been shown to determine areas of hypoperfusion, cerebral blood volume, and time-to-peak measures as markers of tissue viability.[12] Intervention criteria based on time-based measurements (mean transit time and time-to-peak) using CT perfusion are currently being determined. MR perfusion studies have been shown to be a quantitative tool to determine cerebral blood flow and can be used to determine the utility of intervention. It has been shown in a small case series that the zone of hypoperfused tissue (salvageable ischemic penumbra) immediately surrounding the DWI abnormality (infarcted tissue) in acute stroke can be returned to a state of normal perfusion with intraarterial recanalization.[13] Setting thresholds for core and penumbral tissue has been a major issue in MRI-guided interventional stroke therapy. The development of this modality is at a more advanced stage than CT, and its utility is being tested in the NIH-funded MR REcanalization of Stroke Clots Using Embolectomy (MR RESCUE) trial.

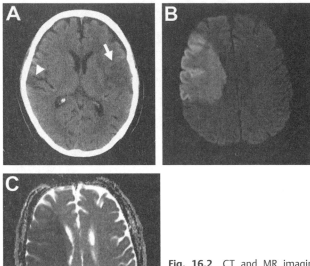

Fig. 16.2 CT and MR imaging of stroke. **(A)** CT image of the head demonstrating a chronic (*arrowhead*) and a subacute (*arrow*) area of ischemia. **(B,C)** MR images of acute stroke: diffusion-weighted **(B)** and apparent diffusion coefficient **(C)** images.

The analysis of clot composition is another potential application of MRI technology to acute stroke intervention. The gradient echo vessel susceptibility vessel sign (GRE-SVS) has been shown to be a very sensitive and specific marker of intravascular thrombus. The intensity of signal on this sequence relates to the amount of paramagnetic deoxyhemoglobin present within red cells and therefore can give some indication of whether the thrombus is composed predominantly of red cells and fibrin (red clot) or is more likely to represent a well organized, platelet-rich thrombus (white clot). Red clot is generally thought to be more susceptible to chemical thrombolysis; therefore, one might select this intraarterial modality in the case of a large-artery occlusion that demonstrated a high GRE-SVS signal. On the other hand, white clot (a low GRE-SVS signal thrombus) may require mechanical disruption or extraction. The preliminary studies testing this hypothesis have been mixed.[14]

Additional Testing

Once all possible acute treatment has been provided, the focus shifts to identifying the etiology of stroke and therefore preventing recurrence. Transthoracic and/or transesophageal echocardiography is performed to look for vegetations, mural thrombus, valve abnormalities, cardiomyopathy, akinetic or hypokinetic segments, and intracardiac shunt. Transthoracic studies are noninvasive and effective at evaluating the left ventricular system, while the transesophageal route is invasive and is preferred for the evaluation of the left atria.[14,15] Carotid duplex Doppler

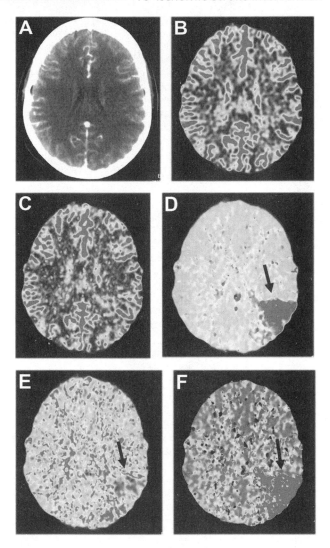

Fig. 16.3 CT perfusion in acute intracranial stroke. Even in this black and white set of images, differences in perfusion images can be delineated. **(A)** Baseline CT with contrast image, demonstrating relative symmetry in the hemispheres. This is supported by the cerebral blood flow **(B)** and cerebral blood volume **(C)** maps. However, in both the mean transit time (MTT, **D**), correlation map **(E)**, and time-to-peak **(F)** maps, there is a clear wedge of parenchyma (*arrows*) in the left parieto-occipital watershed territory representing an acute infarct.

ultrasonagraphy may be used to assess quickly and inexpensively carotid stenosis or dissection if no arterial imaging was performed in the acute phase. Continuous cardiac monitoring (such as telemetry or Holter monitoring) is useful in identifying occult arrhythmias. A fasting lipid profile is performed to evaluate patients for hypercholesterolemia. A hemoglobin A1C is obtained in diabetics to assess the degree of long-term blood glucose control. If stroke occurs in the young and in patients with a strong family history of cerebrovascular disease or a history of venous coagulopathy (for example, deep vein thrombosis), with or without imaging suggestive of venous infarct, the patients should undergo a coagulation work-up. This typically includes the screening laboratory tests listed in **Table 16.6**.

Defining Restoration of Blood Flow

Cerebral revascularization is the only maneuver that provides proven benefit to stroke patients. However, revascularization has two components that are often confused in the literature and in the definitions of restoration of cerebral blood flow. Local recanalization of an occluded segment is often referred to as arterial occlusive lesion (AOL) recanalization (**Table 16.7**). Once the local occlusion is eliminated or diminished, the distal circulation and terminal branches also demonstrate reperfusion, which is often expressed as the thrombolysis in myocardial infarction (TIMI) score (**Table 16.7**). Other scores have been developed that describe recanalization and revascularization based on varying determinations and it is important for neurointerventionists to be aware of them (**Table 16.8**).

Evidence-Based Medicine

Chemical Thrombolysis

Prolyse in Acute Cerebral Thromboembolism Trial II

Prolyse in Acute Cerebral Thromboembolism Trial II (PROACT II) was a randomized, controlled, multicenter trial with an open-label design and blind follow-up. Patients with early signs of infarction in greater than one-third of the MCA terri-

Table 16.6 Special Diagnostic Tests of Coagulation to Screen for Prothrombotic Causes of Ischemic Stroke

Antiphospholipid antibodies (Lupus anticoagulant)
Sickle cell screen and hemoglobin electrophoresis
Serum fibrinogen
D dimer
Fibrinogen degradation products
Proteins C and S
Antithrombin III
Factor V Leiden
Prothrombin gene mutation

Table 16.7 Recanalization and Revascularization Scores

Score	AOL recanalization	Score	TIMI reperfusion
0	No recanalization of the primary occlusive lesion	0	No perfusion
I	Incomplete or partial recanalization of the primary occlusive lesion with no distal flow	1	Perfusion past the initial occlusion but no distal branch filling
II	Incomplete or partial recanalization of the primary occlusive lesion with any distal flow	2	Perfusion with incomplete or slow distal branch filling
III	Complete recanalization of the primary occlusive lesion with any distal flow	3	Full perfusion with filling of all distal branches, including M 3, 4

Abbreviations: AOL, arterial occlusive lesion; TIMI, thrombolysis in myocardial infarction.

Table 16.8 TICI Reperfusion Score Terminology and Definition of TICI Reperfusion (I) and AOL Recanalization Scores (II)*

I. Posttreatment TICI reperfusion grade
0 = No perfusion
1 = Perfusion past the initial obstruction but limited distal branch filling with little or slow distal perfusion
2A = Perfusion of less than half of the vascular distribution of the occluded artery (e.g., filling and perfusion through 1 M2 division)
2B = Perfusion of half or greater of the vascular distribution of the occluded artery (e.g., filling and perfusion through 2 M2 divisions)
3 = Full perfusion with filling of all distal branches
II. Posttreatment AOL recanalization grade
0 = No recanalization of the occlusion
1 = Incomplete or partial recanalization of the occlusion, with no distal flow
2 = Incomplete or partial recanalization of the occlusion, with any distal flow
3 = Complete recanalization of the occlusion with any distal flow

*The modified TICI reperfusion score was essentially equivalent to TIMI score applied in IMS I, with grade 2 further divided into A and B for post hoc analysis
Abbreviations: AOL, arterial occlusive lesion; TICI score, thrombolysis in cerebral infarction score.

tory on the initial CT scan were excluded. A total of 180 patients with MCA, M1 or M2 occlusions were randomized 2:1 to receive either 6 mg of IA r-proUK or intra-aterial saline placebo into the proximal thrombus. All patients received low-dose IV heparin. The patients in PROACT II had a very high baseline stroke severity, with a median NIHSS of 17. The median time from onset of symptoms to initiation of IA thrombolysis was 5.3 hours. For the r-pro-UK treated group, there was a 15% absolute and 58% relative increase (p = 0.043) in good outcome (defined as modi-fied Rankin score of 2 at 90 days). The benefit was most noticeable in patients with a baseline NIHSS between 11 and 20. On average, 7 patients with MCA occlusion would require IA thrombolysis for one to benefit. Recanalization rates were 66% at 2 hours for the treatment group and 18% for the placebo group (p < 0.001). Symp-tomatic brain hemorrhage occurred in 10% of the r-proUK group and 2% of the con-trol group at 24 hours. Considering the later time to treatment and greater baseline stroke severity in PROACT II, the symptomatic brain hemorrhage rate compared favorably with the IV tPA trials.

Despite the scientific evidence of benefit, the FDA did not approve intra-arterial pro-urokinase for the treatment of acute stroke, due to the regulatory requirement for additional confirmatory evidence of benefit. However, on the basis of this trial the American Heart Association Stroke Council's 2003 guidelines for treatment of acute stroke changed the status of intra-arterial thrombolysis from an experimen-tal treatment, provided in a research setting only, to an accepted treatment option for stroke less than 6 hours. As pro-urokinase is no longer available, other throm-bolytics are currently used, such as recombinant tissue plasminogen activator (r-tPA), reteplase (rPA), tenecteplase (TNKase), and urokinase.[17]

Emergency Management of Stroke Trial

The Emergency Management of Stroke (EMS) trial was the first randomized trial, involving 35 patients, to combine the use of IV rt-PA and IA rt-PA. The exclusion criteria included those used in the NINDS study, plus age greater than 84 and NI-HSS less than 6. Intravenous treatment was initiated on average 2.5 hours after the onset of symptoms, and intra-arterial treatment was initiated approximately 3 hours after the onset of symptoms. Patients were either given 0.6 mg/kg of rt-PA intravenously (15% as a bolus over 1 minute and the remainder over 30 minutes) with up to 0.3 mg/kg given intra-arterially, or given a placebo intravenously, fol-lowed by IA treatment. The intra-arterial component of the procedure included placement of a microcatheter distal to the thrombus, followed by infusion of 1mg of r-tPA. The catheter was then retracted into the thrombus, and 1mg of r-tPA was administered. This was followed by an infusion of 10 mg/hour. No difference was seen in either the primary clinical outcome (NIHSS >7) or the 90-day clinical out-come. TIMI 2 or 3 flow was achieved in 54% of patients in the IV/IA group and in 10% of patients in the placebo/IA group. There was a strong correlation between NIHSS and the presence of a clot on angiography. The rate of symptomatic ICH was 11.8% in the IV/IA group and 5.5% in the placebo/IA group.[16]

Interventional Management of Stroke Trial

The Interventional Management of Stroke (IMS) trial followed shortly after the EMS trial. It involved a similar protocol and used an NIHSS score of 10 or greater to screen for patients with large-artery occlusions. All patients received IV r-TPA and underwent angiography. If a large-artery occlusion was identified, IA r-TPA was administered according to the EMS protocol. In this trial there was no placebo arm. Instead, the patients enrolled were compared with a historical control extracted from the NINDS r-tPA trial that had similar ages and NIHSS scores. Two mg of rt-PA was injected through the catheter beyond the thrombus over a period of two minutes. The catheter was then retracted into the thrombus, and 2 mg of rt-PA was injected over two minutes directly into the thrombus. Infusion of rt-PA was then started at the rate of 9 mg/h for up to two hours of infusion time, using an infusion pump. Eighty patients were enrolled. The number of symptomatic intracerebral hemorrhages was similar to the NINDS study (7.5% versus 6%). However, the number of asymptomatic hemorrhages was significantly greater, at 43%. Clinical efficacy was similar to IV tPA alone, but in patients with a median NIHSS score of 18 as compared with 14 in the IV tPA NINDS trial. A direct head-to-head comparison of IV tPA to combined IV-IA tPA is currently under way in an NIH-sponsored study, IMS-III.[17]

Gycoprotein (GP) IIb-IIIa Inhibitors

Gycoprotein (GP) IIb-IIIa inhibitors have become a standard adjunct in percutaneous coronary interventions. One GP IIb-IIIa inhibitor that is frequently used during these procedures is abciximab, starting with a loading dose of 0.25 mg/kg that is followed by a 12 hour infusion of 0.125 mcg/kg/minute. Disappointingly, this agent was associated with an excess incidence of intracranial hemorrhage when used intravenously between three and six hours after the onset of acute stroke; this result halted an industry-sponsored randomized trial designed to test its efficacy.[18] The role of smaller doses of these agents administered intra-arterially for acute stroke has yet to be studied prospectively. Several case series have described success in using these agents as part of a multimodal approach (see below).

Mechanical Thrombolysis

Mechanical Embolus Removal in Cerebral Ischemia (MERCI) Trial

The Mechanical Embolus Removal in Cerebral Ischemia (MERCI) trial was a prospective, single-arm, multicenter, industry-sponsored trial that tested whether a mechanical embolectomy device could safely restore vascular patency in acute stroke. This device is a nitinol corkscrew-shaped snare device, with which the clot is engaged and removed from the arterial system. The mechanical embolectomy is done through an 8 Fr or 9 Fr guide catheter with a balloon at the tip, allowing occlusion of the common carotid artery and reversal of flow through aspiration during clot extraction. A total of 141 patients had the device deployed. Patients were treated between 3 and 8 hours after the onset of stroke symptoms or between 0 and 3 hours and a contraindication for intravenous tissue plasminogen activator (tPA). The average NIHSS score was 20, and the majority of the occlusions were in the M1 segment. Recanalization was achieved in 48% of treated patients with the embolectomy device alone, a significantly higher percentage than expected using historical controls from the NINDS trial (18%; p = 0.0001). Seven percent of patients suffered a clinically significant procedure-related complication (unaffected vessel embolization, subarachnoid hemorrhage due to vessel perforation, vessel dissection, and groin hemorrhage). Four percent of participants suffered clinically significant intraparenchymal hemorrhages. Patients who were successfully recanalized had a three times greater chance of a favorable neurological outcome at thirty days when compared with those whose vessel remained occluded. Based on the results of this trial, the MERCI device received FDA approval in August 2004. However, many stroke neurologists feel that more robust data on clinical outcomes should be collected prior to widespread use of this device. These data may come from the ongoing NIH-sponsored MR RESCUE trial.[19]

Multi-MERCI

A second generation of the Concentric MERCI retriever device called L5 was modified to add Prolene (Ethicon, Inc.) filaments to the nitinol helix, which was thought to ensnare the thrombus and decrease stretching of the device during clot retraction. Data regarding efficacy of the L5 device were published in the report on the Multi-MERCI Phase I trial. The L5 device achieved recanalization in 58% of cases when it was deployed as the first device, as compared with 46% recanalization when the older generation X5/X6 devices were deployed as the first device.[20] The V-series has just been released, which is firmer and intended to provide better pulling force; empiric data suggest that there is a higher recanalization rate with fewer passes.

Penumbra

A recent addition to the acute ischemic stroke armamentarium is the Penumbra system (Penumbra, Inc.). Similar to the MERCI device, this system was studied in a prospective, single-arm, multicenter, industry-sponsored trial (Penumbra Pivotal Stroke Trial). The Penumbra system is composed of two main components: a reperfusion catheter and a separator. For aspiration, the reperfusion catheter is used in parallel with the separator and an aspiration source to separate the thrombus and aspirate it from the occluded vessel. A total of 125 patients were enrolled. Patients were treated between 3 and 8 hours after onset of stroke symptoms, or between 0 and 3 hours and a contraindication for intravenous tissue plasminogen activator (tPA). Recanalizatation was achieved in an impressive 82% of treated patients. Three percent of patients suffered a clinically significant procedure-related complication. The number of patients with little or no disability at 90 days was a disappointing 25%, however. Despite this, the Penumbra device received FDA approval in 2008.[21]

Balloon Angioplasty and Stenting

The use of angioplasty and stenting to treat acute myocardial infarction has been shown to be superior to intravenous thrombolysis. Based on this finding, there is great interest in attempting to use these modalities in treatment of acute stroke. In one case series, 19 patients underwent intracranial stent placement after failing various combinations of thrombolysis and clot retrieval.[22] A 79% recanalization rate was achieved. Recanalization was associated with a "good" outcome. Six patients died, four of whom were not recanalized. One patient developed intracranial hemorrhage. This modality has become even more promising with the introduction of self-expanding stents designed for intracranial use. Many intracranial stent systems are currently in use, but only two such devices have been approved by the

FDA for intracranial atherosclerosis, the Wingspan stent (Boston Scientific, Boston, MA) and the Enterprise (Cordis Endovascular, Miami Lakes, FL).

Ultrasound

The success of the CLOTBUST intravenous t-PA with ultrasound augmentation trial has renewed interest in the use of intra-arterial (IA) ultrasound in combination with IA chemical thrombolysis.[23] It is thought that high-frequency low-intensity sonography can accelerate fibrinolysis. The stable cavitation believed to result from the sonography pulse wave generates local convection currents and microstreaming, which increases diffusion of the thrombolytic agent into the clot and thus the effective surface area for the drug. The EKOS MicroLys US infusion catheter (EKOS Corporation, Bothell, WA) is designed to deliver a local ultrasound pulse within the clot while a thrombolytic agent is infused through a central port. It is a 2.5 Fr standard microinfusion catheter with a 2 mm, 2.1 MHz ring sonography transducer (average power, 0.21–0.45 W) at its distal tip. The catheter accepts a 0.010-inch guidewire and can be placed coaxially through a sheath-catheter system chosen by the operator (a 5 Fr angiographic or 6 Fr guide catheter). This device has been tested in a safety trial involving 14 patients. In this trial, the catheter tip was positioned in the thrombus, and a chemical thrombolytic (either t-PA or retaplase) was infused. Recanalization was achieved in 8 of 14 patients. No device-related adverse outcomes were observed. The average NIHSS went from 18 before the procedure to 7 after it.[24] The use of this device has been incorporated into the ongoing, NIH-funded Emergency Management of Stroke Trial III trial, the results of which should give additional information about its clinical efficacy.

Other Devices

Numerous other modalities have been explored, with disappointing early results: clot maceration and aspiration, rheolytic thrombectomy, primary angioplasty, laser, snare retrievers, and nitinol capture baskets.

The Multimodal Approach

Due to the lack of a consistently effective mode of endovascular recanalization in acute stroke, many neurointerventionists have adopted a "multimodal" approach (**Fig. 16.4**). Abou-Chebl et al. described an approach patterned on that used during percutaneous coronary intervention for acute myocardial infarction. This approach involves the use of fibrinolytics, anticoagulants, and platelet glycoprotein IIb/IIIa (GP IIb/IIIa) receptor antagonists. Angioplasty and stenting were preferentially used in patients with atherosclerotic lesions, while snare and rheolytic devices were used in patients whose lesion appeared to be due to an embolized clot. Twelve patients were treated using this approach, with recanalization being achieved in 11. The average NIHSS score decreased from 19 to 10 after the procedure. There were two procedure-related complications (one symptomatic and one asymptomatic). Two patients died due to their stroke.[25] Gupta et al. conducted a retrospective review of 168 patients with acute stroke treated endovascularly. The general approach involved the use of IA pharmacologic agents (tissue plasminogen activator or urokinase) if the patient arrived within six hours of the onset of symptoms. If recanalization did not occur with the use these agents, then mechanical maneuvers were used with either balloon angioplasty or a snare/MERCI device. If

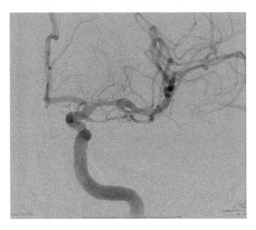

Fig. 16.4 Recanalization with "multimodal" approach.

these interventions failed, then a stent was placed across the lesion. Extracranial carotid occlusions were primarily treated with angioplasty and stenting. Patients arriving beyond six hours from the onset of symptoms were primarily treated using mechanical modalities. Recanalization was achieved in 106 (63%) of patients. Twenty-four patients (14%) suffered symptomatic intracranial hemorrhage. Thirty-five patients (21%) had a four point or greater drop in their NIHSS 24 hours after intervention. The likelihood of recanalization increased with the number of modalities used, and the only predictor of a four point or greater drop in NIHSS at 24 hours was recanalization.[26]

Preprocedural Preparation

It is crucial that the interventionist be involved in the clinical evaluation of the patient prior to beginning any thrombolysis procedure. This evaluation includes a review of the focused history and physical examination described above, with confirmation of the key findings. Relevant laboratory data, especially that pertaining to kidney function, should also be reviewed. At a minimum, a non-contrast head CT should be performed and reviewed to rule out intracranial hemorrhage or extensive ischemic changes. Additional imaging modalities may also be included to provide a more comprehensive preprocedure evaluation at the discretion of the interventionist. It is important to review the treatment plan and equipment being used with the support personnel, including the anesthesiology team. We prefer to perform all such procedures under general anesthesia, given the need to minimize patient movement and the difficulty of communicating with acute stroke patients. In addition, the anesthesiology team is better able to focus on making hemodynamic adjustments as the artery is recanalized.

There is often a delay in obtaining thrombolytic agents and glycoprotein IIb/IIIa agents prepared and delivered from the pharmacy. If the use of these agents it being considered, it is advisable to notify the pharmacy prior to beginning the intervention.

Equipment

Chemical Thrombolysis

Sheath

A 6 Fr sheath is generally adequate. It is attached to a heparinized flush. You may increase the size the sheath to allow continuous intra-arterial blood pressure monitoring if a radial arterial line is not available. In patients with abdominal aortic aneurysmal dilation, aorto-iliac stenosis, or severe vessel tortuosity, a long (35 cm or greater) sheath may allow greater catheter control. Furthermore, larger sheaths are often necessary for mechanical thrombolytic devices.

Diagnostic and Guide Catheters

We generally select a 6 Fr guide catheter. It is large enough to allow high-quality angiography around coaxially inserted devices. It also allows the use of several mechanical devices, such as an angioplasty balloon. We generally use a 45-degree angle (default) or Simmons II tip (in patients with more severe arch angulation) diagnostic catheter through the guide catheter. A heparinized flush is connected to the guide catheter via a three-way stopcock and a rotating hemostatic valve (Tuohy-Borst) adaptor, with one or two additional ports.

Access Glide Wires

A standard hydrophilic 0.035″ glide wire is used to select and catheterize the great vessels. At times a wire with more body and shapeability, such as a 0.035″ Stiff Glidewire (Terumo, Japan), is useful to access tortuous vessels.

Microcatheter

At our institution, the Excelsior SL-10 or Excelsior 1018 (Boston Scientific, Boston, MA) microcatheter is preferred for catheterization of intracranial vessels; however, there are many equally effective microcatheters on the market. A standard flush is connected also to the microcatheter, again via a three-way stopcock and a Tuohy-Borst adaptor, with one or two additional ports.

Microwire

At our institution we utilize a variety of 0.014 microwires. We frequently use the X-pedion 14 (ev3, Irvine, CA) because of its ability to maintain a shaped "J" tip, allowing atraumatic passage through the thrombus into the non-visualized distal vessel. If vessel selection becomes difficult, we rely on the Synchro 14 microwire (Boston Scientific, Boston, MA) due to its excellent 1:1 torque.

Thrombolytic/Antiplatelet Agents

- tPA: We typically utilize up to 30 mg intra-arterially, with several milligrams administered distal to the clot and several within the clot. The remainder is slowly infused into the proximal ⅓ of the clot. It is important to frequently image the thrombus and to advance the microcatheter as the clot lyses.

- Urokinase: This agent was not available for several years but has recently been re-introduced to the market. At most institutions, it is no longer utilized for intracranial thrombolysis.
- Glycoprotein IIb/IIIa Inhibitors: The two most frequently used agents are abciximab (Reopro) and eptifibatide (Integrilin). The dosing of these agents for intracranial procedures is not standardized. They are generally used as an adjunct to mechanical interventions, such as angioplasty and/or stenting.

Mechanical Devices

Sheath

For most modes of mechanical thrombolysis, a 6 Fr sheath is adequate. If you anticipate an attempt to place an intracranial stent, the use of a long sheath (90 cm) may provide additional support. The exception is the MERCI device. The guiding catheter used with the MERCI comes in 8 and 9 French sizes and requires a correspondingly sized sheath.

Guiding Catheter

- MERCI Balloon Guide: As mentioned, this specially designed guiding catheter comes in 8 Fr and 9 Fr. It has a balloon at its distal tip, allowing the operator to produce flow arrest by inflating the balloon in the proximal internal carotid. Flow reversal can then be achieved by attaching a large-volume syringe and aspirating while withdrawing the snare.
- Neuron Delivery Catheter: Designed for use with the Penumbra system, this catheter has a unique distal end that is flexible (to minimize the risk of intimal injury) and tapers from 6 Fr proximally to 5 Fr distally. It also comes in lengths of 105 to 115 cm. These features allow it to be positioned in the petrous and even cavernous internal carotid segments. It can be combined with the Neuron Select Catheter to access more easily the great vessels from the arch.

Access Glide Wire

A standard hydrophilic 0.035″ wire is typically used to select and catheterize the great vessels. It is sometimes easiest to select the target vessel with a diagnostic catheter and use an exchange-length (300 cm) 0.035″ wire to exchange for the guiding catheter. This is especially true when using the Merci Balloon guide and if you do not have the Neuron Select Catheter available.

Microcatheter

There are a variety of catheters that may be used to access the clot. Which to select is largely an operator preference. Three exceptions are listed below.

- 14X: Designed for use with the older generation of Merci devices, the X-series. It has a 0.017″ inner diameter.
- 18L: Designed for use with the two more recent incarnations of the Merci device: the L series and the V series. It has a 0.022″ inner diameter.

Reperfusion Catheter

Designed for use with the Penumbra system. There are 3 sizes (0.026″/2.8 Fr, 0.032″/3.4 Fr, and 0.041″/4.1 Fr inner/outer diameter), allowing their use to be tailored to the size of the target vessel.

Microwire

As described above, there are a variety of 0.014″ microwires that may be used to access and cross the target clot. The Penumbra system comes with an especially designed "Separator" wire. The wire comes in three diameters (0.022″, 0.028″, and 0.035″) and has a bead fused to the distal end that allows clot fragmentation.

Devices

- MERCI: approved by the FDA in 2004, the Mechanical Embolus Removal in Cerebral Ischemia (MERCI) device (Concenctric Medical, Inc., Irvine, CA) is offered in various models (X series, L series, V series, and K Mini). All are constructed of a nitinol coil that is either tapered or cylindrical and, except for the X6 and K Mini, all have attached Prolene filaments. MERCI retrieval devices are designed for use with the proprietary Merci Balloon guide catheter and microcatheters described above.

- Penumbra: The Penumbra System (Penumbra, Inc., Almeda, CA) is a mechanical clot disruptor utilizing a reperfusion catheter and a separator. Once the reperfusion catheter is advanced just proximal to the thrombus, the reperfusion catheter is attached to an aspirator. The aspirator is activated and a series of passes antegrade into the thrombus are made with the separator. The disrupted clot is then aspirated into the reperfusion catheter.

- Angioplasty: Most interventionists use angioplasty as an adjunct once a primary therapy (IA thrombolytic, Merci, etc.) has failed to achieve recanalization. Its use in the circle of Willis is limited by the vessel tortuosity and the fear of vessel injury in distal branches. There is also a high rate of re-occlusion if antiplatelet agents are not used as adjuncts. A short over-the-wire balloon is generally preferred over a monorail device because it is easier to push and provides the ability to perform microcatheter angiograms through the balloon. Several coronary balloons are available (such as the Maverick Balloon, Boston Scientific, Boston, MA). There is also a neuro-specific balloon, the Gateway (Boston Scientific, Boston, MA) that can be used.

- Stent: Several stents have been approved for intracranial use, starting with the Neuroform stent (Boston Scientific, Boston, MA) in 2002, the Wingspan stent (Boston Scientific, Boston, MA) in 2005, and finally the Enterprise (Cordis Neurovascular, Miami Lakes, FL) stent in 2007. Before 2002, most intracranial stenting was limited to off-label use of coronary stents, which are often balloon mounted and more rigid. All three FDA-approved intracranial stents are self-expanding nitinol stents. They were designed to treat either intracranial aneurysms or atherosclerotic stenosis, but they have been used off-label in the setting of acute stroke. While these stents are more navigable than their coronary counterparts, some have the disadvantage of requiring an exchange process, which is cumbersome at best. The requirement for adjunctive use of antiplatelet agents after implantation may also increase the risk of hemorrhagic conversion.

Postprocedural Care

Imaging

At our institution, we routinely obtain an MRI, including only the gradient echo, diffusion weighted, and ADC sequences. This allows early detection of procedure-related hemorrhages. Alternatively, a noncontrast CT may be obtained; however, care must be taken not to confuse contrast staining of ischemic tissue with hemorrhage. An additional noncontrast CT scan is obtained within 24 hours of the event, sometimes before the initiation of antiplatelet or anticoagulation agents. However, most patients are already being administered an antiplatelet agent. Most of the contrast enhancement typically resolves on the 24-hour scan.

Blood Pressure

Aggressive blood pressure control is crucial within the first 24 hours after vessel recanalization. We attempt to keep systolic blood pressure below 160 during this time period. In our experience there is an association between spikes in blood pressure above this value and hemorrhagic conversion. Furthermore, some patients do not perfuse well below their baseline levels, which may be above normal systolic blood pressure. Therefore, individualized therapy should be taken into consideration in patients who are dependent on high systolic baseline pressures.

Acute Neurological Change

Acute neurological change after the procedure can result from several events: (1) Mechanical vessel damage secondary to instrumentation, such as vessel dissection or perforation is possible. (2) Hemorrhagic conversion of an acutely ischemic/infarcted territory secondary to reperfusion injury or from hyperperfusion of a chronically underperfused region may also occur. These hemorrhagic complications in the presence of anticoagulation or the use of antiplatelet agents can be challenging to manage, because their reversal may lead to rethrombosis of the recanalized or stented vessel. Aggressive blood pressure control may also help mitigate the extent of such hemorrhages. Additional reasons for an acute neurological change are re-occlusion of the previously treated vessel and, rarely, cardioembolism to another vascular territory.

Secondary Stroke Prevention

We generally will initiate antiplatelet therapy after vessel recanalization. However, this may be altered if hemorrhage is evident on a postprocedure noncontrast head CT with no originally identified cardioembolic source. For patients with an embolic source, the timing of initiation of anticoagulation is dependent on the volume of infarcted tissue and the thromboembolic potential of the source (for example, mechanical heart valve versus atrial fibrillation). Patients in whom a stent has been placed may require immediate use of antiplatelet agents, such as a combination of clopidogrel and aspirin. An eptifibatide drip is substituted for oral antiplatelet agents if the potential for hemorrhagic conversion is judged to be high due to the short half-life of this agent.

Alternative Treatments

Intravenous tPA

It is important to bear in mind that intra-arterial thrombolysis is not considered the primary treatment of acute ischemic stroke. The standard treatment guideline remains intravenous tPA given within three hours, which is based upon the National Institutes of Neurological Disorders and Stroke tPA study published in 1995. This placebo-controlled trial demonstrated a 30% reduction in disability at 90 days post-treatment.[27]

The window for IV tPA use may be extended in the near future, based on the recently published European Cooperative Acute Stroke Study (ECASS) III. In this placebo-controlled trial, there was a statistically significant benefit to the use of IV tPA between 3 and 4.5 hours after symptom onset. The odds ratio of a functional recovery was 1.3 times higher in the treatment arm.[28] A recent meta-analysis of stroke studies examining patients treated within 4.5 hours after the onset of symptoms demonstrated that IV rt-PA therapy improved functional outcomes in these patients without significantly increasing patient mortality, but increasing symptomatic intracranial hemorrhages (J Emerg Med Jun 2010 Carpenter et al.).

NeuroFlo Catheter

The NeuroFlo catheter (CoAxia, Inc., Maple Grove, MN) is currently in clinical trials (SENTIS; Safety and Efficacy of NeuroFlo for Treatment of Ischemic Stroke) at over 30 participating centers. It is a dual balloon catheter designed to restrict blood flow intra-renally and in doing so, to open collateral pathways to ischemic penumbral tissue. A balloon is placed in the suprarenal and infrarenal aorta (**Fig. 16.5**), inflated to 70% of the vessel diameter for 45 minutes, and then removed.[29]

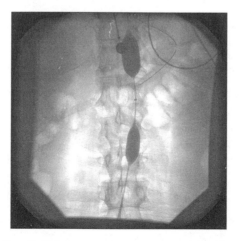

Fig. 16.5 NeuroFlo catheter.

Other Strategies

No medical maneuvers, other that intravenous tPA, have proven efficacy in reducing the severity of acute ischemic stroke. Several areas are being targeted, however. These include blood pressure augmentation and the early administration of potentially neuroprotective agents, such as magnesium sulfate. Finally, another strategy is to augment the effect of IV tPA through focused transcranial ultrasonogarphy.[23]

Technical Pearls and Pitfalls

1. Large-artery ischemic stroke is a high morbidity and mortality disease—don't expect miracles and don't be easily discouraged.
2. Resist the temptation to persist until the angiogram looks perfect. Remember that time is the most crucial factor and that recanalization at greater than nine hours is probably not beneficial in the anterior circulation. Well-selected patients with posterior circulation occlusion can benefit from therapy up to 24 hours after the onset of symptoms.
3. Remember that most successful stroke interventions are "multi-modal."
4. Postprocedurally, use an arterial line and maintain strict blood pressure control for at least 24 hours.
5. Not all that is bright on CT is blood. Contrast staining is often present after intra-arterial thrombolysis, but it usually clears within 24 hours.
6. Smoking has been shown to be the single most important life-style-related risk factor contributing to cardiovascular and cerebrovascular disease.[30,31] Aggressive medical management of atherosclerotic risk factors in the modern age includes targeting an LDL cholesterol level <70 mg/dL in symptomatic patients.[32]

Recommended Reading

Brott T, Bogousslavsky J. Treatment of acute ischemic stroke. N Engl J Med 2000; 343(10):710–722

Chimowitz MI, Lynn MJ, Howlett-Smith H, et al. Warfarin-Aspirin Symptomatic Intracranial Disease Trial Investigators. Comparison of warfarin and aspirin for symptomatic intracranial arterial stenosis. N Engl J Med 2005;352(13):1305–1316

Furlan A, Higashida R, Wechsler L, et al.; Intra-arterial Prourokinase for Acute Ischemic Stroke. Intra-arterial prourokinase for acute ischemic stroke. The PROACT II study: a randomized controlled trial. Prolyse in Acute Cerebral Thromboembolism. JAMA 1999;282(21):2003–2011

References

1. Brott T, Bogousslavsky J. Treatment of acute ischemic stroke. N Engl J Med 2000; 343(10):710–722
2. Chimowitz MI, Lynn MJ, Howlett-Smith H, et al.; Warfarin-Aspirin Symptomatic Intracranial Disease Trial Investigators. Comparison of warfarin and aspirin for symptomatic intracranial arterial stenosis. N Engl J Med 2005;352(13):1305–1316
3. Fisher CM. Lacunar strokes and infarcts: a review. Neurology 1982;32(8):871–876
4. Bonita R, Beaglehole R. Recovery of motor function after stroke. Stroke 1988; 19(12):1497–1500

5. Bonita R, Ford MA, Stewart AW. Predicting survival after stroke: a three-year follow-up. Stroke 1988;19(6):669–673
6. Brott T, Adams HP Jr, Olinger CP, et al. Measurements of acute cerebral infarction: a clinical examination scale. Stroke 1989;20(7):864–870
7. Adams HP Jr, del Zoppo GJ, von Kummer R. *Management of Acute Stroke: A Practical Guide for the Prevention, Evaluation, and Treatment of Acute Stroke*, 3rd ed. Professional Communications, Inc.; 2006:352
8. Culebras A, Kase CS, Masdeu JC, et al. Practice guidelines for the use of imaging in transient ischemic attacks and acute stroke. A report of the Stroke Council, American Heart Association. Stroke 1997;28(7):1480–1497
9. Von Kummer R, Bourquain H, Bastianello S, et al. Early prediction of irreversible brain damage after ischemic stroke at CT. Radiology 2001;219(1):95–100
10. Lev MH, Farkas J, Rodriguez VR, et al. CT angiography in the rapid triage of patients with hyperacute stroke to intraarterial thrombolysis: accuracy in the detection of large vessel thrombus. J Comput Assist Tomogr 2001;25(4):520–528
11. Josephson SA, Dillon WP, Smith WS. Incidence of contrast nephropathy from cerebral CT angiography and CT perfusion imaging. Neurology 2005;64(10):1805–1806
12. Wintermark M, Flanders AE, Velthuis B, et al. Perfusion-CT assessment of infarct core and penumbra: receiver operating characteristic curve analysis in 130 patients suspected of acute hemispheric stroke. Stroke 2006;37(4):979–985
13. Hjort N, Butcher K, Davis SM, et al.; UCLA Thrombolysis Investigators. Magnetic resonance imaging criteria for thrombolysis in acute cerebral infarct. Stroke 2005; 36(2):388–397
14. Cohen A, et al. Value of transesophageal echocardiography in the cardiovascular assessment of an ischemic cerebral accident of suspected embolic origin. Ann Radiol 1994;37(1–2):29–40
15. Albers GW, et al. Transesophageal echocardiographic findings in stroke subtypes. Stroke 1994;25(1):23–28
16. Lewandowski CA, Frankel M, Tomsick TA, et al. Combined intravenous and intra-arterial r-TPA versus intra-arterial therapy of acute ischemic stroke: Emergency Management of Stroke (EMS) Bridging Trial. Stroke 1999;30(12):2598–2605
17. IMS Study Investigators. Combined intravenous and intra-arterial recanalization for acute ischemic stroke: the Interventional Management of Stroke Study. Stroke 2004;35(4):904–911
18. Adams HP. Abciximab in Emergent Stroke Treatment Trial – II. Presented at the 30th International Stroke Conference February 2005.
19. Smith WS, Sung G, Starkman S, et al.; MERCI Trial Investigators. Safety and efficacy of mechanical embolectomy in acute ischemic stroke: results of the MERCI trial. Stroke 2005;36(7):1432–1438
20. Smith WS, for the Multi MERCI investigators. Safety of mechanical thrombectomy and intravenous tissue plasminogen activatro in acute ischemic stroke. Results of the Multi MERCI Trial, Part I. AJNR Am J Neuroradiol 2006;(27):1177–1182
21. McDougall C, Clark W, Mayer T, et al. The Penumbra Stroke Trial: Safety and effectiveness of a new generation of mechanical devices for clot removal in acute ischemic stroke. Presented at the International Stroke Conference, New Orleans, LA, Feb 2008.
22. Levy EI, Ecker RD, Horowitz MB, et al. Stent-assisted intracranial recanalization for acute stroke: early results. Neurosurgery 2006;58(3):458–463
23. Alexandrov AV, Molina CA, Grotta JC, et al.; CLOTBUST Investigators. Ultrasound-enhanced systemic thrombolysis for acute ischemic stroke. N Engl J Med 2004; 351(21):2170–2178
24. Mahon BR, Nesbit GM, Barnwell SL, et al. North American clinical experience with the EKOS MicroLysUS infusion catheter for the treatment of embolic stroke. AJNR Am J Neuroradiol 2003;24(3):534–538
25. Abou-Chebl A, Bajzer CT, Krieger DW, Furlan AJ, Yadav JS. Multimodal therapy for the treatment of severe ischemic stroke combining GP IIb/IIIa antagonists and angioplasty after failure of thrombolysis. Stroke 2005;36(10):2286–2288

26. Gupta R, Vora NA, Horowitz MB, et al. Multimodal reperfusion therapy for acute ischemic stroke: factors predicting vessel recanalization. Stroke 2006;37(4):986–990

27. The National Institute of Neurological Disorders and Stroke rt-PA Stroke Study Group. Tissue plasminogen activator for acute ischemic stroke. N Engl J Med 1995; 333(24):1581–1587

28. Hacke W, Kaste M, Bluhmki E, et al.; ECASS Investigators. Thrombolysis with alteplase 3 to 4.5 hours after acute ischemic stroke. N Engl J Med 2008;359(13):1317–1329

29. Atkinson R, Austin L. Safety and Efficacy of NeuroFlo™ for Treatment of Ischemic Stroke (SENTIS): A Multi-center Evaluation of Cerebral Perfusion Augmentation via Partial Aortic Occlusion. 2006.

30. Inoue T, Oku K, Kimoto K, et al. Relationship of cigarette smoking to the severity of coronary and thoracic aortic atherosclerosis. Cardiology 1995;86(5):374–379

31. Wolf PA, D'Agostino RB, Kannel WB, Bonita R, Belanger AJ. Cigarette smoking as a risk factor for stroke. The Framingham Study. JAMA 1988;259(7):1025–1029

32. LaRosa JC, Grundy SM, Waters DD, et al.; Treating to New Targets (TNT) Investigators. Intensive lipid lowering with atorvastatin in patients with stable coronary disease. N Engl J Med 2005;352(14):1425–1435

33. Rovira A, Orellana P, Alvarez-Sabin J, Arenillas JF, Aymerich X, Grive E, Molina C, Rovira-Gols A. Hyperacute ischemic stroke: middle cerebral artery susceptibility sign at echoplanar gradient-echo MR imaging. Radiol 2004;232(2):466-473.

34. Intra-arterial Prourokinase for Acute Ischemic Stroke. The PROACT II Study: A Randomized Controlled Trial. JAMA 1999;282:2003–2011

17

Extracranial Arterial Occlusive Disease

Ramachandra P. Tummala and Fotis G. Souslian

Etiology

Atherosclerosis, the most common cause of arterial occlusive disease, is a chronic inflammatory response mediated or directed by the endothelial cells, which begins with the deposition of lipids from the blood into the subendothelium (**Fig. 17.1**). Once the atherosclerotic plaque forms and enlarges, it causes the arterial lumen diameter to decrease in size.

Atherosclerotic plaques can be classified broadly as uncomplicated and complicated. The composition of uncomplicated plaques is relatively uniform, and they are covered by the fibrous cap. Complicated plaques contain areas of hemorrhage, necrosis, ulceration, and calcification (**Fig. 17.2**). Plaque rupture results from disruption of the endothelium and fibrous cap and leads to embolization through direct release of plaque contents or through the aggregation of platelets to the exposed plaque surface. The posterior wall of the internal carotid artery (ICA) just distal to the common carotid artery (CCA) bifurcation is usually the most susceptible part of the carotid artery to atherosclerosis, and this region is therefore most vulnerable to significant stenosis. Risk factors associated with the advancement of atherosclerosis are diabetes mellitus, dyslipidemia, smoking, and hypertension.[1]

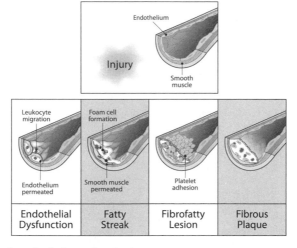

Fig. 17.1 Genesis of atherosclerotic plaque.

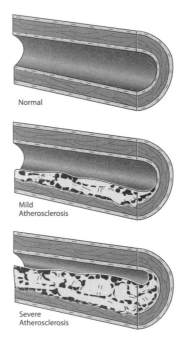

Fig. 17.2 Complicated plaque morphology.

Less common pathological causes of extracranial arterial stenosis include fibromuscular dysplasia (FMD) and certain collagen vascular diseases, such as systemic lupus erythematosus and rheumatoid arthritis. FMD is a nonatherosclerotic, noninflammatory condition that typically affects women aged 15–50 years (**Fig. 17.3**). It can affect almost every systemic arterial territory, most commonly the renal arteries, followed by the internal carotid arteries.[2] The classic angiographic appearance is a "string of beads." Many times, FMD is discovered incidentally, but it can be symptomatic and lead to arterial dissections and pseudoaneurysm formation.

With increased disease-free survival from head and neck cancers, there is an increasing incidence of radiation-induced carotid stenosis. The specific lesion location depends on where the radiation was targeted. This is in contrast to the normal location of atheromatous plaques, which are usually at arterial bifurcations. A segment of radiation-induced stenosis typically appears long and smooth as compared with its purely atherosclerotic counterpart. The mechanism of stenosis is likely related to direct endothelial injury followed by intimal proliferation, necrosis of the media, periadventitial fibrosis, and acceleration of atherosclerotic changes. An interval of more than five years from irradiation seems to be a predictor for developing significant carotid stenosis.[3]

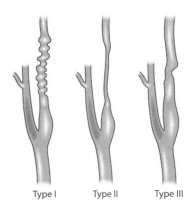

Type I   Type II   Type III

Fig. 17.3 Fibromuscular dysplasia in the carotid artery.

Diagnosis

Neurological Examination

Carotid stenosis can cause ischemic neurological symptoms, usually from embolism from the plaque and less commonly from hemodynamic compromise. The common neurological symptoms due to carotid stenosis can range from transient and mild to permanent and fatal. These include transient ischemic attacks (TIA), which are neurological deficits that last for less than 24 hours, reversible ischemic neurologic deficit (RIND), in which symptoms last from one to seven days, and stroke, which implies permanent neurologic dysfunction. The specific symptoms that can arise are dependent on the part of the brain that has decreased blood flow. Another symptom associated with unstable carotid stenosis is transient monocular vision loss. The clinical examination for a patient suspected of having a stroke should be done in a rapid yet thorough manner. If carotid stenosis is suspected as the cause, any of the imaging modalities listed below can be used, depending on their availability and feasibility. It is imperative, however, that intracranial hemorrhage should be ruled out in the acute period of presentation. Asymptomatic carotid stenosis is often discovered in the presence of a neck bruit, although a bruit is not highly predictive of the presence of a significant stenosis. However, care must be taken when applying a stethoscope or a carotid ultrasound probe on the neck, because some patients may have unstable carotid plaques, which have been reported to embolize during examination.

Diagnostic Imaging Studies and Grading Systems

Four common imaging modalities are used to evaluate carotid stenosis: magnetic resonance (MR) and CT angiography, carotid duplex ultrasound, and catheter-based angiography (**Fig. 17.4**). Each modality has its advantages and disadvantages. Each one, however, is used to determine the percentage of carotid stenosis. The major clinical trials studying the benefit of carotid endarterectomy developed two of the most commonly used techniques to determine the percentage of carotid ste-

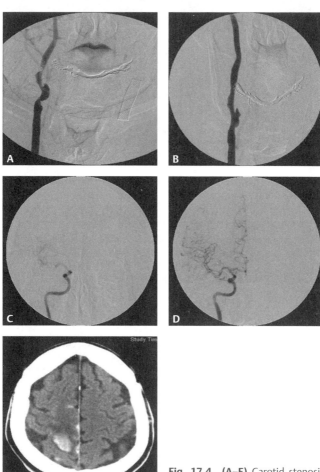

Fig. 17.4 (A–E) Carotid stenosis using various imaging modalities: CTA, MRA, CUS, Angio.

nosis. The North American Symptomatic Carotid Endarterectomy Trial (NASCET) and the European Carotid Surgery Trial (ECST) both use the minimal residual luminal diameter as the numerator. As the denominator, the ECST method uses the imagined vessel diameter at the same point if the stenosis were not present. The NASCET method, which tends to yield lower degrees of stenosis compared with the ECST method, uses the diameter of a disease-free distal segment of the artery where the walls of the vessel are parallel (**Fig. 17.5**).[4,5]

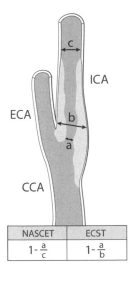

NASCET	ECST
$1 - \dfrac{a}{c}$	$1 - \dfrac{a}{b}$

Fig. 17.5 Determination of carotid stenosis using NASCET/ECST.

Magnetic Resonance Angiography

Magnetic resonance angiography (MRA) is used mostly to evaluate the extracranial carotid arteries. It provides good sensitivity (91–99%) and specificity (90–99%) for high-grade stenosis but is less sensitive for the detection of moderate stenosis[6] (**Fig. 17.4A**). However, MRA is costly and time-consuming, and it requires significant patient cooperation. We have found that MRA tends to overestimate the degree of stenosis if the plaque has significant calcifications. There has been recent attention to nephrogenic systemic fibrosis (NSF) with gadolinium-based contrast agents. Although this is a rare but serious skin disorder, it must be taken into account in patients with compromised renal function.

Computed Tomography Angiography

Computed tomography angiography (CTA) is particularly useful for evaluating vessel lumen diameter in the setting of moderate calcification, high carotid bifurcation or extremely tortuous vessels where conventional duplex ultrasonography is not reliable (**Fig. 17.4B**). The source images obtained in CTA are useful in studying the cross-sectional anatomy of the artery. However, we have found it difficult to evaluate the lumen diameter with CTA in the setting of severe calcification. According to one meta-analysis, CTA had roughly 99% sensitivity in the detection of carotid occlusion.[7] The source image reconstructions are helpful in assessing the tortuousity of the artery and the origins if endovascular intervention is anticipated. CTA should therefore be performed with caution in patients with impaired renal function; however, injection protocols have improved so that lower volumes (approximately 80 mL) and non-ionic contrast agents can be used.

Duplex Ultrasound

Ultrasound is a noninvasive, inexpensive test whose accuracy is highly user dependent (**Fig. 17.4C**). Several parameters, including ICA peak systolic velocity, ICA end diastolic velocity, and carotid ratio (ICA peak systolic velocity divided by the CCA peak systolic velocity), are used to determine the degree of vessel stenosis. Changes in blood flow velocities are typically noted with >50% stenosis. Peak systolic velocity in the ICA ranges from 54 to 88 cm/sec in normal adults. Depending on how the values are adjusted, results can be either very sensitive or very specific. Duplex ultrasonography can be used for higher grades of stenosis, that is, 70–99%, with a sensitivity of 94% and specificity of 89%. False-positive results range from 20% to 41%. Carotid duplex also does not provide information on anatomical configuration, true location, or other areas of distal or tandem stenoses. A set of criteria has been established for ultrasonic classification of carotid stenosis[1] (**Table 17.1**). Care must be taken when applying the carotid ultrasound probe on the neck, as some patients have unstable carotid plaques, which have been reported to embolize during examination.

Angiography

Catheter-based angiography is still considered the gold standard for evaluation of carotid vessels, despite its invasive nature, increased costs, and the potential for procedural morbidity (**Fig. 17.4D**). As a result, diagnostic angiography is often reserved for cases where noninvasive studies give inconclusive or discordant results or when patients have contraindications to CTA and MRA. For example, patients with both pacemakers and renal insufficiency/failure are often evaluated using diagnostic angiography. In experienced hands, carotid angiography can generally be performed with much less contrast than that needed for CTA. The amount of contrast can be reduced further by injecting only the targeted artery and by using biplane fluoroscopy. If available, rotational three-dimensional angiography is useful for optimal viewing that delineates the arterial stenosis. However, this requires an increased contrast load and is not always necessary.

Table 17.1 Criteria for Carotid Duplex Ultrasound

Grade stenosis	Comment
Normal ICA	PSV <125 cm/sec; ICA/CCA <2; no visible plaque on grayscale/color imaging
<50%	PSV <125 cm/sec; ICA/CCA <2; visible plaque or intimal thickening
50–69%	PSV 125–230 cm/sec; ICA/CCA 2–4; visible plaque
>70%	PSV >230 cm/sec; ICA/CCA >4; visible plaque
>99%	Variable velocities due to turbulent flow; may appear occluded on grayscale; color Doppler should show narrow lumen
Occluded	No patent lumen or flow on grayscale or color Doppler imaging

Abbreviations: ICA, internal carotid artery; CCA, common carotid artery; PSV, peak systolic velocity.

Evidence-Based Medicine

Several major trials have shown clear benefits for carotid revascularization in carefully chosen patients. Most of these trials compared carotid endarterectomy to medical therapy. More recent trials have attempted to compare carotid angioplasty and stenting (CAS) and carotid endarterectomy (CEA). These trials are summarized in **Table 17.2** and **Table 17.3**. Indications for CAS are evolving, but patients considered high risk for CEA seem to be appropriate for CAS. The high-risk criteria (**Table 17.4**) seem intuitive, and clinical experience has confirmed these suspicions. We have also learned that high-risk criteria exist for CAS. As experience with CAS and technology is evolving, we see that the high-risk criteria for CAS can be divided into patient-related factors and vascular anatomical factors (**Table 17.5**).

Preprocedural Preparation

Antiplatelet Therapy

The processes of angioplasty and stenting create intimal injury that promotes thrombosis. Therefore, antiplatelet agents are recommended in the perioperative period. For elective CAS, patients are placed on dual antiplatelet therapy, typically aspirin 325 mg daily and clopidogrel 75 mg daily. Ideally, patients should have started both agents five to seven days prior to the procedure. Patients can also receive 650 mg aspirin and up to 600 mg clopidogrel as a load if more urgent CAS is considered. The onset of action is 20 minutes for aspirin and 4 hours for clopidogrel. Up to 25% of patients are considered "non-responders" to antiplatelet medications, as demonstrated on a variety of platelet function assays. However, there is no general consensus on what level of platelet function must be dysfunctional before thromboembolic risks from stent placement are significantly reduced. Despite this, it is recommended that platelet function be assessed so that patients may be reloaded before their procedure in cases where platelet function is still present.

If CAS is performed on an emergency basis, a glycoprotein IIb/IIIa inhibitor can be administered intravenously once the stent has been deployed and can be followed by a continuous infusion, depending on when the patient can initiate oral antiplatelet agents. (For example, if a patient is loaded orally on aspirin and clopidogrel in the angiography suite during or immediately following CAS, an intravenous bolus of a IIb/IIIa inhibitor may suffice as the onset of action of clopidogrel coincides with the duration of the effect of the IV bolus.)

Anesthesia

CAS is usually performed under conscious sedation because the duration of the procedure is relatively short, the patient's neurological examination can be assessed readily, and a small amount of patient motion is tolerable. If a patient is uncooperative or does not tolerate conscious sedation, performing the procedure under general anesthesia is an option.

Table 17.2 Summary of Major Trials Comparing CEA and Medical Therapy for Carotid Stenosis

	Purpose	Eligibility	Results	Criticism
Asymptomatic Carotid Atherosclerosis Study (ACAS)[11]	Randomized prospective 5-year multicenter study comparing medical management to CEA for asymptomatic patients with carotid stenosis (via ultrasound and arteriogram) in 1662 patients.	Patients had at least 60% asymptomatic carotid stenosis and were randomized to aspirin only (325 mg daily) or aspirin plus CEA. Barred further participation of some surgeons who had adverse outcomes during the trial.	For the CEA group, the risk of death, any perioperative stroke or ipsilateral stroke over 5 years was half that of the aspirin-only group (5.1% in the surgery group versus 11% in the non-surgical group). There was no significant benefit of CEA in women.	(1) Absolute risk reduction with CEA was only ~1% per year. (2) The low operative risk may not be matched in "real world" practice. (3) Non-significant absolute risk reduction of disabling or fatal stroke with surgery (2.7%). (4) The trial had insufficient power for subgroup analysis compared with ACST.
Asymptomatic Carotid Surgery Trial (ACST)[12]	A 5-year prospective, randomized trial that included 126 hospitals and randomized 3120 asymptomatic patients with carotid stenosis (by ultrasound) to either receive immediate CEA or deferral of CEA until treatment was indicated.	At least 60% unilateral or bilateral carotid stenosis without any TIA or stroke within 6 months prior to the study. Very few exclusion criteria.	Similar results to ACAS. Absolute reduction in 5 year stroke risk was 6.4% in the CEA group versus 11.8% in the deferral group. Unlike ACAS, there was a significant absolute reduction with CEA in risk of disabling or fatal stroke. Because of larger enrollment, the study had sufficient power for subgroup analysis.	(1) Medical management in the deferral group was variable. (2) The study excluded patients who had neurological symptoms or stroke for up to 6 months prior to the study; however, around 300 patients were admitted into the study who had neurological symptoms more than 6 months prior to the study onset.

North American Symptomatic Carotid Endarterectomy Trial (NASCET)[4]	One of the original multicenter, randomized, controlled prospective trials designed to compare CEA to medical therapy for secondary stroke prevention in patients with symptomatic carotid stenosis. The trial studied 2885 patients at 106 centers. Primary outcome was fatal or nonfatal stroke ipsilateral to the stenosis for which patient was treated. Secondary outcome was all strokes and deaths.	Hemispheric or retinal TIA or nondisabling stroke within 120 days prior to enrollment. Patients were divided into two categories based on severity of carotid stenosis: 30–69% and 70–99%. 659 patients were randomized in the high-grade category, and 858 patients were in the 50–69% category. The remainder were in the <50% stenosis group.	The 2-year ipsilateral stroke risk was significantly lower in the CEA group compared with medical group (9% in the surgery group versus 26% in the medical group, p < 0.001). The moderate stenosis group achieved a statistically significant 5-year stroke risk reduction with CEA (15.7% versus 22.2% in medical group). CEA was clearly beneficial for symptomatic high-grade (≥70%) stenosis. CEA was beneficial in carefully selected patients with symptomatic moderate stenosis. There was no benefit with CEA for stenosis <50%.	(1) There were no standardized guidelines for the medical management group. (2) Patients ≥80 years and medical comorbidities were excluded; study population not reflective of entire population at risk of stroke from carotid stenosis. (3) The low surgical complication rates in the trial are not reflective of "real world" practice. (4) Medical management has improved since this trial and the results in the medical arm may no longer be applicable.
European Carotid Surgery Trial (ECST)[5]	ECST was a randomized, multicenter, prospective trial that compared CEA to medical management in 3024 patients with symptomatic carotid stenosis. The trial was conducted at 100 centers in 14 countries.	Similar to NASCET. Patients with any degree of carotid stenosis were eligible for ECST. 501 patients had stenosis ≥70% and 684 patients were in the moderate stenosis category. Method of measurement of stenosis was different than in NASCET. The ECST method resulted in higher degrees of stenosis compared with NASCET. Very few exclusion criteria.	Results were similar to NASCET with regard to high-grade (≥70%) stenosis. Two-year risk of ipsilateral stroke was 7% for CEA compared with 19.9% for medical therapy. ECST showed negative benefit with CEA in patients with moderate stenosis (50–69%). There was no benefit with CEA for stenosis <50%.	(1) When stenosis was remeasured using NASCET criteria, CEA reduced 5-year stroke and death risk by 5.7%, a modest reduction similar to the results seen in NASCET. (2) ECST defined follow-up stroke as a deficit persisting more than 7 days and did not include retinal TIAs. (3) Medical management has improved since this trial was conducted.

Abbreviations: CEA, carotid endarterectomy; TIA, transient ischemic attack.

Table 17.3 Major CAS Trials

	Purpose	Eligibility	Results	Criticism
Stent-Protected Angioplasty versus Carotid Endarterectomy Trial (SPACE)[13]	Prospective, randomized trial, designed to establish non-inferiority of CAS compared with CEA for symptomatic extracranial carotid stenosis in low surgical risk patients.	Inclusion criteria—patients from 35 different centers throughout Europe with symptomatic severe carotid stenosis (≥70% on duplex ultrasound, ≥50% by NASCET criteria, ≥70% by ECST criteria). 1183 patients were randomized within 6 months of a TIA or stroke to receive either CAS or CEA. High-risk surgical candidates were excluded from the study. Primary endpoint was stroke or death, with follow-up at 30 days and at 2 years following treatment.	The 30-day post-treatment results failed to support non-inferiority of CAS compared with CEA. The rate of ipsilateral stroke or death was 6.34% in the CEA group and 6.84% in the CAS group, which was not statistically significant. The 2-year post-treatment results showed that the rates of ipsilateral stroke between the two modalities are similar (8.8% in the CEA group and 9.5% in the CAS group, p = 0.62).	(1) Enrollment was halted well short of intended enrollment of 1900 patients. Interim analysis suggested that 2500 patients would be needed to demonstrate significance. The trial did not have funds to meet this goal and was terminated early. (2) Use of embolic protection devices was not required and was used in 27% of the CAS cases.

Endarterectomy versus Angioplasty in Patients with Symptomatic Severe Carotid Stenosis (EVA-3S)[14]	Prospective, randomized, assessor-blinded trial designed to compare CEA versus CAS in patients with symptomatic extracranial carotid stenosis.	527 patients with symptomatic severe carotid artery stenosis (≥60% on angiography or duplex ultrasound and MRA) from 30 different centers in France were randomized within 4 months of stroke. Primary endpoint was stroke or death within 30 days following treatment. The trial was stopped prematurely after it was estimated that at least 4000 patients would have to be enrolled to test the non-inferiority of carotid stenting. As in the SPACE trial, high-risk surgical candidates were excluded from this trial.	30-day rate of death or any stroke was 3.9% in the CEA group versus 9.6% in the CAS group (significant). 6-month rate of death or stroke was 6.1% for CEA and 11.7% for CAS. 30-day rate of disabling stroke was 1.3% for CEA and 3.4% for CAS (not significant).	(1) The inexperience of the operators performing CAS in this trial has been cited as one factor for the high complication rate for CAS. The complication rate for CAS was much higher than described in previously published papers. (2) Embolic protection devices were recommended after half the trial duration was completed. (3) Dual antiplatelet therapy was used in fewer than 50% of the CAS patients. (4) Rates of MI were not assessed.
Stenting and Angioplasty with Protection in Patients at High Risk for Endarterectomy (SAPPHIRE)[15]	A prospective observational randomized trial that included 29 centers throughout North America. This study compared high-risk surgical patients who were symptomatic with ≥50% carotid stenosis (with duplex ultrasound or angiography) to high-risk surgical patients who were asymptomatic with ≥80% stenosis. Primary endpoints were major adverse events that included stroke, death, and MI (unlike EVA-3S and SPACE).	Only high-risk surgical candidates were included in the study. They defined high-risk as having one or more of the co-morbidities listed in Table 15.3.	This trial demonstrated that CAS was not inferior to CEA in high-risk patients. The 30-day rates of death, stroke, or MI were 5.8% for CAS and 12.6% for CEA. At 6 months, combined major adverse events rate was 12.2% with CAS and 20.1% in the CEA group. There was a significant decrease in cranial nerve injuries with CAS.	(1) Almost 29% of patients in both treatment groups had recurrent arterial stenosis, which favors carotid stenting. This is because repeat surgery is associated with a higher complication rate. (2) Many patients were lost to follow-up at 3 years. (3) The inclusion of MI as an endpoint was not part of the NASCET or ECST trials.

(Continued on page 334)

Table 17.3 (*Continued*) Major CAS Trials

	Purpose	Eligibility	Results	Criticism
Carotid Revascularization Endarterectomy versus Stenting Trial (CREST)[16]	CREST was a randomized, multicenter, prospective trial that compared CEA to CAS in 2502 patients with symptomatic and asymptomatic carotid stenosis. The trial was conducted at 117 centers in the US and Canada.	Symptomatic: transient ischemic attack (TIA), amaurosis fugax (AF), or non-disabling stroke within the past 180 days, and who have an ipsilateral carotid stenosis ≥50% by angiography or ≥70% by ultrasound or ≥70% by CTA or MRA. Asymptomatic subjects: Patients who have carotid stenosis ≥60% by angiography or ≥70% by ultrasound or ≥80% by CTA or MRA are eligible for this study. (Subjects with symptoms beyond 180 days are considered asymptomatic.) Outcome: Mortality, stroke, or myocardial infarction at 30 days postoperatively; ipsilateral stroke at 30 days postoperatively.	For 2502 patients (median follow-up 2.5 years), there was no significant difference in the estimated 4-year rates of the primary endpoint between the CAS group and the CEA group (7.2% and 6.8%, respectively; hazard ratio with CAS, 1.11; 95% confidence interval, 0.81 to 1.51; $p = 0.51$). There was no differential treatment effect with regard to the primary endpoint according to symptomatic status ($p = 0.84$) or sex ($p = 0.34$). The 4-year rate of stroke or death was 6.4% with CAS and 4.7% with CEA (hazard ratio, 1.50; $p = 0.03$); the rates among symptomatic patients were 8.0% and 6.4% (hazard ratio, 1.37; $p = 0.14$), and the rates among asymptomatic patients were 4.5% and 2.7% (hazard ratio, 1.86; $p = 0.07$), respectively. Periprocedural rates of individual components of the endpoints differed between the CAS group and the CEA group: for death (0.7% versus 0.3%, $p = 0.18$), for stroke (4.1% versus 2.3%, $p = 0.01$), and for myocardial infarction (1.1% versus 2.3%, $p = 0.03$). After this period, the incidences of ipsilateral stroke with CAS and with CEA were similarly low (2.0% and 2.4%, respectively; $p = 0.85$).	N/A

Table 17.4 High-Risk Criteria for Carotid Endarterectomy[15]

CHF (class III/IV) and/or known severe LV dysfunction LVEF <30%
Open-heart surgery within 6 weeks
Recent MI (>24 hours and <4 weeks)
Unstable angina (CCS class III/IV)
Coexistent severe cardiac and carotid disease requiring open-heart surgery and carotid revascularization
Severe pulmonary disease
Abnormal stress test
Age ≥80 years as a single risk factor
Contralateral carotid occlusion
Post radiation treatment
Previous CEA recurrent stenosis
High cervical CCA bifurcation or CCA lesions below the clavicle
Severe tandem lesions

Abbreviations: CCA, common carotid artery; CEA, carotid endarterectomy; MI, myocardial infarction.

Table 17.5 High-Risk Criteria for Carotid Angioplasty and Stenting

Symptomatic carotid stenosis
Age >80 years
Renal failure
Multiple (overlapping) stent placements
Duration of embolic protection device deployment
Tortuousity/calcification of aortic arch and great vessels

Equipment and Technique of CAS

Vascular Access

Typically, the procedure begins with diagnostic cervical carotid and cerebral angiograms to evaluate the carotid stenosis and vascular access route for any excessive tortuosity and for tandem stenoses, whether extracranially or intracranially. A 4 or 5 Fr diagnostic catheter, which is advanced through a 4 or 5 Fr groin sheath over a 0.035″ glide wire, is used for this purpose. Occasionally, an aortic arch injection is useful to visualize the tortuousity of the proximal great vessels. The operator must note not only the severity of carotid stenosis but also the tortuosity of the CCA and ICA, along with the degree of calcification in the stenotic segment. Measurements of the diameter of the ICA at the intended landing zone of the embolic protection device and the diameters of the native ICA and distal CCA are taken. These factors help determine the choice and size of the stent, balloons, and embolic protection device.

After completion of the angiogram, the diagnostic catheter and groin sheath are exchanged over a stiff 0.035-inch wire for a 6 Fr, 90 cm long introducer. The exchange-length stiff wire is positioned in the distal external carotid artery branches for stability during the exchange maneuver. The 6 Fr introducer is positioned in the distal half of the common carotid artery. The introducer is advanced over a dilator (obturator) that may be radiolucent; care must be taken not to advance the introducer too far and potentially disrupt the carotid plaque. The dilator and exchange length wire are removed and back-bleeding through the introducer is confirmed. The patient then receives a sufficient dose of intravenous heparin (typically, 50–70 units/kg) to achieve an activated coagulation time (ACT) between 250 and 350 seconds. The appropriate devices for the intervention can then prepared while the ACT is pending.

Preparation of Devices

To increase the efficiency of the procedure, all the necessary devices (embolic protection device, angioplasty balloon, stent, embolic protection device retrieval catheter, and balloon inflator) can be prepared and placed at the foot of the angiography table in the order of anticipated use. This preparation is done during the several minutes after the administration of intravenous heparin and while waiting for the ACT results. The choice of stent and distal protection device may be limited if the patient has been enrolled in a specific study or registry. If the lesion involves the internal carotid artery (ICA) origin, the patient receives intravenous glycopyrrolate (0.4 mg) or intravenous atropine (0.75 mg) just before angioplasty in anticipation of bradycardia that may result from manipulation of the carotid bulb.

Crossing the Stenosis and Deployment of the Distal Embolic Protection Device

Almost all carotid interventions use distal embolic protection. Most distal embolic protection devices have filters attached to a microwire. After the ACT is in the appropriate range, we cross the stenotic lesion with the distal embolic protection device under roadmap guidance. Crossing the lesion should be smooth, and buckling of the wire tip should not occur. If traversing the lesion proves difficult, especially in cases of ulcerated or calcified plaques, the fluoroscopic views are changed to visualize the lesion better, or the shape of the wire tip is altered. Frequently, these maneuvers will result in a successful crossing. Once beyond the lesion, the embolic protection device is navigated distally and deployed in a straight segment in the distal cervical ICA. This usually positions the wire tip in the horizontal petrous segment of the ICA. Alternatively, if the anatomy proves to be too tortuous for deployment of a distal protection device, a distal balloon can be used as a distal protection device. In some cases in which the carotid is markedly tortuous or nearly occluded, a 0.014 inch diameter wire can be advanced across the lesion first as a "buddy wire" to keep access to the distal carotid in case advancing the distal protection device causes a dissection or occludes the carotid artery.

Angioplasty Prior to Stent Placement

Some operators perform this step routinely, although it is not necessary in all cases. Presenting angioplasty ("predilatation") can be reserved for lesions too stenotic for safe passage of the stent delivery system (typically <2 mm). The need for predilatation is assessed based on the appearance of the stenosis and the difficulty in crossing the lesion with the filter. An undersized balloon (e.g., 3 mm in diameter) typically is used for this step, as the goal is simply to facilitate the next step, which is positioning and deployment of the stent.

Deployment of the Stent

We typically use one of the carotid stents approved by the United States Food and Drug Administration. The type (closed cell versus open cell, large porosity versus small porosity) and length of stent chosen depend on several factors, such as calcification of the plaque, vascular tortuosity, and navigability of the delivery system (**Table 17.6**). An angiographic roadmap or run is made just prior to crossing the lesion with the stent delivery system. A roadmap may not be necessary if the lesion is calcified and can be easily visualized without the use of contrast material. A roadmap or run performed before stent deployment will identify alterations in the arterial tortuosity made by the wire of the distal embolic protection device. Once the stent delivery system is positioned, we slowly begin the deployment. Because most delivery systems release their inherent forward energy as the stent is deployed, caution must be exercised not to place the stent too distally. As the forward energy is released, the operator must keep negative tension or pull the system proximally before completing the stent deployment. In cases of very severe stenosis, the stent may spring too proximally or distally (a phenomenon colloquially known as "watermelon seeding"). Therefore, slow stent deployment and proper visualization are important to adjust the stent position appropriately. Use of a longer stent may also prevent this phenomenon.

Table 17.6 Stent Selection in Carotid Artery Disease

Stent design	Pro	Con
Closed cell	Can completely cover and stabilize plaque, decreasing distal embolization risk	Cannot cross into the CCA if plaque extends into CCA; cannot be used in the ECA; difficulty with navigation in tortuous anatomy
Open small cell	Improved navigation in tortuous anatomy; can be used in CCA-ICA plaques	Should not be used in CCA-ECA due to small perforating vessels off ECA; some reports of "watermelon seeding"; can erode into plaque, causing distal embolization
Open large cell	Improved navigation in tortuous anatomy; can be used in CCA-ICA and CCA-ECA plaques	Erosion into plaque can cause distal embolization

Abbreviations: CCA, common carotid artery; ECA, external carotid artery; ICA, internal carotid artery.

Angioplasty Following Stent Placement

If residual stenosis exists following placement of the stent, it will appear on fluoro-scopic imaging as an impression within the stent resembling the waist of an hour-glass. An angiographic run can confirm the residual stenosis. A balloon sized to or slightly undersized to the diameter of the normal ICA is advanced into the stent. Because the stent is radiopaque, the angioplasty is done under fluoroscopy alone. The balloon is purged of air, and the inflation device is filled with half-strength contrast material. The balloon should be positioned completely within the stent. Care must be taken to avoid angioplasty of the native ICA distal to the stent. The balloon is then inflated quickly to its nominal pressure and deflated just as rapidly. The stenotic impression within the stent can usually be seen to resolve during the angioplasty. Despite the prophylactic use of atropine or glycopyrrolate, some patients may still develop severe bradycardia and hypotension. In addition to in-travenous administration of bolus doses of fluid, a dopamine infusion is started immediately. In the event of asystole, we find that a deep cough by the patient (and a deep breath by the operator) results in rapid return of normal cardiac rhythm.

Retrieval of Distal Embolic Protection Device

Most of the commercially available distal protection devices come with a retrieval catheter. This catheter is used to capture the filter. Prior to filter retrieval, a final intracranial run and neurological examination should be performed. Normally, the retrieval catheter can pass beyond the struts of the stent to capture the protection device. Some retrieval catheters have an angled tip, allowing rotation of the cath-eter, to prevent being caught on the struts of the stent. If there is difficulty going beyond the stent, turning the neck can significantly aid in traversing the stent. Other techniques include redilating the stent or using a more rigid wire, such as a buddy wire, for distal access. After the filter has been retrieved, it is removed and checked for any trapped debris. The final run is compared with the baseline views to check for any irregularities in the carotid artery and any evidence of thromboembolic occlusions in the cerebral circulation.

Postoperative Care

General Care

The groin puncture site is closed percutaneously with a closure device in most cases. Otherwise, the 6 Fr introducer is exchanged for a short, 7 Fr groin sheath that is removed several hours later. If the closure device fails and manual compression has to be employed, one can use a compression device, such as the FemStop (St. Jude's Medical), to hold prolonged pressure with a pressurized system, gradually decreasing over time to prevent localized bruising and ischemia. The patient is monitored overnight on telemetry and maintained on intravenous fluids and vasopressor infusion if hypotension persists. Typically, the blood pressure normalizes by the next day, especially if the patient becomes ambulatory promptly. If hypotension occurs, any antihypertensive medications that the patient was taking preoperatively, except β-blockers, should be withheld for two days after discharge. Baseline carotid ultrasound imaging is obtained before discharge on the first postoperative day. The patient remains on aspirin (325 mg daily) and clopidogrel (75 mg daily) for four to twelve weeks, followed by daily aspirin thereafter. Alternatively, we use ticlopidine 250 mg daily if the patient has an allergy or intolerance to clopidogrel.

Acute Neurological Changes in the Postoperative Period

If the patient's neurological status changes acutely, one must consider the differential diagnosis of hypoperfusion, embolism, hemorrhage, or hypotension. If the neurological deficit occurs during the procedure, the operator should complete the current maneuver, such as deployment of the stent, inflation of the balloon, etc. Then the etiology of the neurological deficit can be sought. An immediate angiogram should be performed to evaluate the carotid artery and the intracranial circulation. In addition to perfusion defects, the angiogram should be evaluated for vessel displacement and other signs of mass effect. Acute vessel displacement is likely due to hemorrhage, whether it is in the neck or intracranial.

If a neurological change is highly suspicious for an embolism but there is no angiographic evidence of vascular occlusion or intracranial hemorrhage, a CT scan of the brain is useful for evaluating intracranial hemorrhage. If no hemorrhage is identified, the degree of neurological deficit determines how aggressive we are in treating the patient. MR imaging can be used to examine for diffusion-weighted lesions. For significant neurological deficits (such as moderate to severe weakness, or dysphasia) without evidence of hemorrhage or contrast leakage, an intravenous or intraarterial bolus of a glycoprotein IIb/IIIa inhibitor can be used. Luckily, mild deficits (for example, pronator drift, dysarthria) usually recover favorably with only conservative management.

If an intracranial arterial occlusion is noted, the patient's neurological condition and the location of the occlusion determine how aggressively revascularization is attempted. Thus, an intraprocedural embolism is generally managed using the same endovascular techniques that we would apply to any other appropriately selected acute stroke. Typically, the occlusion occurs in distal branches such as the angular artery. The distal embolic protection device is retrieved, and we advance a navigable guide catheter past the stent. Selective microcatheterization of the occluded branch is performed when possible. Since most occlusions in this setting involve smaller branches, thrombolysis with local intra-arterial thrombolytics or glycoprotein IIb/IIIa inhibitors or mechanical disruption of the embolus with the microcatheter is performed. If there is a large embolus in a proximal artery, mechanical thrombectomy can be attempted. As with many intra-arterial stroke interventions, a combination of strategies may be necessary. Cautionary measures should be taken when selecting the MERCI retrieval system for mechanical thrombolysis. Many have the nylon filament for better clot retrieval but can get caught on the carotid stent, resulting in damage or migration.

Reperfusion (Hyperperfusion) Syndrome

Reperfusion syndrome is an uncommon complication that usually occurs in the first few days, but may occur up to two weeks following carotid revascularization. Although several explanations exist for reperfusion syndrome, the common theme is impaired cerebral autoregulation. The ipsilateral smaller cerebral arterioles are usually maximally vasodilated in the setting of hemodynamically significant carotid stenosis. Immediately following revascularization, the previously vasodilated arterioles are unable to autoregulate in the setting of re-established normal reperfusion. This syndrome occurs most often in the setting of increases of more than 100% in cerebral perfusion compared with the baseline after carotid revascularization[8] (**Table 17.7**).

The resultant elevated cerebral blood flow induces cerebral white matter edema that may result in a wide spectrum of findings. These include simple partial or secondarily generalized seizures, focal neurological deficit, ipsilateral or bilateral headaches, and subarachnoid or intracerebral hemorrhage. Although some symptoms are nonspecific and can be easily overlooked, one must consider reperfusion injury following carotid revascularization, particularly for severe, flow-limiting stenoses. Early recognition and aggressive blood pressure control are critical to prevent severe sequelae. Noncontrast CT with perfusion imaging would determine if hemorrhage had occurred and may demonstrate hyperperfusion of the affected hemisphere. Transfer of the patient to the intensive care unit and intravenous administration of antihypertensives is recommended. If seizures occur, appropriate antiepileptics, such as phenytoin, should be initiated.

Table 17.7 Signs and Symptoms of Cerebral Reperfusion Syndrome

Although it can present in patients up to one month postprocedure, most patients present within the first week
Usually presents as a triad of ipsilateral headache, seizure, and contralateral neurological deficits
Headache is the most common feature (62%) and is usually migrainous in nature
Neurological deficits are usually cortical in nature, e.g., hemiplegia, neglect, aphasia, or present as worsening of preexisting deficits
Seizures usually present as focal or generalized

Recurrent Carotid Stenosis

The long-term durability of CAS remains unknown. Because of its noninvasiveness, duplex ultrasound is commonly used to follow patients with CAS for possible development of in-stent stenosis. The frequency of follow-up is variable depending on the institution and the type of CAS trial or registry. A typical scenario would be to obtain a baseline ultrasound immediately following CAS and then at 1 month and 6 months, and then yearly. Recurrent stenosis following CEA or CAS is typically described as ≥50% by ultrasound. Neointimal hyperplasia seems to be responsible for early restenosis following carotid revascularization, whether CEA or CAS. The early restenosis rate for CAS seems to be comparable to that for CEA. The cumulative incidence of restenosis in the first year following CEA is approximately 10%. Compared with angioplasty alone, the placement of a stent clearly reduces restenosis rates, recently reported as 6–8% within the first two years after CAS.[9] Similar to CEA, the risk of recurrent stenosis seems to be greatest in the first year after CAS and then deceases with time. In the same report, roughly 1% of all patients underwent retreatment for restenosis within the first two years of CAS.[9] Similar to CEA, the natural history of recurrent stenosis following CAS seems to be benign, but long-term follow-up is necessary.

Treatment options for in-stent stenosis include repeating angioplasty with a standard balloon, cutting balloon angioplasty, and placement of a second stent in addition to angioplasty. A cutting balloon has equally spaced atherotomes mounted on a balloon, and the resulting cutting balloon incises the stenotic lesion as the balloon is inflated. Cutting balloon angioplasty in conjunction with stent placement has been suggested as first-line endovascular treatment for severely calcified carotid lesions, but no large series studies exist to support this practice currently.

Subclavian and Vertebral Artery Angioplasty and Stenting

Stenosis involving the subclavian artery (SCA) or vertebral artery (VA) may cause posterior circulation ischemic symptoms. The mechanism of ischemia may be embolic or hemodynamic. Angioplasty and stenting of these arteries are typically reserved for symptomatic stenosis ≥50% (**Fig. 17.6**). The natural history of stenosis in these arteries is poorly understood, and there are no established guidelines to treat asymptomatic disease of these arteries. SCA stenosis may also cause upper extremity ischemia, particularly with exertion. Subclavian steal involves a stenosis of the SCA proximal to the VA origin and manifests as vertebrobasilar ischemia exacerbated by upper extremity exertion. Another variant of subclavian stenosis is subclavian-coronary steal, in which a proximal SCA stenosis may cause coronary ischemic symptoms in patients with coronary bypass graft with an internal mammary artery donor. The technique is similar to that of CAS. Usually a shorter (70 or 80 cm) introducer or guide catheter will suffice. A brachial or radial approach may be superior to the femoral approach in cases of excessive tortuosity of the SCA that may compromise stability of the guide catheter. A support wire placed in the axillary artery may give greater support for the guide catheter. For stenosis of VA origin, the lesion is crossed with a 0.014″ wire, and the tip is positioned around the first curve of the V2 segment. The stent is advanced under road map guidance. A balloon-mounted stent is optimal for stenoses of VA or SCA origin, because it allows more precise stent placement compared with the self-expanding stents, which have some inherent forward energy in their delivery systems. This feature

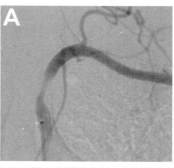
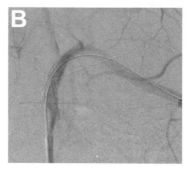
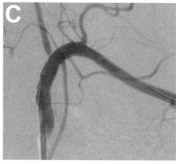

Fig. 17.6 Subclavian stenosis. **(A)** Significant stenosis in the left subclavian artery and absence of vertebral artery filling. **(B)** Placement of subclavian stent. **(C)** Improved blood flow in the left subclavian artery and filling of the vertebral artery.

is particularly important at the VA origin, where a large overhang of the stent into the SCA should be avoided. The stent should be sized as closely to the artery diameter as possible. Balloon-mounted coronary artery stents are convenient for vertebral arteries ≤3.5 mm in diameter. While there are high rates of technical success with these procedures, the restenosis rate for VA origin stents has been reported as high as 43%.[10] One reason for this high rate of restenosis may be mechanical stress from artificially straightening the normally tortuous VA origin with a stent. More recently, investigators have reported using distal protection devices during stent placement, drug-eluting stents, and self-expanding stents in the VA with hopes of reducing restenosis.

Clinical Pearls

1. Atherosclerosis, the most common cause of arterial occlusive disease, is a chronic inflammatory disease.
2. The common neurological symptoms that are due to carotid stenosis can range from transient ischemic attacks (TIA, with neurological deficits <24 hours), reversible ischemic neurologic deficit (RIND, symptoms last from 1–7 days), and stroke (permanent neurologic dysfunction).
3. Prestenting angioplasty ("predilatation") can be reserved for lesions too stenotic for safe passage of the stent delivery system (typically <2 mm).
4. Reperfusion syndrome is an uncommon complication that usually occurs in the first few days, but may occur up to two weeks following carotid revas-

cularization; this syndrome occurs most often with increases of more than 100% in cerebral perfusion.

5. Recurrent stenosis following CEA or CAS is typically described as ≥50% by ultrasound and is most commonly caused by neointimal hyperplasia early on.

6. The cumulative incidence of restenosis in the first year is approximately 10% after CEA and 6–8% within the first two years after CAS, and it is greatest for each within the first year after treatment.

Recommended Reading

Executive Committee for the Asymptomatic Carotid Atherosclerosis Study. Endarterectomy for asymptomatic carotid artery stenosis. JAMA 1995;273:1421–1428

MRC European Carotid Surgery Trialists. Randomised trial of endarterectomy for recently symptomatic carotid stenosis: final results of the MRC European Carotid Surgery Trial (ECST). Lancet 1998;351:1379-1387

North American Symptomatic Carotid Endarterectomy Trial Collaborators. Beneficial effect of carotid endarterectomy in symptomatic patients with high-grade carotid stenosis. N Engl J Med 1991;325(7):445–453

Yadav JS, Wholey MH, Kuntz RE, et al.; Stenting and Angioplasty with Protection in Patients at High Risk for Endarterectomy Investigators. Protected carotid-artery stenting versus endarterectomy in high-risk patients. N Engl J Med 2004;351(15):1493–1501

Zwiebel WJ, Pellerito JS. *Introduction to Vascular Ultrasonography*, 5th ed. Elsevier Saunders; 2005

References

1. Zwiebel WJ, Pellerito JS. *Introduction to Vascular Ultrasonography*, 5th edition. Elsevier Saunders; 2005

2. Olin JW, Pierce M. Contemporary management of fibromuscular dysplasia. Curr Opin Cardiol 2008;23(6):527–536

3. Cheng SW, Wu LL, Ting AC, Lau H, Lam LK, Wei WI. Irradiation-induced extracranial carotid stenosis in patients with head and neck malignancies. Am J Surg 1999;178(4):323–328

4. Barnett HJ, Taylor DW, Eliasziw M, et al. Benefit of carotid endarterectomy in patients with symptomatic moderate or severe stenosis. North American Symptomatic Carotid Endarterectomy Trial Collaborators. N Engl J Med 1998;339(20):1415–1425

5. European Carotid Surgery Trialists MRC. Randomised trial of endarterectomy for recently symptomatic carotid stenosis: final results of the MRC European Carotid Surgery Trial (ECST). Lancet 1998;351(9113):1379–1387

6. Debrey SM, Yu H, Lynch JK, et al. Diagnostic accuracy of magnetic resonance angiography for internal carotid artery disease: a systematic review and meta-analysis. Stroke 2008;39(8):2237–2248

7. Koelemay MJ, Nederkoorn PJ, Reitsma JB, Majoie CB. Systematic review of computed tomographic angiography for assessment of carotid artery disease. Stroke 2004;35(10):2306–2312

8. van Mook WN, Rennenberg RJ, Schurink GW, et al. Cerebral hyperperfusion syndrome. Lancet Neurol 2005;4(12):877–888

9. Gröschel K, Riecker A, Schulz JB, Ernemann U, Kastrup A. Systematic review of early recurrent stenosis after carotid angioplasty and stenting. Stroke 2005;36(2):367–373

10. Albuquerque FC, Fiorella D, Han P, Spetzler RF, McDougall CG. A reappraisal of angioplasty and stenting for the treatment of vertebral origin stenosis. Neurosurgery 2003;53(3):607–614, discussion 614–616

11. Executive Committee for the Asymptomatic Carotid Atherosclerosis Study. Endarterectomy for asymptomatic carotid artery stenosis. JAMA 1995;273:1421–1428

12. Halliday A, Mansfield A, Marro J, et al.; MRC Asymptomatic Carotid Surgery Trial (ACST) Collaborative Group. Prevention of disabling and fatal strokes by successful carotid endarterectomy in patients without recent neurological symptoms: randomised controlled trial. Lancet 2004;363(9420):1491–1502

13. Ringleb PA, Allenberg J, Brückmann H, et al.; SPACE Collaborative Group. 30 day results from the SPACE trial of stent-protected angioplasty versus carotid endarterectomy in symptomatic patients: a randomised non-inferiority trial. Lancet 2006; 368(9543):1239–1247

14. Mas JL, Chatellier G, Beyssen B, et al.; EVA-3S Investigators. Endarterectomy versus stenting in patients with symptomatic severe carotid stenosis. N Engl J Med 2006;355(16):1660–1671

15. Yadav JS, Wholey MH, Kuntz RE, et al.; Stenting and Angioplasty with Protection in Patients at High Risk for Endarterectomy Investigators. Protected carotid-artery stenting versus endarterectomy in high-risk patients. N Engl J Med 2004;351(15):1493–1501

16. Brott TG, Hobson RW II, Howard G, Roubin GS, et al. Stenting versus endarterectomy for treatment of carotid-artery stenosis. N Engl J Med 2010 Jul 1;363(1):11–23. Epub 2010 May 26. Erratum in: N Engl J Med 2010 Jul 29;363(5):498. N Engl J Med 2010 Jul 8;363(2):198.

Intracranial Arterial Stenosis

Raymond D. Turner IV, M. Imran Chaudry, and Aquilla S. Turk

Etiology

Intracranial stenosis is responsible for approximately 10% of all strokes. The most common etiologies for intracranial stenosis are intracranial atherosclerotic disease (ICAD) and intracranial vasculitides.[1,2] ICAD often occurs in patients with widespread vasculopathy and is more common in the Asian, Hispanic and African American populations.[3–6] Increased age, hypertension, hyperlipidemia, smoking, and diabetes are also risk factors.[3–7] Intracranial vasculitides have a variety of causative factors.

Fibromuscular dysplasia (FMD) is an arteriopathy of medium and large arteries and can be unifocal or multifocal. The precise cause of FMD is unknown. Histological studies demonstrate that the dysplasia presents as intimal fibroplasia, medial fibroplasia, or adventitial hyperplasia.[8] FMD is more common in women, which may be explained by a role of estrogen and progresterone or by an inheritable trait with poor penetrance in men.[9–11] Angiographically, FMD appears as irregularly spaced regions of constriction, having a "string of beads" appearance.[8]

Moyamoya disease is an intracranial occlusive disease that is more common in the Japanese population and involves stenosis and occlusion of the supraclinoid arteries. The etiology of moyamoya is unknown.[12] These occlusions result in poor cerebral perfusion and the development of arterial collaterals, most commonly located at the distal supraclinoid and proximal M1 and A1 segments. Angiographically, they resemble a "puff of smoke," which is the English translation of the Japanese word moyamoya, first coined by Suzuki and Takaku.[13] The early appearance of moyamoya can be easily mistaken for ICAD; however, moyamoya usually appears in a younger population (bimodal distribution: <10 years old and at the fourth decade) and can be bilateral. However, a subgroup of patients was discovered in the U.S. Wingspan registry who were younger than 55 years old with symptomatic supraclinoid internal carotid artery stenosis, due to their high propensity to develop recurrent stenosis (nearly 89%) despite stenting.[14] These patients may represent either another form of the disease or simply be a part of the ongoing pathogenesis. A four-stage development of moyamoya disease, which incorporates the multitude of presentations, has been proposed and each should be taken into consideration in young people who present with intracranial stenosis (**Table 18.1**).

Table 18.1 Stages of Moyamoya Disease

Stage	Findings
I/II	1. Only mild stenosis of the carotid fork
	2. All main cerebral arteries dilated
III	Marked luminal narrowing in MCA and ACA
IV	Occlusion of the ICA to the posterior communicating artery
V	1. Occlusion of the ICA and the siphon region of the ICA
	2. Almost complete disappearance of all the main arteries from the internal carotid artery supply
VI	Complete disappearance of the ICA siphon region

Diagnosis

Clinical Presentations

It is important to understand the functional implications of vascular ischemia in any given arterial territory (**Table 18.2, Table 18.3,** and **Table 18.4**). For example, anterior cerebral artery ischemia would manifest with contralateral leg weakness as the most prominent symptom, whereas middle cerebral artery ischemia presents primarily with contralateral face and arm weakness, along with aphasia if it occurs in the dominant hemisphere. It is uncommon for anterior circulation stroke to present with cranial nerve palsies, such as peri-oral numbness, a sign of dysfunction in the chief sensory nucleus of cranial nerve V. It is important to note that it is not uncommon for patients with ICAD to present with a stuttering presentation of waxing and waning symptoms. Dominant hemisphere, anterior circulation stroke differs from the nondominant hemisphere stroke in the profound loss of language abilities (**Table 18.3**). Posterior circulation hypoperfusion typically presents with brainstem and cerebellar abnormalities, such as ataxia, vertigo, and cranial nerve findings (**Table 18.4**).

A comprehensive understanding of stroke physiology will not only assist in the diagnosis of an ischemic event (as opposed to other neurological causes of dysfunction, such as the post-ictal state of a seizure) but also in determining whether or not a given stenosis or occlusion can cause the patient's current symptomatology.

Table 18.2 Non-Dominant Hemisphere Anterior Circulation Stroke Symptoms

Contralateral hemiparesis and sensory loss
Extinction to contralateral stimuli
Neglect of contralateral visual field
Poor contralateral conjugate gaze
Dysarthria
Spatial disorientation

Table 18.3 Dominant Hemisphere, Anterior Circulation Stroke Symptoms

Expressive aphasia, receptive aphasia, or both
Loss of language abilities
Alexia, agraphia, acalculia
Contralateral weakness, sensory loss, and visual field deficits

Table 18.4 Posterior Circulation Stroke Symptoms

Dizziness
Vertigo
Syncope
Cranial nerve palsies
Extremity weakness
Visual changes
Gait ataxia
Cerebellar dysfunction
Locked-in syndrome

Clinical Examination

Although a thorough medical history and physical examination are always important, a patient with acute neurological change must be triaged in a different manner than a patient who presents to your outpatient clinic with longstanding complaints.

- In the acute setting, it is critical to determine the onset of symptoms, a medication history (with close attention to antiplatelet and anticoagulation medications), and allergies; in addition, a focused neurological examination should be performed in concordance with the National Institutes of Health Stroke Scale (NIHSS).
- Once initial evaluation is completed, the patient should be taken for emergent imaging, with preference given to a non-contrast, non-spiral CT scan, CT angiogram (CTA), and CT perfusion (CTP), since these can typically be done more expeditiously than MRI at most institutions.
  - At this point, the physician can determine whether or not the neurological decline is related to a stroke or not, as well as whether the stroke is secondary to an occlusion or a stenosis.
  - A decision must then be made of whether or not to implement emergency stroke therapy.
  - Once that decision point is reached, the remainder of the history must be obtained, a review of systems completed, past medical and surgical history obtained, and a thorough physical and neurological examination performed by the physician or mid-level provider.

○ It is important to emphasize that in the acute setting, it is impossible to determine whether the acute decline in neurological status will require emergency intervention until the focused history, neurological exam, and imaging have been completed.

The American Stroke Association recommends that the target time from presentation to CT scan should be within 25 minutes, which justifies the need for a more focused triage approach up front.[15]

Diagnostic Imaging Studies

- Computed tomography (CT) is the first line of imaging.
  ○ CT is widely available and faster than magnetic resonance (MR) imaging, while also being less expensive. However, there may be issues with contrast and radiation exposure.
  ○ Non-contrast CT can provide information related to the presence or absence of early infarct signs (for example, hypodensity, loss of insular ribbon) as well whether or not the patient's deficits are related to a hemorrhagic stroke.
  ○ Most centers are able to provide CT angiography and CT perfusion data.
    ▪ CT angiography provides images of the intracranial and extracranial vasculature.
    ▪ CT perfusion evaluates blood flow, volume, and mean transit time to identify territories of decreased perfusion. Diamox imaging can test a patient's reserve or ability to provide additional blood flow to a territory that has been vasodilated.
  ○ An alternative to CT is single photon emission computed tomography (SPECT), which allows for a better evaluation of the posterior circulation and does not require contrast.
- MR imaging
  ○ Although MR is a superior imaging modality that provides better sensitivity and specificity for stroke along with improved imaging of the surrounding tissues and requires no iodinated contrast agents or radiation, it is more costly, less available, and requires more time for image acquisition.
- Positron emission tomography (PET) evaluations of oxygen extraction fractions are useful in determining areas of hypoperfusion and at risk of stroke; however, PET imaging is expensive and has very limited availability.

Grading Systems

Several grading systems have been developed to measure the severity of intracranial arterial stenosis. However, the two most commonly used systems were developed to measure extracranial carotid artery stenosis in the the following studies: (1) the North American Symptomatic Carotid Endarterectomy Trial (NASCET) and (2) the European Carotid Surgery Trial (ECST).

The warfarin-aspirin symptomatic intracranial disease (WASID) grading scheme (**Fig. 18.1**) was designed to measure intracranial arterial disease and uses the measured area of greatest stenosis (b) in reference to the diameter of the proximal segment of the same artery that is disease free (a): stenosis = $1 - (a - b)/a$.[13] If the proximal por-

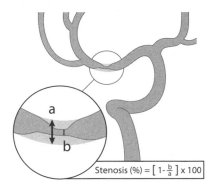

$$\text{Stenosis (\%)} = \left[1 - \frac{b}{a} \right] \times 100$$

Fig. 18.1 WASID grading scheme.

tion of the artery that contains the target lesion is also diseased, the distal normal segment is substituted as the reference diameter. The third option, if the artery proximal and distal to the target lesion is diseased, is the proximal parent artery.

Evidence-Based Medicine

The natural history of ICAD was evaluated by Akins et al., who studied 21 patients with 45 intracranial stenoses via cerebral angiography with average interval of 26.7 months. In their study, based on a minimum change of 10%, 20% of intracranial internal carotid artery lesions progressed, while 61% of anterior cerebral artery, middle cerebral artery, and posterior cerebral artery lesions progressed.[16]

Many patients with ICAD are treated with oral anticoagulation based on the data from the EC-IC Bypass study, which showed poor clinical outcomes in the surgical arm of the trial for patients with middle cerebral artery stenosis.[17] In this study, 1377 patients with recent hemispheric stroke, retinal ischemia, or transient ischemic attacks were randomized to either best medical management (n = 714) or that plus superficial temporal artery to middle cerebral artery bypass (n = 663). Patients needed to have either ipsilateral internal carotid artery or middle cerebral artery stenosis or occlusion. The mean follow-up was 55.8 months. The conclusions were that the surgical group had a higher incidence of fatal and non-fatal stroke (20%) compared with the medical group (12.5%). However, with recent advances in imaging modalities and better selection criteria, EC-IC bypasses appear to be useful in selected patients with intracranial arterial stenosis, and the results of this trial are pending. Posterior circulation bypass has also been associated with high morbidity and mortality.[18,19]

The Warfarin-Aspirin Symptomatic Intracranial Disease (WASID) study,[12] a double-blind randomized control trial, compared a dose of 1300 mg daily of aspirin to warfarin. 569 patients had suffered stroke or transient ischemic (TIA) attack within the last 90 days and had angiographic evidence of 50–99% stenosis of a major intracranial artery that supplied the territory of the stroke or TIA; these patients were randomized either to 1300 mg of aspirin daily or warfarin (goal INR of 2.0–3.0). The trial was halted early after the warfarin group demonstrated a higher rate of death, major hemorrhage, myocardial infarction (MI), sudden death, and non-vascular related death. The risk of major intracranial hemorrhage or death with Coumadin was significantly greater than with aspirin, without any significant difference in stroke prevention.

WASID also demonstrated three subgroups of patients; those with 70–99% stenosis presenting with a stroke, those enrolled within 17 days of their qualifying event, and women had a higher risk of additional stroke in the same vascular territory as the stenosis.[20] The one-year stroke risk in patients with 50–69% stenosis is 6%, while the 70–99% stenosis group had a one-year stroke risk approaching 17%.[15]

Given the poor outcomes with EC-IC bypass and with medical management of ICAD, many investigators began to experiment with angioplasty, with and without the use of stents, for treatment of this difficult disease and reported technical success with the procedure.[21-24] Until 2001, the only stents available in the United States that were small enough for intracranial use were coronary stents. In 2005, the FDA granted humanitarian device exception (HDE) approval for the Gateway PTA Balloon Catheter/Wingspan Stent system (Boston Scientific, Fremont CA), an open-cell, self-expanding stent with an angioplasty balloon system designed for the treatment of intracranial atherosclerotic lesions of >50% stenosis. More recently, the FDA granted an investigational device exception (IDE) clearance for the Pharos Vitesse balloon-mounted angioplasty and stent system (Micrus Endovascular, San Jose CA).

The U.S. Wingspan Registry, an industry-sponsored multicenter prospective registry, evaluated the Gateway balloon/Wingspan stent system in patients with symptomatic ICAD >50% refractory to medical therapy[25]: 158 consecutive patients with 168 intracranial atherosclerotic lesions of at least 50% stenosis and failed medical therapy were included in this registry. There was a periprocedure stroke and stroke-death rate of 5.4%, and a long-term (mean follow-up 14.2 months) stroke and stroke-death rate of 9%.

This registry provided important data that was used to help shape the SAMM-PRIS Study—Stenting vs. Aggressive Medical Management for Preventing Recurrent Stroke in Intracranial Stenosis. SAMMPRIS is an NIH-funded, multicenter randomized trial comparing stenting to medical management with enrollment beginning in November 2008. This study was halted prematurely in 2011 due to preliminary data suggesting that the maximal medical therapy arm is superior to stenting plus maximal therapy. Long-term results and final analysis are forthcoming.

Stenting for Symptomatic Atherosclerotic Lesions in the Vertebral or Intracranial Arteries (SSYLVIA)[21] is an industry-funded, non-randomized, prospective international study evaluating the Neurolink stent (Guidant Corp) for treatment of intracranial atherosclerotic lesions and extracranial vertebral artery atherosclerotic lesions in patients with at least 50% stenosis and greater than seven days from last stroke or TIA. Sixty-one patients enrolled; 43 had intracranial lesions and 18 had extracranial vertebral artery lesions. The overall 30-day stroke and death rate was 6.6%, and the one-year stroke rate was 11.5%. The intracranial atherosclerotic group had a 6-month stroke and death rate of 14% and a 6-month restenosis (>50%) rate of 32%, with 14% being symptomatic.

Wojak et al. reported on 62 consecutive angioplasty and 22 stent procedures for intracranial stenosis and found a 4.8% stroke and death rate[26] and a 90.5% complication-free success rate. The annualized stroke rate was 1.8%. The procedure was technically successful in reducing stenosis by 20% in all patients; however, in 13% of all patients, there was had a residual stenosis of >50%. There was a 27.4% restenosis rate and a 6% symptomatic restenosis rate. The mean follow-up for this series was 62.5 months.[26] The shortcomings of angioplasty alone are acute lesion recoil, dissection, acute occlusion, and recurrent stenosis. Combining stenting with angioplasty has focused on trying to prevent these complications.

Preprocedure Preparation

Antiplatelet Agents

Appropriate antiplatelet activity is essential for reducing the risk of the thromboembolic complications associated with stenting. Patients who cannot tolerate antiplatelet medications, have a contraindication to antiplatelet medication, or demonstrate a high risk of noncompliance are suitable for angioplasty but not for stenting. For details about the mechanisms of antiplatelet agents, refer to Chapter 4.

With regard to antiplatelet treatment for intracranial stenosis, there is a paucity of data in the neurointerventional literature regarding the appropriate use of these medications. However, several key points can be extrapolated from the coronary stent literature.

1. Use of dual antiplatelet therapy is better than single therapy. Though each interventionist may have specific preferences, after placement of intracranial stents, patients typically receive aspirin and clopidogrel for three months, then aspirin alone indefinitely. If there is evidence of in-stent stenosis, the dual regimen is maintained until the stenosis resolves. Issues arise when patients require warfarin long term for cardiac issues such as atrial fibrillation. Most thromboembolic events occur within two weeks of stent placement, so regardless of other anticoagulation requirements, one should consider using aspirin and clopidogrel for at least two weeks. After that time, warfarin can be restarted, clopidogrel can be discontinued once the warfarin is therapeutic, and then the patient is maintained on aspirin and warfarin.

2. There is a significant variability to antiplatelet medication response. Diligent use of platelet function tests will assist in identifying poor responders and non-responders. Though preferences may vary, we typically load patients with 650 mg of non-enteric aspirin and then use a 325 mg per day maintenance dose. Clopidogrel is loaded at 600 mg, and then a 75 mg per day maintenance dose is administered. We chose this regimen based on the above literature, to minimize the number of poor responders and non-responders.

3. The coronary stent literature has shown that poor response to antiplatelet medication has clinical implications and should not be ignored. In patients who are poor responders, we reload the patients based on the above doses and use the same maintenance regimen. However, if the patients are able to achieve appropriate inihibition after the load but are unable to maintain therapeutic response, those patients then require higher maintenance doses.

4. In the emergency setting, where a patient cannot be loaded prior to the procedure (which is an extremely rare event), we prefer to use abciximab because of its rapid onset, reliable dissociation curve, and longer activity. We typically will not load the patient until the stent is in the parent vessel proximal to the stenosis. This decreases the risk of hemorrhage if there is an adverse event prior to stenting. Once the inhibition is adequate, the stent is deployed, the angiogram is concluded, and the patient is given the load of aspirin and clopidogrel. The reliable antiplatelet effect of abciximab will bridge the patient until the aspirin and clopidogrel achieve therapeutic levels. This is most important for clopidogrel, which, as stated above, is a prodrug and requires time to become active. Reversible GP IIb/IIIa inhibitors will not reliably bridge the patient long enough for clopidogrel to be therapeutic unless the patient is maintained on an intravenous infusion of the inhibitor.

Equipment

Sheath and Catheter

A standard 6 Fr sheath is used, or if significant tortuosity is anticipated, an arrowflex sheath is used for added support. Standard guide catheters provide good support.

Glide Wires

Standard 0.035 or 0.038 hydrophilic glide wires are usually sufficient for exchanging out a diagnostic catheter for the guide catheter. In some situations, shapeable or extra-stiff guide wires, such as the Amplatz Ultra Stiff guide wire (Cook Medical, Bloomington, IN), may be needed.

Microcatheter

- A straight microcatheter, such as the Excelsior SL-10 (Boston Scientific, Fremont CA) or Echelon 10 (Microtherapeutics Inc, Irvine, CA), is sufficient to cross the stenosis and set up for an exchange for the balloon catheters.
- Straight-tipped microcatheters (as opposed to the pre-shaped angled ones) are favorable for crossing stenotic lesions because they provide the lowest profile; angled microcatheters may dig into the plaque during passage.
- The commonly used 0.014″ exchange microwires are usually more robust, such as the Transcend (Boston Scientific, Fremont, CA). In some situations, coronary wires, such as the Balanced Middleweight (BMW, Guidant Corp.), Prowater (Asahi, Japan), or Luge (Boston Scientific, Fremont, CA), are preferred by some.
- A slightly curved 0.014-inch microwire is usually sufficient to guide the microwire across the lesion.

Balloon Angioplasty (Fig. 18.2)

Balloons can be classified as compliant and noncompliant. Compliant balloons are generally unable to generate enough force in angioplasty to open an atherosclerotic lesion. Noncompliant balloons are stiffer and are able to generate enough outward radial force not only to open an atherosclerotic lesion by angioplasty but also to rupture the vessel if one is not careful. The Maverick (Boston Scientific, Fremont CA), a coronary balloon, and the Gateway (Boston Scientific, Fremont CA), a neurovascular balloon, are two examples of noncompliant balloons that are commonly used in angioplasty of intracranial stenosis.

Stents (Fig. 18.2)

Before neurovascular stents came onto the market, bare metal coronary stents were used off-label in the cerebral circulation. These stents were stiff and difficult to navigate. In 2002, the Neuroform stent (Boston Scientific, Fremont, CA), a self-expanding stent designed to assist in coiling of wide-necked aneurysms, came onto the market as the first intracranial cerebral stent. Boston Scientific modified this stent to obtain greater outward radial force and introduced it in 2005 as the

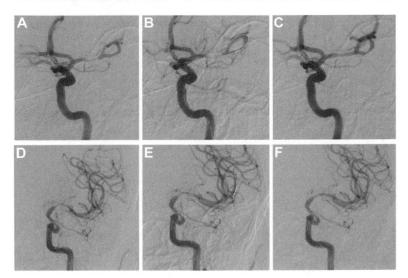

Fig. 18.2   Intracranial stenosis. **(A,D)** Both patients presented with multiple TIAs, involving transient weakness of the right arm and face. Diagnostic angiography demonstrated significant M1 left stenoses, as seen on these AP views of the left internal carotid artery injection. **(B,E)** Both lesions were traversed with a microcatheter and microwire, followed by removal of microwire, placement of an exchange-length microwire, navigating a balloon across the lesion and performing angioplasty. **(C,F)** After angioplasty, the balloon was removed and an intracranial stent was navigated across the lesion and deployed.

Wingspan Stent, combining it with the Gateway Balloon. It was released with a HDE from the FDA for the specific indication of treatment of ICAD. More recently, Micrus Corporation (San Jose, CA) and Boston Scientific have developed balloon-mounted stents, the Pharos Vitesse and Neurolink, respectively. These stents were both approved as balloon-expandable intracranial stents for the treatment of ICAD.

Drug-eluding stents (DES) for the coronary circulation are also available on the market. A DES is designed to decrease the rate of in-stent stenosis. Recent evidence has shown delayed intimal healing and late in-stent thrombosis, which have led to the recommendation of life-long dual antiplatelet therapy.[27,28] The use of DES in the intracranial circulation, particularly since there is little evidence that it is superior to bare metal stents, should be considered with caution.

Postprocedure Care

After balloon angioplasty or intracranial stent placement, patients usually recover in a unit where blood pressure can be monitored closely and neurological examinations performed regularly; this typically is an intensive care or step-down unit. Recommendations are to maintain systolic blood pressure in the 120–140 mmHg range. It is important during the procedure to have strict blood pressure control and not to allow the patient to become hypotensive during induction or during the procedure. After revascularization, it is important to avoid hypertension, which can cause reperfusion injury. Specific laboratory studies should include checking renal function (creatinine) because of the procedural contrast load, hematocrit to assess for a potentially developing retroperitoneal hematoma, and platelet count. Serial neurological examinations must be performed to evaluate for deterioration, which may be a sign of an intracerebral hemorrhage, reperfusion syndrome, or stroke from stent thrombosis.

Acute Neurological Change

Acute neurological deficits after revascularization procedures most commonly result from ischemic stroke, hemorrhage, or seizure.

Stroke after angioplasty or stent placement typically is the result of in-stent thrombosis or a thromboembolic event. Adequate anticoagulation with heparin during the procedure and the use of antiplatelet agents before and after the procedure will decrease the risk of these clotting complications.

Hemorrhage during or after an ICAD procedure can occur because of arterial perforation or dissection during the procedure and systemic hypertension after the procedure. During the procedure, a pre-stent placement angiogram should be performed to evaluate for evidence of vascular injury, because once the stent is placed, the patient is committed to antiplatelet therapy. Postprocedural hypertension in the setting of a newly reperfused brain can lead to impaired autoregulation of the cerebral vasculature and a significant intracranial hemorrhage, particularly in the setting of antiplatelet agents.

Seizures can also be a sign of dysregulation of the cerebral blood flow and cause an acute change in neurological condition. Headaches, focal neurological deficits, and altered mental status can also be warning signs of hyperperfusion syndrome. Detailed work-up, including non-contrast CT to look for hemorrhage, CTA and CTP to evaluate blood flow and brain perfusion, and an electroenchephalogram (EEG) to look for seizure activity, should all be considered adjuncts in treating the correct inciting event of any acute neurological change.

Alternative Therapies

Anticoagulation

The WASID trial has shown that patients do poorly with medical therapy alone. It is unknown whether or not angioplasty with stenting will be a more durable and efficacious treatment option; SAMMPRIS will attempt to answer that question.

Extracranial-Intracranial Bypass

The EC-IC Bypass trial showed that the surgical group had a higher incidence of fatal and non-fatal stroke compared with the medical group. Some will argue that the patients who would receive the most benefit from a bypass were not included in the trial, based on a fear that the patient would be randomized to the non-surgical arm. In addition, with newer perfusion technology, it was thought that perhaps the patients were not selected properly; this was the basis for the ongoing COSS trial, which has recently ceased enrollment. Although not published at this time, the initial results from the halted COSS trial seems to indicate that the data will not reach significance to recommend revascularization. As such, while the evidence for revascularization is still not positive, careful patient selection has resulted in reportedly good outcomes in small case series, but not for ICAD, however.

Technical Pearls

1. It is paramount to have high-quality imaging detailing the anatomy of the atherosclerotic lesion so that accurate measurements of the stenosis can be performed.
2. Appropriate patient selection will minimize complication rates and maximize clinical benefit for the patient.
3. Diligent use of antiplatelet medications, with a thorough understanding of platelet aggregometry, will help reduce complications.
4. A baseline angiogram just prior to stent deployment to assess vessel anatomy and evaluate for vessel injury is the last opportunity to abort the procedure prior to placing the stent, which, once deployed, commits the patient to antiplatelet agents for approximately 3 months.
5. Balloon angioplasty may be required prior to stent placement if the vessel lumen is too stenotic to pass the stent through safely.

Recommended Reading

Akins PT, Pilgram TK, Cross DT III, Moran CJ. Natural history of stenosis from intracranial atherosclerosis by serial angiography. Stroke 1998;29(2):433–438

Caplan LR, Gorelick PB, Hier DB. Race, sex and occlusive cerebrovascular disease: a review. Stroke 1986;17(4):648–655

Chimowitz MI, Lynn MJ, Howlett-Smith H, et al.; Warfarin-Aspirin Symptomatic Intracranial Disease Trial Investigators. Comparison of warfarin and aspirin for symptomatic intracranial arterial stenosis. N Engl J Med 2005;352(13):1305–1316

The EC/IC Bypass Study Group. Failure of extracranial-intracranial arterial bypass to reduce the risk of ischemic stroke. Results of an international randomized trial. N Engl J Med 1985;313(19):1191–1200

Suzuki J, Takaku A. Cerebrovascular "moyamoya" disease. Disease showing abnormal net-like vessels in base of brain. Arch Neurol 1969;20(3):288–299

Wojak JC, Dunlap DC, Hargrave KR, DeAlvare LA, Culbertson HS, Connors JJ III. Intracranial angioplasty and stenting: long-term results from a single center. AJNR Am J Neuroradiol 2006;27(9):1882–1892

References

1. Wityk RJ, Lehman D, Klag M, Coresh J, Ahn H, Litt B. Race and sex differences in the distribution of cerebral atherosclerosis. Stroke 1996;27(11):1974–1980
2. Sacco RL, Kargman DE, Gu Q, Zamanillo MC. Race-ethnicity and determinants of intracranial atherosclerotic cerebral infarction. The Northern Manhattan Stroke Study. Stroke 1995;26(1):14–20
3. Craig DR, Meguro K, Watridge C, Robertson JT, Barnett HJ, Fox AJ. Intracranial internal carotid artery stenosis. Stroke 1982;13(6):825–828
4. Moossy J. Pathology of cerebral atherosclerosis. Influence of age, race, and gender. Stroke 1993;24(12, Suppl):I22–I23, I31–I32
5. Caplan LR, Gorelick PB, Hier DB. Race, sex and occlusive cerebrovascular disease: a review. Stroke 1986;17(4):648–655
6. Leung SY, Ng TH, Yuen ST, Lauder IJ, Ho FC. Pattern of cerebral atherosclerosis in Hong Kong Chinese. Severity in intracranial and extracranial vessels. Stroke 1993;24(6):779–786

7. Ingall TJ, Homer D, Baker HL Jr, Kottke BA, O'Fallon WM, Whisnant JP. Predictors of intracranial carotid artery atherosclerosis. Duration of cigarette smoking and hypertension are more powerful than serum lipid levels. Arch Neurol 1991;48(7):687–691

8. Osborn AG, Anderson RE. Angiographic spectrum of cervical and intracranial fibromuscular dysplasia. Stroke 1977;8(5):617–626

9. Stanley JC, Gewertz BL, Bove EL, Sottiurai V, Fry WJ. Arterial fibrodysplasia. Histopathologic character and current etiologic concepts. Arch Surg 1975;110(5):561–566

10. Mettinger KL, Ericson K. Fibromuscular dysplasia and the brain. I. Observations on angiographic, clinical and genetic characteristics. Stroke 1982;13(1):46–52

11. Mettinger KL. Fibromuscular dysplasia and the brain. II. Current concept of the disease. Stroke 1982;13(1):53–58

12. Fukui M. Current state of study on moyamoya disease in Japan. Surg Neurol 1997;47(2): 138–143

13. Chimowitz MI, Lynn MJ, Howlett-Smith H, et al.; Warfarin-Aspirin Symptomatic Intracranial Disease Trial Investigators. Comparison of warfarin and aspirin for symptomatic intracranial arterial stenosis. N Engl J Med 2005;352(13):1305–1316

14. Turk AS, Levy EI, Albuquerque FC, et al. Influence of patient age and stenosis location on Wingspan in-stent restenosis. AJNR Am J Neuroradiol 2008;29(1):23–27

15. American Stroke Association. *Get With The Guidelines—Stroke*. American Stroke Association; 2008

16. Akins PT, Pilgram TK, Cross DT III, Moran CJ. Natural history of stenosis from intracranial atherosclerosis by serial angiography. Stroke 1998;29(2):433–438

17. The EC/IC Bypass Study Group. Failure of extracranial-intracranial arterial bypass to reduce the risk of ischemic stroke. Results of an international randomized trial. N Engl J Med 1985;313(19):1191–1200

18. Hopkins LN, Budny JL. Complications of intracranial bypass for vertebrobasilar insufficiency. J Neurosurg 1989;70(2):207–211

19. Hopkins LN, Budny JL, Castellani D. Extracranial-intracranial arterial bypass and basilar artery ligation in the treatment of giant basilar artery aneurysms. Neurosurgery 1983;13(2):189–194

20. Kasner SE, Chimowitz MI, Lynn MJ, et al.; Warfarin Aspirin Symptomatic Intracranial Disease Trial Investigators. Predictors of ischemic stroke in the territory of a symptomatic intracranial arterial stenosis. Circulation 2006;113(4):555–563

21. SSYLVIA Study Investigators. Stenting of Symptomatic Atherosclerotic Lesions in the Vertebral or Intracranial Arteries (SSYLVIA): study results. Stroke 2004;35(6):1388–1392

22. Mori T, Mori K, Fukuoka M, Arisawa M, Honda S. Percutaneous transluminal cerebral angioplasty: serial angiographic follow-up after successful dilatation. Neuroradiology 1997;39(2):111–116

23. Levy EI, Horowitz MB, Koebbe CJ, et al. Transluminal stent-assisted angioplasty of the intracranial vertebrobasilar system for medically refractory, posterior circulation ischemia: early results. Neurosurgery 2001;48(6):1215–1221, discussion 1221–1223

24. Connors JJ III, Wojak JC. Percutaneous transluminal angioplasty for intracranial atherosclerotic lesions: evolution of technique and short-term results. J Neurosurg 1999; 91(3):415–423

25. Fiorella D, Levy EI, Turk AS, et al. US multicenter experience with the Wingspan stent system for the treatment of intracranial atheromatous disease: periprocedural results. Stroke 2007;38(3):881–887

26. Wojak JC, Dunlap DC, Hargrave KR, DeAlvare LA, Culbertson HS, Connors JJ III. Intracranial angioplasty and stenting: long-term results from a single center. AJNR Am J Neuroradiol 2006;27(9):1882–1892

27. Bavry AA, Kumbhani DJ, Helton TJ, Borek PP, Mood GR, Bhatt DL. Late thrombosis of drug-eluting stents: a meta-analysis of randomized clinical trials. Am J Med 2006;119(12):1056–1061

28. Pfisterer M, Brunner-La Rocca HP, Buser PT, et al.; BASKET-LATE Investigators. Late clinical events after clopidogrel discontinuation may limit the benefit of drug-eluting stents: an observational study of drug-eluting versus bare-metal stents. J Am Coll Cardiol 2006;48(12):2584–2591

Vascular Injuries of the Head and Neck

Eric M. Deshaies and David Padalino

This chapter will focus on the more commonly seen traumatic injuries to the great vessels of the neck and intracranial circulation, including dissections, pseudoaneurysms, and lacerations. The etiology, diagnosis, and management of these injuries will be discussed as well.

Arterial Dissection

Etiology

Traumatic arterial dissections occur as a result of shearing forces between the layer of luminal endothelial cells (intima) and the smooth muscle layer deep to it (tunica media). This tear results in a tissue flap within the arterial lumen, creating a false passage for blood to propagate into the subintimal space (**Fig. 19.1**). Enlargement of this false lumen can narrow or obstruct the true arterial lumen, resulting in diminished blood flow at, and distal to, the site of injury. The torn endothelium and exposed basement membrane are thrombogenic, and platelet adhesion to these damaged layers places the patient at risk for cerebral hypoperfusion and thromboembolic events. Additionally, a pseudoaneurysm can form at the dissection site secondary to further weakening of the arterial wall.

Arterial dissections are more commonly seen in the cervical segment of the external carotid (ECA), internal carotid (ICA), and vertebral (VA) arteries than in the intracranial segments.[1,2] Spontaneous dissections are much less common than traumatic ones and are often associated with connective tissue disorders (**Table 19.1**). If the dissection spreads into the intracranial space, where the arterial wall is thinner, subarachnoid hemorrhage can result.[3] Rapid rotation or extension of the head or neck, a fracture through the skull base or cervical vertebrae, and facial trauma are the most common causes of traumatic arterial dissections of the ICA and VA; occasionally, however, there is no apparent inciting event.

Diagnosis

Extracranial carotid artery (CA) dissections most commonly occur 2–3 cm above the common carotid artery (CCA) bifurcation and are seen in up to 0.45% of blunt neck trauma patients, with an associated mortality of 40%.[4] Symptomatic vertebral artery injury is diagnosed in up to 1% of blunt neck trauma cases. Screening studies have shown that the incidence of asymptomatic vertebral artery injury from blunt trauma in patients with mid-cervical spine fractures or subluxations is as high as

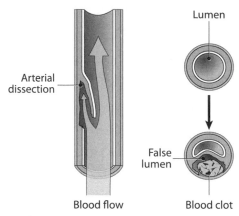

Fig. 19.1   Anatomy of an arterial dissection.

46%. Many arterial dissections go undiagnosed because they are often asymptomatic. However, the onset of neurological deficits from CCA, ICA, and VA dissections can occur any time from immediately after the injury to days later; most occur within 24 hours. Carotid dissections may present with ipsilateral neck pain over the carotid artery (carotidynia) or neurological deficits (**Table 19.2**).

Vertebral artery dissections can present with pain in the posterior neck and symptoms of posterior circulation ischemia (**Table 19.3**). These dissections are more commonly seen in the first segment of the VA (cervical segment) at its origin from the subclavian artery and the third segment as the VA exits C2. Ten percent of these dissections extend intracranially, with a risk of subarachnoid hemorrhage (SAH) associated with high morbidity.

Angiography remains the gold standard for detecting arterial dissections in both the neck and skull base, although CT angiograms (CTA) are being utilized in an increasing number of cases, particularly in the setting of trauma, where CTA of the head and neck can be rapidly obtained as part of the trauma evaluation. The characteristic angiographic appearance of an arterial dissection is a smooth tapering of the true vessel lumen called a "string sign," (**Fig. 19.2A**) or in severe dissections, an abrupt cessation of contrast filling representing an occlusion (**Fig. 19.2B**).

Ultrasonography is a useful tool for rapidly evaluating a patient for cervical arterial dissections, particularly for the carotid artery, since it does not lie in a bony canal like the VA. Arterial lumen narrowing from a dissection is suggested by abnormally high blood flow velocities on ultrasound. However, occasionally a dissection can be difficult to differentiate from hypoplasia with ultrasonography,

Table 19.1   Connective Tissue Disorders

Ehlers-Danlos syndrome
Polycystic kidney disease
Marfan syndrome
Loeys-Dietz syndrome

Table 19.2   Anterior Circulation Exam Findings in Patients with Carotid Dissection

Contralateral hemiparesis
Hemisensory deficits
Aphasias
Agnosias
Hemineglect
Ipsilateral Horner syndrome

Table 19.3   Posterior Circulation Exam Findings in Patients with Vertebral Artery Dissection

Cortical blindness
Vertigo
Vomiting
Cranial nerve deficits
Coma or death

in which case magnetic resonance angiography (MRA), CTA, or catheter-based angiography (CBA) is more helpful because these modalities can demonstrate the intimal flap. Ultrasonography is less useful for detecting intracranial arterial dissections because the bone density interferes with the sonar waves, resulting in poorer quality images. In these situations, CBA, CTA, or MRA is preferred.

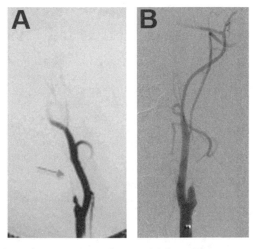

Fig. 19.2   Angiographic appearance of an arterial dissection.

Evidence-Based Medicine

To date, there have been no randomized controlled trials evaluating arterial dissections. At the time of this writing, the Cervical Artery Dissection in Stroke Study (CADISS) has been initiated.[5] We look forward to the results of this study, which is assessing medical treatment of cervical arterial dissections.

Stroke Rates

Cervical dissection, whether spontaneous or traumatic, accounts for approximately 2% of all ischemic strokes.[6]

Management

Conservative Therapy

The natural history of dissection is somewhat unclear. Asymptomatic carotid artery and VA dissections frequently heal with anticoagulation or antiplatelet agents alone. However, for CA or VA dissections, no randomized clinical trials have compared antiplatelet or anticoagulant agents to each other or to no treatment at all.[7,8] Yet, during the healing period, the patient is at risk for two potential complications: (1) extension of the arterial dissection, and (2) thromboembolic infarcts. Some studies have shown that 50–90% of these tears will heal completely.[6] Others report that the rate of spontaneous healing of the dissection is much lower and that early intervention is imperative.[9] Morbidity from stroke ranges between 8% and 80%.[6,9]

Despite the absence of data supporting or refuting the use of antiplatelet and anticoagulant agents, they are commonly used during the healing phase (generally up to six months) to lower the risk of thromboembolic events. Once an arterial dissection is diagnosed, urgent treatment with intravenous heparin and oral warfarin (Coumadin) or antiplatelet agents should be initiated to prevent thromboembolic infarcts after all other potential sources of bleeding have been identified and treated. Intracranial hemorrhage on CT is a contraindication to anticoagulation. In the absence of intracranial hemorrhage, intravenous heparinization (with the goal of a partial thromboplastin time [PTT]/control ratio of 2.0–2.5) and oral warfarin (Coumadin) should be initiated urgently until the International Normalized Ratio (INR) is 2.0–2.5, at which time the heparin can be stopped; initial use of heparin reverses the early hypercoagulability seen with warfarin. If antiplatelet agents are used, heparin does not necessarily need to be started in conjunction, but this is also debatable and left to individual physician preferences.

Treatment with antiplatelet or anticoagulant agents should be continued for a minimum of six months, at which time imaging should be performed to assess whether or not the luminal stenosis from the dissection is stable or improved, suggesting that the intimal tear has healed. If the dissection has healed, the agents can be discontinued; if the stenosis is worse or if the patient becomes symptomatic, then a stent is recommended for definitive treatment.[9]

It is important to recognize the small group of patients who complain of vague or intermittent neurological symptoms that cannot clearly be attributed to an arterial dissection. In such circumstances, there are two studies that we find helpful: CT or MR perfusion study and continuous transcranial Doppler (cTCD). Perfusion studies are useful when deciding whether or not the dissection is causing cerebral hypoperfusion.

Patients with nonspecific neurological symptoms and an abnormal perfusion study should be considered for stent placement across the dissection to improve blood flow to the brain. Patients with normal perfusion studies who complain of intermittent neurological symptoms should undergo cTCD to determine if microembolic showers from the dissection are causing microinfarcts and transient ischemic attacks. If this is the case despite anticoagulation, then the dissection should be stented to tack the thrombogenic intimal flap back against the arterial wall to reduce the risk of further thromboembolic events. If the cTCD and perfusion studies are normal, non-endovascular treatment is recommended. The conservative management of pseudoaneurysms, which can occur with dissections, is discussed later in this chapter.

Surgery

Open surgical treatment of arterial dissections traditionally meant arteriotomy with suturing of the intimal flap against the arterial wall or arterial sacrifice, with or without bypass. The latter surgical method has typically been more successful because the friability of the vessel wall and the length of the dissection usually preclude tacking the intimal flap to the arterial wall as a viable option. Vessel sacrifice can be done via multiple methods, although the most common in the endovascular era is with coil embolization or endovascular arterial occlusion devices. Sacrifice can be done by surgical ligation as well. A balloon occlusion test should be performed first to make sure the patient would tolerate arterial occlusion. If the patient fails the temporary balloon occlusion test, an intracranial to extracranial arterial bypass by a cerebrovascular neurosurgeon is recommended prior to vessel sacrifice.

Pseudoaneurysms

Extracranial Pseudoaneurysms

Etiology and Diagnosis

When there is injury to both the arterial intima and tunica media, a false channel forms between the tunica media and outer adventitia that fills with blood. With only a thin layer of adventitia between the tunica media and surrounding soft tissue of the neck, the false lumen expands and creates a pseudoaneurysm (**Fig. 19.3**). The injury occurs when the neck is hyperextended, causing stretching of the ICA and VA that is similar to that of dissections. Unlike dissections, pseudoaneurysms cannot form in arterial segments that are securely encased in bone, such as the petrous segment of the ICA, since there is no room for the adventitia to expand.

Extracranial pseudoaneurysms are more commonly seen in patients with injury to the neck or skull base after penetrating trauma or complications of otolaryngological surgery. Patients who present with pseudoaneurysms after blunt injury to the neck typically have pain localized to the general area of the injury, a neck mass, or oropharyngeal compromise in the case of larger cervical carotid pseudoaneurysms.

Arterial duplex ultrasound can be used to detect cervical carotid and vertebral artery pseudoaneurysms, the distinguishing feature being an extraluminal mass with slow blood flow. Pseudoaneurysms of the CA and VA appear as a mass on CT and MRI that is consistent with hematoma in the pseudoaneurysm (**Fig. 19.4**). The

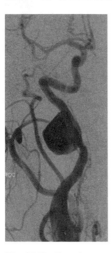

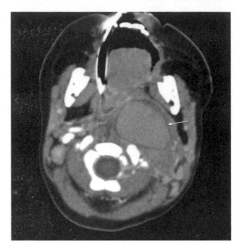

Fig. 19.3 Pseudoaneurysm.

Fig. 19.4 Noninvasive CT-angiography of a pseudoaneurysm.

sensitivity of CTA in diagnosing pseudoaneurysms is 80%. CBA demonstrates flow through the lumen of the parent artery, usually without luminal narrowing. The injured segment of the parent artery can be identified angiographically as it fills the pseudoaneurysm pouch.

Management

Small, asymptomatic, extracranial cervical carotid pseudoaneurysms can be observed with serial imaging studies long term. If the pseudoaneurysm expands or becomes symptomatic (thromboembolic events or soft tissue compression of the airway and oropharynx), then stent placement, stent-coil embolization, or vessel sacrifice may be necessary (**Fig. 19.5**).

Intracranial Pseudoaneurysms

Etiology and Diagnosis

Intracranial pseudoaneurysms are rare and unstable injuries that are associated with a very high risk of rupture if they are left untreated. The mortality rate is reported as high as 50% from re-rupture of untreated lesions, particularly within the first three weeks after diagnosis.[10–12] Pseudoaneurysms account for less than 1% of all intracranial aneurysms, with an estimated incidence of 0.15–0.40% of all diagnosed intracranial aneurysms.[11] A few relatively large case series are reported, evaluating up to 31 patients with cerebral angiography after head trauma, and reporting an associated incidence of traumatic intracranial pseudoaneurysms anywhere from 3.2% to 42%.[10]

Table 19.4 Soft Tissue Structures of the Neck

Neck Zone	Anatomical borders	Soft tissue structure at risk for injury
Zone I (root of the neck)	Clavicle and manubrium (inferiorly) Cricoid cartilage (superiorly)	Arteries: subclavian, brachiocephalic, vertebral, common carotid. Veins: brachiocephalic, subclavian, jugular. Nerves: vagus, recurrent laryngeal, brachial plexus roots. Other: trachea, esophagus, thyroid, lung apex, thoracic duct, lower cervical spine.
Zone II (mid-cervical)	Cricoid cartilage (inferiorly) Mandibular angle (superiorly)	Arteries: common, internal, and external carotid and branches. Veins: jugular and tributaries. Nerves: vagus, recurrent laryngeal, phrenic, hypoglossal, nerve roots to brachial plexus. Other: larynx, oropharynx, thryroid, mid-cervical spine.
Zone III (upper cervical)	Mandibular angle (inferiorly) Skull base (superiorly)	Arteries: vertebral, internal, and external carotid and branches. Veins: jugular Nerves: upper cervical nerve roots, cranial nerves (V,VII, IX–XII branches). Other: salivary glands, oropharynx.

rates were reported as around 7% during World War II and as approximately 11% in World War I.[17] The majority (>95%) of all penetrating neck trauma today results from gun or knife wounds, with the remainder being from motor vehicle, household, and industrial accidents.[16]

There is no role for blind deep probing of the neck wound when one is not in an operating room, as this can disturb fragile tissue or clots that may be the only structures preventing severe uncontrollable hemorrhaging.[16] Great care should be taken to examine the back, abdomen, and extremities, as around 30% of all penetrating neck trauma are associated with serious injuries to other parts of the body, many of which may not be immediately apparent until identified on a thorough exam.

If adjacent arteries and veins are injured, delayed vascular lesions can also include arteriovenous fistula formation such as carotid-jugular or carotid-cavernous fistulae. The treatment of these lesions depends on the location and size of the pathologic conduit.

Evidence-Based Medicine

As early as 1552, Ambroise Paré, a sixteenth-century surgeon to the kings of France, recorded the first described case of carotid ligation as the most effective treatment available for penetrating neck trauma resulting in carotid vascular injury.[17] This clearly resulted in serious complications, such as stroke and death, as a result of the treatment of these types of injuries, with mortality rates around 60% and neurologic impairment from stroke in approximately 30% of cases. Because of the severity of many of these iatrogenic complications, a trend toward conservative management, including external pressure for vascular injuries and simple observation, was adopted prior to World War II, when a more aggressive surgical exploration of these injuries was again proposed.[17]

In 1956, Fogelman and Stewart reported a 65% mortality rate for early mandatory exploration of all penetrating neck injuries deep to the platysma, compared with 35% for selective delayed neck exploration.[17,18] Additionally, mandatory early exploration was associated with a 40–60% rate of negative intraoperative findings and therefore unnecessary surgeries.[17,18] This resulted in significant controversy regarding early versus delayed neck exploration.

Recently, the use of diagnostic cerebral angiography has been suggested as a screening modality to rule out serious vascular injuries before surgical exploration for stable patients with deep penetrating neck trauma and no clear surgical indication based on physical exam alone. Diagnostic angiography for zones I and III, particularly, is indicated for a variety of reasons, such as injuries that may not be readily apparent on physical exam and the high risk of injury to other structures in these zones. The advent of interventional radiological endovascular procedures, such as endovascular embolization and stent placement, for the treatment of these vascular injuries has helped to reduce the morbidity of open neck dissection techniques in appropriately selected patients.

Traumatic Carotid-Cavernous Fistulae

Traumatic and spontaneous carotid-cavernous fistulae (CCF) are described in detail in Chapter 15 and are not discussed in this chapter.

Preprocedural Preparation

Dissection and Extracranial Pseudoaneurysm

In the majority of cases, patients with dissections and/or pseudoaneurysms are seen in the post-trauma setting. In cases of severe, symptomatic arterial injury that requires endovascular management, the patient should be loaded with aspirin 325 mg and clopidogrel 300–600 mg orally unless their use is contraindicated (for example, by intracranial pseudoaneurysm, acute blood on head CT, other system bleeding, or presurgical trauma). In such a setting, close communication with the trauma team about the plans for antiplatelet use is mandatory to optimize the care and safety of the patient. While most recommend the use of an antiplatelet agent periprocedurally, the exact timing—pre-stent versus post-stent—is somewhat controversial in this setting, but we recommend using it pre-stenting unless it is contraindicated, as mentioned above.[19]

During stent placement, compression of the intimal flap against the carotid sinus can induce bradycardia and hypotension. For this reason, atropine and dopamine should be readily available to prevent or reverse these symptoms.

Intracranial Pseudoaneurysm

Once identified, these lesions should be treated before further hemorrhaging occurs. As mentioned earlier, these lesions have a very high risk of bleeding and are associated with a high rate of morbidity and mortality. Treatment requires embolization of the lesion, usually with coils, but if the pseudoaneurysm is small or on a very distal branch of the arterial tree, parent vessel occlusion may be necessary. Antiplatelet and anticoagulating agents must not be given in this setting, and normotension should be maintained to avoid severe bleeding. If endovascular treatment cannot be performed, then a neurosurgeon should be consulted for surgical obliteration of the pseudoaneurysm.

Penetrating Neck Injuries

Penetrating neck injuries should be managed with a trauma team; it is necessary to evaluate the patient completely for other injuries while following ACLS and ATLS protocols. Once it has been determined that there is a penetrating arterial injury and the decision has been made to treat it by endovascular means, the patient should be brought emergently to the interventional suite, intubated and ventilated, to protect the airway. Compression of the source of bleeding, blood transfusion as necessary, and management of blood pressure are critical components of pre-treatment protocol to reduce mortality. Antiplatelet and anticoagulant agents should not be given in this situation until after the bleeding has been controlled in the endovascular suite.

Potential Complications

Dissection and Pseudoaneurysm

Thromboembolic Complications

Thromboembolic complications are reported to be as high as 9% without an antiplatelet preload, which reduces this risk to less than 2%. Heparinization (with an ACT of 200–350) during the procedure reduces this complication rate even further. After heparinization, care should be taken to control the patient's blood pressure to prevent hemorrhagic complications.

Bradycardia

Stretching of the parasympathetic fibers in the carotid sinus by the dissection or pseudoaneurysm can cause bradycardia. An atropine bolus or a dopamine infusion can reverse or prevent bradycardia.

Ischemic Insult

The goals of treating vascular injuries are to restore normal flow through the vessel quickly and to preserve neurological function. Extensive, irreparable vascular injury may require vessel sacrifice by direct surgical ligation or endovascular embolization. However, arterial bypass may be required to restore adequate perfusion if vessel occlusion results in neurological deficits or the patient does not tolerate a balloon occlusion test. Endovascular treatment options, including stent placement and coil embolization in appropriately selected patients, can often repair arterial injury with minimal invasiveness to the patient. This is especially helpful for vascular injuries in neck zones I and III, where surgical morbidity is high.[16]

The evaluation and treatment of penetrating neck trauma remain a challenge because of the many different critical structures found in this region, including vascular, tracheal, esophageal, and spinal structures. Injuries to these structures can result in some of the most devastating consequences, and every case should be evaluated for their presence.

Intracranial Pseudoaneurysms

The major potential complications with treating intracranial pseudoaneurysms are ischemic insult and hemorrhage. As mentioned earlier, in many cases the bleeding from these aneurysms is stopped by surrounding brain tissue, so that the arterial wall is actually open. Attempts at coil embolization of the pseudoaneurysm can result in a lethal hemorrhage. Endovascular occlusion of the parent artery from which the pseudoaneurysm arises can result in ischemic stroke in that vessel territory and also incomplete occlusion of the aneurysm if the vessel is not occluded distal to the pseudoaneurysm as well. Such a situation would allow for retrograde filling of the pseudoaneurysm, with a persistent risk of hemorrhage.

Equipment

Sheath and Catheter

At least a 6 Fr diameter guide catheter and sheath are needed to access the vessel proximal to the dissection or pseudoaneurysm and to have enough room to deliver the extracranial stents and obtain angiograms as needed during placement. In cases of severe proximal vessel tortuosity, particularly in the aorta-great vessel junction, larger, stiffer sheaths, such as the 6 Fr 90 cm shuttle or Brite Tip sheaths inserted primarily (without a sheath), will allow greater stability during stent placement. If the shuttle sheath is used, a 6 Fr "special catheter," which is stiffer and longer than most guide catheters, can be used to access the proximal vessel with the shuttle sheath. A dissection usually precludes the safe use of a distal embolic protection device, but one can be used during treatment of pseudoaneurysms.

Glide Wire

Generally, angled glide wires will allow catheterization of the ICA and VAs. Shapeable glide wires are helpful for tortuous proximal arteries, and the authors also like to use this wire to access the right vertebral artery when the origin acutely angles leftward. A stiff glide wire provides better support when stiff catheters and sheaths are used, particularly in vessels with an acutely left-angled origin from the brachiocephalic or subclavian arteries, where the stiff wire will straighten the vessel out and make it easier to advance the guide catheter.

Microwire

Many microwires are available, each having its own advantages, but it is important to have one soft enough to pass the dissection flap without causing further injury yet stiff enough to navigate past the dissection into the true lumen of the artery (see Chapters 7 and 8). We usually prefer a Synchro 14 or Fathom 16 microwire for this purpose. When a microcatheter is used to help pass a dissection, a 300 cm exchange length microwire is preferable so that access across the lesion is not lost during equipment exchanges.

Microcatheter

The microcatheter will be used to navigate through the true lumen of dissection or past the pseudoaneurysm with the microwire. In some instances, the stent and the microwire can be used primarily, but in most instances, the microcatheter is used first with a 300 cm exchange microwire to pass the lesion, followed by exchanging the microcatheter for the stent. This allows the microwire to pass far enough past the lesion to maintain wire support when the stiffer stent is advanced.

Distal Protection Device

If possible, placement of a distal protection device prior to stent placement may lower the risk of thromboembolic events, but this is controversial. Unfortunately, especially when the vessel is completely occluded from a dissection, it may be difficult to navigate the device up the true lumen of the dissection safely.

Stents

Selection of a stent depends on the diameter and length of the area to be stented. For dissections, the stent should be 1 to 2 mm larger than the normal diameter of the artery to allow for the radial forces of the stent to compress the dissection. Balloon-expandable stents should be avoided, due to the theoretical risk of extending the dissection during inflation.[7] In the case of a pseudoaneurysm, oversizing the stent is not necessary. Covered stents can be used to treat arterial lacerations.

Embolic Agents

A covered stent or stent-coil embolization can be used to occlude pseudoaneurysms. Onyx 500 with balloon protection could also be considered, but there currently are no data to support this technique. Additionally, since the Onyx 500 is less compressible than the coil mass, Onyx 500 embolization could theoretically result in more mass effect in the neck than coil embolization.

Coils can also be used for arterial sacrifice. They should be oversized so that they pack the artery tightly. Sometimes a balloon will need to be placed distal to the site of coil embolization to prevent the coils from traveling distally and to form the initial coil plug in the arterial lumen. Detachable balloons formerly were commonly used for vessel occlusion, but they have fallen out of favor due to complications, the most frequent being a failure of the balloon to lodge where it was placed and its traveling distally after release. Other vascular occlusion devices are currently available on the market for this purpose as well.

Intracranial pseudoaneurysms are usually embolized with coils or occluded with Onyx or n-BCA glues; the reader is referred to Chapters 7 and 8 for details on how to prepare and use these glues.

Technique

The nuances of extracranial and intracranial stent placement and embolization are described in detail elsewhere in this handbook (Chapters 7 and 8). Here, we will only highlight the techniques pertinent to stent placement for arterial dissections and extracranial pseudoaneurysms and to vessel occlusion for intracranial pseudoaneurysms and arterial lacerations. Extracranial arterial dissections and pseudoaneurysms can be managed either under conscious sedation or general anesthesia, depending on the medical stability of the patient. Though intracranial procedures are performed be some interventionists under conscious sedation, it is not our preference to do so; in these instances, we prefer general anesthesia to minimize motion artifact, maintain strict blood pressure parameters, and optimize patient comfort and safety.

Stent Placement for Dissections and Lacerations

ICA and VA dissections causing neurological deficits should be revascularized with endovascular stent placement. The goals of stent placement are three-fold: (1) to tack down the intimal flap to prevent extension of the dissection, (2) to restore the normal luminal diameter to improve cerebral perfusion, and (3) to reduce the risk of thromboembolic events.[5]

It is very important that particular care be taken neither to enter the false lumen nor to puncture through the dissection flap by first entering the false lumen and then puncturing the intimal flap to enter the true lumen. This through-and-through would lead to stent deployment within the false lumen, resulting in occlusion of the true lumen.

Once across the dissection and in the true lumen, a microcatheter angiogram can be done to ensure that the microcatheter is in the true lumen and to determine the patency of the distal vasculature. The microcatheter, now distal to the dissection, can be exchanged for a 300 cm exchange-length microwire, if this was not used at the beginning, and the microcatheter exchanged for the stent. Care should be taken to ensure that enough microwire is distal to the dissection to avoid losing access when the equipment is manipulated during device exchanges.

Once the stent is aligned across the dissection or neck of the pseudoaneurysm, it can be deployed across the dissection flap to tack it against the arterial wall; overlapping stents can be placed for long dissections. After the stent has been deployed, revascularization needs to be confirmed angiographically before the guide catheter is removed from the patient.

For lacerated arteries, a covered stent can be placed across laceration to stop the bleeding.

Stent Placement for Extracranial Pseudoaneurysms

The technique for stenting extracranial pseudoaneurysms is similar to that for stenting extracranial arterial dissections. It is not uncommon for dissections and pseudoaneurysms to occur simultaneously. Before crossing the lesion, the interventionist should perform a baseline angiogram of the cervical and intracranial circulation to visualize the dissection or pseudoaneurysm and to determine the presence of collateral intracranial blood flow in case arterial sacrifice is needed. A roadmap can then be used to visualize the pseudoaneurysm and to guide the microwire and microcatheter past the lesion. The lesion is generally passed fairly readily, and it is normally easy to visualize where the stent needs to be placed. Further occlusion of the pseudoaneurysm with coils may be required. If a dissection is also present, care must be taken to stent within the true lumen, as discussed above.

Intracranial Pseudoaneurysms

Microcatheterization and coil embolization of intracranial pseudoaneurysms should be done very carefully, more so than for berry aneurysms, because typically there is no arterial wall to the pseudoaneurysm, placing it at a very high risk of rebleeding during treatment. Sometimes glue embolization of the parent artery with n-BCA or Onyx is the preferred method of treatment if the pseudoaneurysm is in a very distal segment of the parent artery and difficult to access with a microcatheter. It is important to make sure that both arterial segments proximal and distal to the pseudoaneurysm are occluded during embolization to stop flow into the lesion and to prevent the risk of bleeding.

Postprocedural Care

Stent placement requires long-term antiplatelet therapy to prevent platelet adhesion to the metal tines of the stent. Aspirin (325 mg) and clopidrogel (75 mg) are recommended for a minimum of six weeks after stent placement to prevent platelet adhesion to the bare metal tines while the endothelium is healing over the stent. After this time period, clopidrogel is typically stopped and aspirin (81 mg or 325 mg) is continued indefinitely to reduce the risk of thromboembolic complications. This also abates the healing response, which, if left unchecked, can result in in-stent stenosis from overgrowth of the endothelial lining and scar tissue over the metal tines of the stent. If this occurs, the in-stent stenosis may need to be treated with a cutting balloon angioplasty or re-stenting if the narrowing of the vessel lumen becomes hemodynamically significant (usually greater than or equal to 70% stenosis for extracranial vessels).

In circumstances where there were no technical complications or adverse anesthesia events, stenting of an arterial dissection is typically straightforward, with a short hospital course and basic postprocedural care.

Blood Pressure Control

After treatment of traumatic arterial lesions, blood pressure control is paramount. Immediately after treatment, normotensive therapy is usually satisfactory, as long as adequate revascularization has been established in patients with arterial dissections, lacerations, and extracranial pseudoaneurysms. The same principle holds true for intracranial pseudoaneurysms that have been completely embolized. However, if a large parent artery was embolized to occlude the pseudoaneurysm completely, then one may consider hypertensive therapy to maintain adequate collateral perfusion to that area.

Imaging

Noninvasive imaging studies after treatment of traumatic lesions typically include CTA and MRA. Carotid duplex can be used after extracranial stent placement and pseudoaneurysm embolization, but CTA and MRA provide better visualization of the stent and arterial lumen. However, angiography remains the gold standard.

Acute Neurological Change

In postprocedural patients who have an acute neurological change, one must consider the possibility of a thromboembolic event, vessel dissection, or an intracranial process such as a hemorrhage. CT/CTA or MRI/MRA can quickly evaluate for these pathologies. If these studies are positive, consider emergent angiography and intervention.

Intracranial Hemorrhage

An important consideration in the acute post-treatment period in a patient with a traumatic intracranial hemorrhage (ICH) is the timing of antiplatelet or anticoagulant administration. If the patient has been given heparin, protamine is an effective reversal agent. For aspirin or clopidogrel, there is no true reversal agent, although some feel that platelet administration is a good temporizing measure to reduce bleeding. Other agents, such as recombinant factor VII, desmopressin, and steroids, have been looked at as well. It is the practice of the senior author (EMD) to administer a cocktail of platelets, decadron, DDAVP, and FFP to counteract the effects of clopidrogel; he has found this cocktail to reduce temporarily the hemorrhage rate for emergent neurosurgical procedures (unpublished data presented at the national AANS meeting, April 2011).

Follow-Up Imaging Studies

Guidelines have not been established for follow-up imaging schedules to assess long-term efficacy. Carotid duplex, CTA, and MRA are useful noninvasive modalities for following stent patency. Any suspicion of in-stent stenosis or pseudoaneurysm recurrence on noninvasive imaging should be further evaluated by angiography.

Clinical Pearls

1. Medical treatment of asymptomatic carotid and vertebral artery dissections typically requires long-term treatment with warfarin (Coumadin) or antiplatelet agents, although no prospectively randomized clinical trials have been performed to test if medical management is better than no treatment at all.

2. Proper placement of a stent in a dissected artery requires the correct identification of the true lumen of the vessel.

3. Once the microwire is in the true lumen distal to the dissection, it is imperative to keep the microwire there until the procedure is completed to prevent having to re-access the lumen.

4. Large symptomatic cervical carotid pseudoaneurysms require stent placement, sometimes followed by coil embolization.

5. A balloon occlusion test should be performed before making the decision to sacrifice an artery; if the patient fails the test, then an extracranial-to-intracranial arterial bypass by a cerebrovascular neurosurgeon should be considered prior to vessel sacrifice if time permits.

6. When intracranial pseudoaneurysms are treated, the inflow and outflow zones of the aneurysm need to be occluded to prevent recanalization of the lesion and to prevent it from rebleeding.

7. Patients with penetrating neck injuries should first be evaluated and stabilized by a trauma team before they are brought to the angiography suite for treatment.

Recommended Reading

Diaz-Daza O, Arraiza FJ, Barkley JM, Whigham CJ. Endovascular therapy of traumatic vascular lesions of the head and neck. Cardiovasc Intervent Radiol 2003;26(3):213–221

Kerry S, et al.; Cervical Artery Dissection in Stroke Study Trial Investigators. Antiplatelet therapy vs. anticoagulation in cervical artery dissection: rationale and design of the Cervical Artery Dissection in Stroke Study (CADISS). Int J Stroke 2007;2(4):292–296

Larson PS, Reisner A, Morassutti DJ, Abdulhadi B, Harpring JE. Traumatic intracranial aneurysms. Neurosurg Focus 2000;8(1):e4

Massac E Jr, Siram SM, Leffall LD Jr. Penetrating neck wounds. Am J Surg 1983;145(2):263–265

Reddy SS, Newlands SD. Management of penetrating neck trauma. http://www.utmb.edu/otoref/Grnds/Penetrat-NeckTrauma-2002-0905/Penetrat-Neck-Trauma-2002-0905-slides.pdf. 2009

Uzan M, Cantasdemir M, Seckin MS, et al. Traumatic intracranial carotid tree aneurysms. Neurosurgery 1998;43(6):1314–1320, discussion 1320–1322

References

1. Campos-Herrera CR, Scaff M, Yamamoto FI, Conforto AB. Spontaneous cervical artery dissection: an update on clinical and diagnostic aspects. Arq Neuropsiquiatr 2008;66(4):922–927

2. Schievink WI. Spontaneous dissection of the carotid and vertebral arteries. N Engl J Med 2001;344(12):898–906

3. Conforto AB, Yamamoto F, Evaristo EF, Puglia P Jr, Caldas JG, Scaff M. Intracranial vertebral artery dissection presenting as subarachnoid hemorrhage: successful endovascular treatment. Acta Neurol Scand 2001;103(1):64–68

4. Diaz-Daza O, Arraiza FJ, Barkley JM, Whigham CJ. Endovascular therapy of traumatic vascular lesions of the head and neck. Cardiovasc Intervent Radiol 2003;26(3):213–221

5. Kerry S, et al.; Cervical Artery Dissection in Stroke Study Trial Investigators. Antiplatelet therapy vs. anticoagulation in cervical artery dissection: rationale and design of the Cervical Artery Dissection in Stroke Study (CADISS). Int J Stroke 2007;2(4):292–296

6. Abou-Chebl A. Cervical artery dissection. Curr Treat Options Cardiovasc Med 2009;11(2):167–175

7. Lyrer P, Engelter S. Antithrombotic drugs for carotid artery dissection. Cochrane Database Syst Rev 2010;(10):CD000255

8. Georgiadis D, Arnold M, von Buedingen HC, et al. Aspirin vs anticoagulation in carotid artery dissection: a study of 298 patients. Neurology 2009;72(21):1810–1815

9. DuBose J, Recinos G, Teixeira PG, Inaba K, Demetriades D. Endovascular stenting for the treatment of traumatic internal carotid injuries: expanding experience. J Trauma 2008;65(6):1561–1566

10. Cohen JE, Ben-Hur T, Rajz G, Umansky F, Gomori JM. Endovascular stent-assisted angioplasty in the management of traumatic internal carotid artery dissections. Stroke 2005;36(4):e45–e47

11. Uzan M, Cantasdemir M, Seckin MS, et al. Traumatic intracranial carotid tree aneurysms. Neurosurgery 1998;43(6):1314–1320, discussion 1320–1322

12. Larson PS, Reisner A, Morassutti DJ, Abdulhadi B, Harpring JE. Traumatic intracranial aneurysms. Neurosurg Focus 2000;8(1):e4

13. Massac E Jr, Siram SM, Leffall LD Jr. Penetrating neck wounds. Am J Surg 1983; 145(2):263–265

14. Amirjamshidi A, Rahmat H, Abbassioun K. Traumatic aneurysms and arteriovenous fistulas of intracranial vessels associated with penetrating head injuries occurring during war: principles and pitfalls in diagnosis and management. A survey of 31 cases and review of the literature. J Neurosurg 1996;84(5):769–780

15. Wang X, Chen JX, You C, He M. Surgical management of traumatic intracranial pseudoaneurysms: a report of 12 cases. Neurol India 2008;56(1):47–51

16. Reddy SS, Newlands SD. Management of penetrating neck trauma. http://www.utmb.edu/otoref/Grnds/Penetrat-NeckTrauma-2002-0905/Penetrat-Neck-Trauma-2002-0905-slides.pdf. 2009

17. LeBoeuf HJ, Quinn FB. Penetrating neck trauma. Department of Otolayrngology Grand Rounds. http://www.otohns.net/default.asp?id=15230. 26 January 1999

18. Fogelman MJ, Stewart RD. Penetrating wounds of the neck. Am J Surg. 1956: 91:581-593

19. Edwards NM, Fabian TC, Claridge JA, Timmons SD, Fischer PE, Croce MA. Antithrombotic therapy and endovascular stents are effective treatment for blunt carotid injuries: results from long-term follow-up. J Am Coll Surg 2007;204(5):1007–1013, discussion 1014–1015

Spinal Arteriovenous Malformations

Mohamed Samy Elhammady, Stacey Quintero Wolfe,
and Mohammad Ali Aziz-Sultan

Etiology

Spinal vascular malformations form a diverse group of vascular entities, with disparate etiologies as well as presentation. Three main categories compose the majority of spinal vascular malformations: spinal arteriovenous malformations (sAVMs), spinal cavernous malformations, and spinal vascular tumors. Spinal AVMs have been classified in many ways, based on both their anatomy and pathogenesis; these classifications are discussed below.

Many classification systems for spinal arteriovenous malformations have been proposed, most of which are based on the nidus, the feeding artery, and anatomic location of the lesion. Spinal AVMs can generally be classified into four types (**Fig. 20.1**). Type I represents an arteriovenous fistula between a dural branch of the spinal ramus of a radicular artery and an intradural medullary vein. The fistula is usually located in the dural sleeve of a dorsal spinal nerve root. Type II represents an intramedullary arteriovenous malformation with a compact nidus within the substance of the spinal cord. Type III represents an extensive arteriovenous malformation, often extending into the vertebral body and paraspinal tissues. Type IV represents an intradural perimedullary arteriovenous fistula. This fistula is along the spinal cord and feeds from the spinal arteries, usually the anterior spinal artery.

Type I is the most common type of spinal AVM and accounts for approximately 60–80% of cases. These lesions are also synonymous with spinal dural arteriovenous fistula, the long dorsal AVM, angioma racemosum venosum, and the single-coiled vessel malformation. Type I spinal AVMs have been further classified into lesions with a single arterial feeder (Type I-A) or those with multiple arterial feeders (Type I-B). Failure to visualize all feeders in a Type I-B AVM may make it difficult to localize the draining vein and provide definitive treatment.

The exact etiology of these AVMs is unknown; they are believed to be acquired lesions that may occur either spontaneously or following trauma. They are commonly located in the dural sleeve of the lower thoracic and lumbosacral nerve roots. These malformations are, in fact, arteriovenous fistulas in the dural sheath of a spinal nerve. The fistula is supplied by a radicular artery or arteries, which drain into one and occasionally more veins located on the dorsal pial surface. As a result of the shunt, the coronal venous plexus, which normally drains the posterior two thirds of the spinal cord, becomes arterialized, and the resulting increase in venous pressure impairs spinal cord perfusion and venous drainage. These engorged veins may extend for several spinal levels; since they are valveless, they occasionally drain cranially and arterialize the posterior cranial fossa veins. Despite the high venous pressure, type I AVMs are relatively low-flow fistulas and rarely hemorrhage.

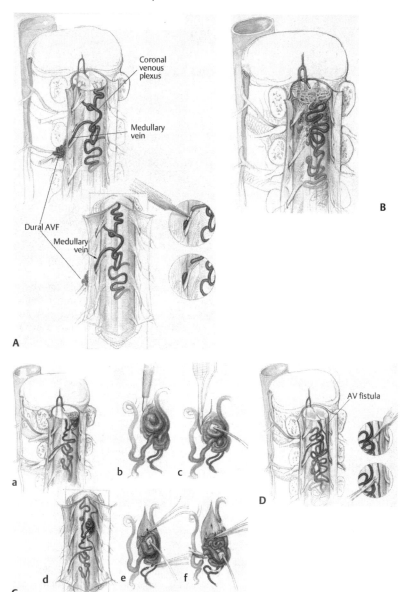

Coronal
venous
plexus

Medullary
vein

Dural AVF

Medullary
vein

A

B

a

b

c

d

e

f

C

AV fistula

D

Type II AVMs (also referred to as glomus AVMs or angioma racemosum arterio-venosum) are the second most common spinal vascular malformation, accounting for ~19–45% of cases, and appear to be congenital lesions. These lesions are true AVMs located within the substance of the spinal cord and can occur anywhere along the spinal axis.

Type III AVMs (also called juvenile or metameric AVMs) are the least common type of spinal vascular malformation and appear to be congenital lesions. They are diffuse lesions that not only involve the spinal cord but may have significant extension into subdural and epidural spaces, as well as into the surrounding soft tissue and bone. In cases with involvement of all embryological layers of a metamere, the condition is known as Cobb's syndrome. They may be associated with cutaneous angiomas and angiomatous phakomatoses, such as Klippel-Trenaunay-Weber syndrome and Rendu-Osler-Weber syndrome. The natural history is not well known; however, most patients do poorly.

Type-IV AVMs (also called perimedullary fistulas) appear to be acquired lesions that are most commonly located in the thoracolumbar region, occasionally are isolated to the thoracic levels, and rarely occur in the cervical region. These AVMs consist of a direct fistulous connection between the anterior or (less commonly) the posterior spinal artery and a spinal vein. As a result of the fistula, there may

---

Fig. 20.1 **(A)** The vascular anatomy of a spinal dural arteriovenous fistula (AVF). The AVF is supplied by a dural artery and drained by a medullary vein. Arterial input into the valveless intradural venous system increases venous pressure within the coronal venous plexus and causes myelopathy. Treatment is to coagulate and divide the arterialized draining vein at the site of the AVF. **(B)** Vascular anatomy of a juvenile intramedullary arteriovenous malformation (AVM) of the spinal cord. The juvenile type of intramedullary AVM is fed by enlarged medullary arteries via dilated anterior and posterior spinal arteries. The nidus of the AVM is extensive, often filling the spinal canal, and contains neural tissue within the interstices of the vessels of the AVM. **(Ca)** Vascular anatomy of glomus intramedullary arteriovenous malformation (AVM). The nidus of the glomus type of intramedullary AVM is a tightly packed nidus of blood vessels confined to a limited segment of the spinal cord. **(Cb)** After separating the arachnoid from the AVM, a diamond knife is used to incise the pia at the edge of the nidus. **(Cc)** To obtain the necessary exposure, the pial incision is extended a few millimeters rostrally and caudally. **(Cd)** Surgical anatomy of spinal AVM. **(Ce)** The superficial feeding vessels are interrupted sharply after they have been coagulated. **(Cf)** Resection of the AVM, using a standard microsurgical technique. **(D)** Vascular anatomy of an intradural or perimedullary arteriovenous fistula (AVF). Medullary arteries provide the arterial supply, in this instance via a posterior spinal artery. Intradural AVFs often have associated arterial or venous aneurysms at the junction of the arterial and venous elements. Note the dilatation of the vein just distal to the AV shunt. The site of arterial to venous transition is identified, and after bipolar coagulation of a 4 to 6 mm segment of the distal portion of the artery(s) to the AVF, the AVF is interrupted on the distal portion of the arterial side of the fistula, beyond the last arterial branch to the spinal cord. In some instances, a small clip or ligature is required, but most feeders can be managed by bipolar coagulation and sharp interruption alone. If an aneurysm or varix is the site of convergence of the feeding vessels, it is excised. Many of these lesions are not as simple as the one illustrated here because these lesions can have more than one simple fistula in the same region of the pia, and the tortuosity and dilatation of the venous drainage often obscure the site of the AVF beneath a nest of blood vessels. (From Macdonald RL. Vascular neurosurgery. In: *Neurosurgical Operative Atlas*, 2nd ed. Thieme Medical Publishers; 2008.)

be massive aneurysmal venous dilatation, which may extend to the craniocervical junction and even into the posterior cranial fossa. The clinical manifestations may be caused by venous hypertension, arterial steal, or compression from dilated venous varicosities. In contrast to type I AVMs, which rarely hemorrhage due to the dural location of the fistula, perimedullary fistulas may occasionally present with subarachnoid hemorrhage.

Presentation of Spinal AVMs

Type I AVMs are most frequently found in males between the ages of 40 to 70 years. The most common clinical syndrome is progressive sensory and motor neurological deterioration. The mode of progression may be continuous, stepladder, or waxing and waning. A history of back or sciatic-like pain at the time of presentation may be seen in 40% of patients. Similarly, a history suggestive of neurogenic claudication with exacerbation of the pain and neurologic symptoms with exercise is not infrequent. Under these circumstances, it is likely that the venous hypertension, which is believed to be responsible for the progressive symptomatology, is exacerbated by foraminal narrowing that compresses exiting draining veins.

Type II AVMs usually present between the ages of 20 to 40 years. The clinical course may be an apoplectic neurological deficit or a gradually progressive change in sensory or motor function. Approximately one third of patients present with hemorrhage. Clinical manifestations may be caused by subarachnoid or intramedullary hemorrhage, arterial steal, compression by distended vessels and varices, or venous hypertension.

Type III AVMs tend to present in adolescents and young adults with apoplectic hemorrhage or progressive neurological decline. In addition to the findings seen with type II spinal AVMs, an MRI will demonstrate extraspinal extension of the vascular lesion. Type III AVMs are fed by multiple spinal and paraspinal arteries and drain diffusely.

Type IV AVMs commonly present in early to middle adulthood as a progressive ascending sensory motor disturbance associated with sphincter dysfunction. An MRI will demonstrate flow voids in the subarachnoid space without intra-axial components. Angiography remains the test of choice to demonstrate the fistulous point.

Imaging of Spinal AVMs (Fig. 20.2)

Imaging of spinal AVMs presents the same challenges as their intracranial counterparts. Most of these lesions involve high-flow hemodynamics, thereby necessitating imaging protocols that not only have high temporal resolution but also must have adequate spatial resolution to provide detailed images of the often small vessel calibers that are involved with these lesions.

CT and CTA have been used, but with limited success, even in the era of multidetector CT scanners. The ill-defined dynamic capabilities, issues with bolus-timing, and limited spatial resolution of CT, in addition to the use of radiation and iodinated contrast agents, make CT a modality that can be used, but it is not the first choice for examining spinal AVMs. MRI and time-resolved MRA are more useful imaging modalities to locate the lesion within the spinal cord, to assess the presence of an intraparenchymal hemorrhage, intravascular thrombosis, a syrinx, and spinal cord edema or atrophy, and to determine the hemodynamic behavior of the lesion. Numerous studies have demonstrated that MR protocols make it feasible to visualize spinal AVMs and provide a useful modality, without the use of radiation or iodinated contrast agents. Despite this, catheter-based digital subtraction angiography (DSA) remains the gold standard, because it provides improved dynamic, high temporal resolution views of hemodynamic flow through the malformation and a more detailed understanding of its angioarchitecture, including the number and source of the arterial feeders arising from both the anterior and posterior spinal circulation, as well as information on the venous outflow system.

When imaging spinal AVMs, several characteristics should be noted during all the hemodynamic phases, whichever modality is used. The arterial phase should be characterized by the location and number of feeders. Often, several levels above and below the lesion should be examined so as to not miss occult feeding arteries. Further, other associated vascular lesions should be identified, such as perinidal aneurysms or venous varicosities. The nidal phase should be characterized by the extent of the lesion, location with respect to spinal level, and its anatomical characteristics, that is, intramedullary, intradural, or other. The venous phase should be characterized by the number and location of venous drainage. Often, there will be a single fistulous connection that is some distance away from the location(s) of the dilated venous complex. Careful angiographic determination of this fistulous point(s) is critical to appropriate therapy and resolution of arteriovenous fistulae.

Evidence-Based Medicine

Our understanding of the natural history of type I AVMs is largely deduced from a retrospective analysis of 60 patients reported by Aminoff and Logue in 1974.[1] Although the study was performed prior to the introduction of selective spinal angiography and before the recognition of spinal dural AVFs as a separate entity, the demographics strongly suggest that the majority of cases were dural AVFs. The study was composed predominantly of adult males older than 40 years, with thoracolumbar lesions that had never hemorrhaged. The clinical course was one of progressive neurological deterioration. From the time of onset of leg weakness, ~20% of the patients required crutches or were non-ambulatory by 6 months, and 50% were non-ambulatory by 3 years. In view of the dismal prognosis, treatment is warranted in all cases to halt the progression of myelopathy.

In 2002, Eskandar et al. reported their experience treating 26 patients with spinal dural AVFs.[2] All patients were evaluated with the intention to treat by embolization and to reserve surgery for those in whom endovascular treatment failed or for whom it was thought to be unsafe. Three (12%) of the patients underwent surgery as a primary modality, because the feeding artery was at the same level as a major arterial supply to the spinal cord. Of the 23 patients treated by embolization, 9 (39%) ultimately required surgery for various reasons: 6 patients had incomplete occlusion of the fistula, 2 patients developed collateral supply to the fistula, and 1 patient developed recanalization of the fistula.

Niimi et al. reported their experience treating 47 Type I dural AVFs with cyanoacrylate embolization.[3] Of the 43 patients with more than one month follow-up, 26 (60%) either had inadequate embolization or recurrence of the fistula.

The natural history of type II AVMs is not as well defined as in type I malformations. Patients who present with progressive myelopathy have a similar prognosis to patients with type I AVMs and tend to do poorly. On the other hand, patients who present with hemorrhage have an unclear natural history. Retrospective analysis of Aminoff and Logue's series in 1974 showed that of 6 patients who suffered subarachnoid hemorrhage, only one had a recurrent hemorrhage.[1]

Although his previous study suggested a low rebleeding rate, Aminoff in 1976 presented a more worrisome natural history.[4] He reported 53 patients with spinal AVMs that presented with hemorrhage, and although he did not differentiate between dural AVFs and true spinal cord AVMs, we can presume that they were true

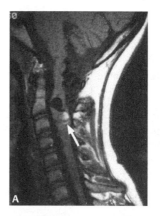
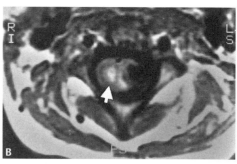
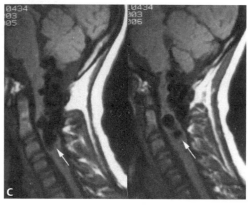

Fig. 20.2 **(A–G)** An intradural arteriovenous fistula (AVF). **(A–C)** T1-weighted sagittal and axial magnetic resonance imaging (MRI) without contrast and **(D)** selective left vertebral arteriography using standard "cut films" (anteroposterior-left and lateral-right views) and **(E)** rapid-sequence (10 frames/s) digital imaging (lateral view) of an AVF at the upper cervical segments of the spinal cord in a 17-year-old female with four hemorrhages but normal neurological function. An MRI scan 11 days after acute neurological changes **(A,B)** shows the patent (areas of low intramedullary and extramedullary signal) and thrombosed (high intramedullary signal, *arrows*) portions on an intramedullary varix and abnormal vessels in the upper cervical subarachnoid space and cisterna magna. Symptoms were attributed to thrombosis of one of the intramedullary varices **(A)**, a thrombosis that was not present on an MRI scan performed 4 months previously **(C)**. Arteriography

spinal AVMs, as dural AVFs rarely hemorrhage. Of the 53 patients, 3 died within a few days of the hemorrhage, 4 were operated on within a month of hemorrhage and in 5 cases no further details were available. Thus, 41 patients remained at risk of rebleeding. Twenty-two of the 41 patients had a second hemorrhage, 4 of whom died. Of the 18 surviving patients, 9 had an additional hemorrhage. The time to rebleeding varied from 24 hours to well over 5 years from the initial hemorrhage. Aminoff further analyzed the data and determined a rebleeding rate of ~10% within the first month and 40% within the first year.

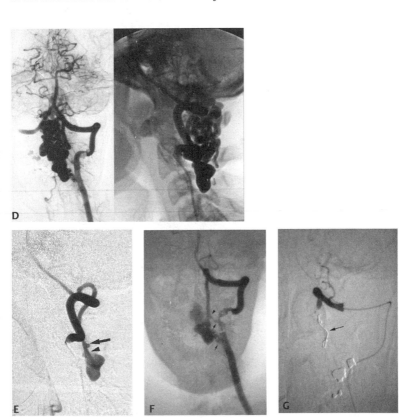

(D) suggested an arteriovenous malformation (AVM) of the spinal cord with extensive blood flow, but rapid-sequence (10 frames/s) imaging in (E) demonstrates that this is a more simple AVF (*arrowhead*) with an aneurysm (*arrow*) proximal to the AVF and a varix distal to the fistula. The varix was visible on the sagittal MRI on the left side of the spinal cord (C, left). (E,F) Multiple feeding vessels converged at the site of the fistula, which was at the upper margin of the large intramedullary varix. In (D) the coiled, dilated arterialized veins conceal the fistula and obscure the aneurysm. (G) To reduce blood flow through the fistula, a coil was positioned in the distal portion of the principal feeding artery (a posterior spinal artery) just proximal to the aneurysm, the day before the fistula was interrupted surgically and the large varix was excised. (With permission from McDonald RL. Vascular neurosurgery. In: *Neurosurgical Operative Atlas,* 2nd ed. Thieme Medical Publishers; 2008.)

In another study, by Hurth and colleagues, the clinical features and evolution of 90 patients with intradural AVMs (20 cervical, 20 thoracic, and 50 thoracolumbar) were analyzed during a period of 15 years.[5] Subarachnoid hemorrhage was the initial manifestation in 35% of cases. Recurrent hemorrhage occurred in 39% of cases.

Biondi et al. reported their experience embolizing 35 patients with thoracic intramedullary AVMs using PVA (mean follow-up 6 years).[6] Although neither complete nor permanent obliteration of the AVM was possible in any patients, 63% of cases showed clinical improvement at the end of the study. Seven patients (20%) deteriorated following embolization. Two patients (6%) suffered subarachnoid hemorrhage; however, both had missed their annual follow-up angiogram for 3 years. The authors recommended routine yearly angiograms and embolization of thoracic AVMs.

Berenstein and Lasjaunias reported their experience with liquid embolics.[7] Thirty-eight of 47 patients with AVMs underwent embolization with NBCA. Complete AVM obliteration was achieved in 25 (53%) cases. A favorable outcome was reached in 36 of 47 patients (77%). There were 10.6% permanent and 10.6% transient complications. No hemorrhages were observed in patients with complete AVM obliteration, whereas two patients suffered recurrent hemorrhage following partial embolization during a follow-up of 7.5 years.

Equipment

Sheath

A short (24 cm) 6 Fr femoral sheath allows the sheath to remain within the iliac artery. This facilitates injection of the iliac arteries, the median sacral artery, and the L4/5 segmental vessels.

Guide Catheter

A diagnostic angiogram is performed using a 5 Fr Cobra or Mickelson catheter. The angle of the segmental vessels decreases from the horizontal plane as they descend from the thoracic to the lumbar spine. Therefore, in the lower spine and sacral arteries, switching to a Simmons catheter may be helpful. Embolization procedures can be performed with a 5 Fr or 6 Fr Simmons 2 or Mickelson catheter. This procedure can also be done with a 5 Fr guide catheter.

Glide Wire

A 0.035″ wire is used to advance the catheter through the aorta and to aid in forming the Simmons catheter. Once the level of interest has been reached, the wire is removed, and very low-volume hand injections of diluted contrast are used to visualize the segmental vessels and to guide the catheter into the vessel origin.

Microcatheter

A 0.010″ catheter navigated over a soft, torqueable wire not only is excellent for distal catheterization but also provides the ability to embolize into the venous drainage of the fistula. A permanent liquid embolic should be used for these lesions, such as n-BCA or Onyx. If Onyx embolization is planned, a DMSO-compatible microcatheter should be used, such as an Ultraflow (0.010″), Marathon (0.013″), or Echelon (0.014″).

Microwire

The softer a microwire is, the safer it is for accessing these small, tortuous vessels; examples include the Synchro-10/14 or Transcend EX 10/14. The Mirage wire (0.008″) may be preferred when using the Ultraflow or Marathon microcatheters to reduce the risk of injuring the microcatheter with the wire.

Technique

General Techniques

Several principles of spinal angiography should be followed (**Table 20.1**). Spinal angiography is performed using AP fluoroscopy, with a radiopaque measuring ruler placed on the table to mark the spinal levels during the procedure. During the diagnostic angiogram, it is important to inject the segmental vessels two levels above and below the lesion to avoid missing arterial feeders. The artery of Adamkiewicz and the feeding arteries with concomitant medullary supply must be recognized prior to embolization. One hallmark appearance of the artery of Adamkiewicz includes a hairpin loop that is made along the anterior aspect of the spinal canal. This is consistent with the anterior spinal artery. The angiogram should be studied to determine the rapidity of flow in order to select the appropriate viscosity of the liquid embolic agent. Visualization of the thoracic vessels may be enhanced if the patient does not breath during image acquisition. If patients are awake, they should be asked to hold their breath, or respiration may be suspended for the ventilated patient. For the lower thoracic and lumbosacral vessels, the administration of glucagon can decrease gastrointestinal motility to improve image quality.

Table 20.1 General Principles of Spinal Angiography

Preoperative imaging (dynamic CTA/MRA) should be done to narrow the area(s) of interest, which will reduce the amount of required radiation during angiography.
Single-plane angiography is normally used to reduce the amount of radiation exposure, as lateral views require more radiation for quality images.
Three-D rotational angiography results in improved depiction of the vascular lesion's relationship to the spinal cord and surrounding structures.
Important anatomic features to note are angioarchitecture, spinal cord normal vasculature, vascular blushes, early venous filling, and signs of venous hypertension.
The origins of the segmental arteries are more symmetric and posterior further caudally down the aorta/iliacs.
A complete spinal angiogram includes catheterization of the vertebrals, carotids, subclavians (and associated trunks), and iliacs. All of these arteries contribute some vascular supply to the spinal cord and its associated vascular pathologies.

Embolization of spinal AVMs is frequently performed under general anesthesia, with neurophysiologic monitoring, such as somatosensory or motor evoked potentials. This allows better control of the patient's respiration to enhance image quality during selective catheterization of feeding arteries and the embolization phases of the procedure. Any patient movement during these phases can distort proper visualization and may increase the chances of inadvertent embolization of vessels supplying normal spinal cord tissue.

During the procedure, systemic heparinization (goal ACT = 200–250 seconds) is used to avoid thrombosis, and Decadron can be administered to decrease inflammation and swelling from embolization. Selective catheterization of feeding arteries is performed using a microcatheter and wire appropriate for the target vessel and embolic agent. Before injection of the embolic agent, a hand-run, superselective angiogram through the microcatheter should always be performed to confirm that the feeding artery supplies only the lesion. For intramedullary lesions, provocative testing prior to embolization with Brevital or lidocaine may be helpful. Once the embolization is complete, a final angiogram should be performed to assess for residual AVM or inadvertent embolization of other vessels.

Specific Techniques

The goal of treatment is to eliminate the fistula or at least to disconnect it from the coronal venous plexus. Given the various types of angioarchitecture, not every type of spinal AVM has an endovascular solution. However, technical considerations regarding each type are discussed below.

Embolization (Table 20.2)

Embolization of Type I AVMs may be attempted, so long as the dural artery supplying the fistula does not originate from branches supplying the spinal cord. However, this is not an infrequent occurrence and may be seen in approximately 15% of cases. The goal of embolization is to inject a column of the embolic agent through the fistula and into the proximal portion of the draining vein. Inability to embolize up to the proximal venous segment of the fistula increases the risk of recurrence of the fistula from collateralization, whereas embolization and occlusion of deep spinal veins may exacerbate venous hypertension or venous infarction. A post-embolization CT scan to detect the presence of intradural embolic material will allow confirmation that the embolic material has reached the draining vein and may be helpful in predicting long-term obliteration.

Endovascular embolization of Type II spinal AVMs (intramedullary) rarely results in complete obliteration. Partial embolization, however, may be used to obliterate angiographically high-risk areas of a malformation, such as arterial or intranidal aneurysms, or to occlude intranidal AVFs or portions of a lesion with outflow restriction to reduce the risk of hemorrhage, arterial steal, or venous congestion. Also, as stated above, gradual embolization, usually over several sessions, can be very effective in reducing flow and hence venous hypertension in patients who present with progressive myelopathy.

Treatment of Type III spinal AVMs is usually palliative and consists of the staged reduction of arterial supply, either by surgical ligation of feeders and partial resection or by endovascular embolization.

Table 20.2 Embolization of Spinal AVMs

Type of spinal AVM	Comments
Type I	The goal is to catheterize as close to the fistulous point as possible and to embolize into the proximal venous segment.
Type II	Rarely results in complete obliteration; serial embolization may reduce venous hypertension.
Type III	Usually palliative and staged embolization has been used to reduce vascular burden.
Type IV-1	Small fistulae that normally cannot be safely embolized; surgery is generally the treatment of choice.
Type IV-2	Depending on arterial supply, embolization and/or surgery can be performed.
Type IV-3	Staged embolization is the typical choice, due to multiple large arterial feeders.

Merland and Rezine further classified Type IV AVMs into three categories (Types 1–3 perimedullary fistulas) according to the size, quantity of flow, and venous drainage.[8]

- Type 1 perimedullary fistulas (Type IV-1) are small fistulas fed by a long and thin spinal artery, with minimal shunting and venous dilatation. Since embolization must be performed as close to the fistulous point as possible to preserve blood flow through the spinal artery, this type of fistula is not amenable to endovascular therapy, and surgery is the therapy of choice.
- Type 2 perimedullary fistulas (Type IV-2) are intermediate-sized fistulas that are fed by one or two dilated arteries and drain into winding, dilated veins. This type of fistula can be treated with embolization, surgery, or both.
- Type 3 perimedullary fistulas (Type IV-3) are giant, high-flow fistulas fed by multiple large-caliber arteries that drain into massively dilated veins. These fistulas require embolization, because surgical resection alone carries a high risk of intraoperative hemorrhage or spinal artery stroke.

Alternative Treatments

Before the advent of endovascular therapy, surgery or observation was the primary mode of management of spinal AVMs. In contrast to endovascular therapy, numerous surgical series report low procedural morbidity and a success rate of nearly 100%.[9] Dural AVFs can be successfully treated by disconnection of the fistula via permanent occlusion of the arterialized vein, which is usually single but in rare cases can be multiple. Surgical exposure of the fistula may be achieved via a laminectomy, hemilaminectiomy, or foraminotomy. The draining arterialized medullary vein, which lies on the posterior aspect of the dorsal root, is identified as it penetrates the dura and is distinguished from the smaller radicular arteries that are intermingled with the nerve and generally run in a more ventral direction.

To ensure that the vessel identified is indeed a medullary vein, the intraoperative anatomy is compared with the venous phase of the preoperative angiogram, and the course of the vessel is followed posteriorly to where it joins the arterialized coronal venous plexus. A useful maneuver is to place a temporary clip on the vein, to observe the arterialized venous coils become soft, and to change to a blue color within 5 to 10 minutes. If this does not occur, it is necessary to search for other arterialized veins above and below the level of the fistula. Once all arterialized draining veins have been indentified, they can be coagulated and divided. If dural resection is necessary, as in cases with both epidural and intradural venous drainage, the dura is coagulated around the nerve root sleeve, and the portion containing the fistula is excised.

It should be emphasized that surgery for type II AVMs is difficult and carries significant morbidity. Yasargil et al. reported a 20% clinical deterioration, 5% mortality rate, and 27% incomplete resection.[10] However, one location in particular, the cervicomedullary region, is frequently amenable to surgical resection, since the arterial supply is usually dorsal from branches of the vertebral artery.

However, not all types of spinal AVMs benefit from surgical resection. Complete surgical resection of Type III AVMs carries a significant risk of neurological deterioration, so it is rarely attempted. Surgery is typically an option only for Type IV-1 and possibly IV-2 lesions, as the type IV-3 carries significant morbidity to any surgical procedure.

Although it is a viable option for the treatment of intracranial AVMs, radiosurgery for spinal AVMs has not been examined rigorously. Until recently, LINAC and gamma knife systems were not capable of safely radiating spinal AVMs below the cervicomedullary junction. In fact, there are very few series on radiosurgical treatment of spinal AVMs. More recently, however, new technology that adapts with the patient's respiratory movements has allowed spinal AVMs to be treated with radiation.

Postprocedure Care

Routine post-angiogram care is followed. Patients are monitored in an intensive care unit. Steroids are administered to minimize post-embolization swelling and inflammation. Regular neurological assessments are required, with particular attention to sensory and motor spinal examination. Any deterioration requires further evaluation with an MRI of the spine to look for spinal cord ischemia, hemorrhage, or edema.

Technical Pearls and Pitfalls

1. Evaluation of spinal AVMs should be done by a multidisciplinary team that includes neurosurgeons, neurointerventionists, and neurointensivists. Treatment algorithms for spinal AVMs frequently may include surgery by a neurosurgeon, either alone or in combination with endovascular embolization.
2. Imaging evaluation of spinal AVMs should include both a vascular study as well as one geared toward resolving the properties of the surrounding spinal tissues. Catheter-based angiography remains the gold standard for assessing spinal AVMs, because it is a dynamic study that defines the anatomy and flow of the lesion.

3. Adequate angiographic assessment of spinal vascular lesions includes catheterization of bilateral segmental arteries at least two levels above and below the level of the lesion.

4. For vascular lesions in the cervical region, catheterization must include the vertebral arteries, external carotid arteries, thyrocervical and costocervical trunks, and the supreme intercostal arteries; in the lumbosacral area, both iliac arteries and the median sacral artery must also be catheterized.

5. Obliteration rates for surgical treatment of Type 1 DAVF approach 100% and should always be considered. If the fistula is considered potentially curable, that is, it has one or more well visualized and appropriately sized arterial feeders that can be catheterized safely by endovascular treatment, it is imperative to get liquid embolic into the venous side of the fistula; this can best be assessed by obtaining a post-embolization CT to confirm intradural glue, signifying that the intradural vein has been reached.

Recommended Reading

Afshar JK, Doppman JL, Oldfield EH. Surgical interruption of intradural draining vein as curative treatment of spinal dural arteriovenous fistulas. J Neurosurg 1995;82(2):196–200

Aminoff MJ, Logue V. Clinical features of spinal vascular malformations. Brain 1974; 97(1):197–210

Berenstein A, Lasjuanias P, ter Brugge K. Spinal dural arteriovenous fistulae. In: *Surgical Neuroangiography*, vol. 2.2. New York: Springer; 2004:849–872

Heros RC, Debrun GM, Ojemann RG, Lasjaunias PL, Naessens PJ. Direct spinal arteriovenous fistula: a new type of spinal AVM. Case report. J Neurosurg 1986;64(1):134–139

References

1. Aminoff MJ, Logue V. The prognosis of patients with spinal vascular malformations. Brain 1974;97(1):211–218

2. Eskandar EN, Borges LF, Budzik RF Jr, Putman CM, Ogilvy CS. Spinal dural arteriovenous fistulas: experience with endovascular and surgical therapy. J Neurosurg 2002;96(2, Suppl):162–167

3. Niimi Y, Berenstein A, Setton A, Neophytides A. Embolization of spinal dural arteriovenous fistula: results and follow-up. J Neurosurg 1997;40:675–683

4. Aminoff M. *Spinal Angiomas*. Oxford: Blackwell; 1976

5. Hurth M, Houdart R, Djindjian R, Rey A, Djindjian M. Arteriovenous malformations of the spinal cord: clinical, anatomical and therapeutic considerations—series of 150 cases. Prog Neurol Surg 1978;9:238–266

6. Biondi A, Merland JJ, Reizine D, et al. Embolization with particles in thoracic intramedullary arteriovenous malformations: long-term angiographic and clinical results. Radiology 1990;177(3):651–658

7. Berenstein A, Lasjuanias P, ter Brugge K. Spinal dural arteriovenous fistulae. In: *Surgical Neuroangiography*, vol. 2.2. New York: Springer; 2004:849–872

8. Merland J, Rezine D. Treatment of arteriovenous spinal cord malformations. Semin Intervent Radiol 1987;4:281–291

9. Afshar JK, Doppman JL, Oldfield EH. Surgical interruption of intradural draining vein as curative treatment of spinal dural arteriovenous fistulas. J Neurosurg 1995; 82(2):196–200

10. Yaşargil MG, Symon L, Teddy PJ. Arteriovenous malformations of the spinal cord. Adv Tech Stand Neurosurg 1984;11:61–102

Vascular Tumors of the Skull Base, Neck, and Spine

Stacey Quintero Wolfe, Mohamed Samy Elhammady, and Mohammad Ali Aziz-Sultan

Etiology

An in-depth discussion of all tumors affecting the skull base, neck, spine, and spinal cord is beyond the scope of this chapter, but we will briefly describe vascular tumors that may benefit from preoperative or primary embolization (**Table 21.1**). Several common indications for tumor embolization exist, namely, (1) to reduce blood loss by control of surgically inaccessible arterial feeders and to increase visualization during resection, (2) to reduce operative times and to increase the chances of complete surgical resection, (3) to relieve intractable pain, and (4) to decrease tumor recurrence. The seven vascular tumors discussed here include glomus tumors, hemangioblastoma, hemangioma, aneurysmal bone cyst (ABC), osteiod osteoma/osteoblastoma, giant cell tumors, and metastatic tumors. The specific etiology of each tumor will be described within each subsection below.

Table 21.1 Vascular Tumors Often Thought Amenable to Preoperative Embolization

Intracranial and skull base tumors
Meningiomas
Hemangioblastomas
Hemangiopericytomas
Neurogenic tumors
Juvenile nasopharyngeal angiofibromas
Esthesioneuroblastomas
Paragangliomas (glomus tumors)
Metastatic tumors (renal cell, myeloma)
Spinal and spinal cord tumors
Hemangioblastoma
Hemangioma
Aneurysmal bone cyst (ABC)
Osteiod osteoma/osteoblastoma
Giant cell tumors
Metastatic tumors (renal cell, thyroid)

Diagnosis

In general, for tumors of the skull base, neck and spine, diagnosis can best be determined by plain radiographs and CT to delineate the extent of bony involvement; by MRI for the extent of soft tissue involvement, which may include cranial nerve or spinal cord compression, as well as enhancement patterns and signal characteristics; and finally by biopsy for definitive histopathological diagnosis. Angiography can demonstrate the pattern and extent of vascularity and provide presurgical identification of the relationship of the tumor blood supply to that of the surrounding structures, cranial nerves, and spinal cord. For an adequate assessment of tumor vascularity, several things must be considered. For glomus tumors of the skull base and neck, specific imaging of the external carotid artery must be done, as this is the most common blood supply. For tumors of the spine, the segmental arteries on both sides must be catheterized at least two levels above and below the level of the tumor. For tumors of the cervical region, the vertebral arteries, external carotid arteries, thyrocervical and costocervical trunks, and the supreme intercostal arteries must also be catheterized and studied. In the lumbosacral area, both iliac arteries and the median sacral artery must be catheterized and studied. Radiographic identification of each of the six specific tumors will be discussed below within each subsection.

Glomus Tumors

Glomus tumors, which are part of the paraganglioma family of tumors, are rare hypervascular tumors that typically occur in three areas: the middle ear (glomus tympanicum), jugular foramen (glomus jugulare), and skull base (glomus vagale). These tumors are thought to arise from chemoreceptor organs derived from the neural crest. Glomus jugulare tumors are thought to originate from the chief cells of the paraganglia, or glomus bodies, located within the jugular bulb adventitia. Other locations occur when the tumor is associated with either the auricular branch of the vagus nerve (glomus vagale) or the tympanic branch of the glossopharyngeal nerve (glomus tympanicum). Glomus tumors are found most commonly in women during the fifth and sixth decades and have an estimated annual incidence of 1 in 1.3 million people. Although most glomus tumors are thought to be sporadic, familial inheritance (autosomal dominant and incomplete penetrance) does occur in 25%–50% of cases. Tumors develop almost exclusively in the children of disease-gene-carrying males. Due to the tumors' slow-growing nature, the clinical presentation is often indolent and delayed. The most common presentations are usually related to the location of the tumor, that is, conductive hearing loss and pulsatile tinnitus for glomus tympanicum, jugular foramen syndrome (paresis of cranial nerves IX-XI) for glomus jugulare, and hoarseness and dysphagia for glomus vagale.

All common imaging modalities may show changes related to the location of the glomus tumor. Plain X-rays may show asymmetric sizes of the middle ear or jugular foramen. CT scans of the skull base will usually demonstrate the extent of bone thinning or bone erosion around the mass lesion. MR images are classically described as having a "salt and pepper" appearance, as the imaging characteristics involve heterogeneous signal intensity on both T1- and T2-weighted sequences with and without contrast.

Angiography is recommended only if surgical resection becomes an option and only if preoperative embolization will benefit the resection. In cases of extensive involvement of the cervical vessels, a trial balloon occlusion may be necessary, given the likelihood of parent artery occlusion.

Hemangioblastomas

Hemangioblastomas are histologically benign tumors located predominantly in the posterior fossa and the cervicothoracic spinal cord. These tumors are composed of densely packed capillaries with intervening stroma and may be confused histopathologically with renal cell carcinoma. Hemangioblastomas compose approximately 2% of spinal cord tumors and are associated with von Hippel Lindau (VHL) disease in approximately 20% of the cases. These lesions often present as a mural nodule with a large cystic component, which may manifest with pain, sensory disturbance, and myelopathy. In cases of VHL, it is important to note that not all lesions necessarily progress. Consequently, strong consideration for treatment should be reserved for symptomatic lesions.

These lesions are most often characterized with MRI. T1-weighted MRI demonstrates an isointense nodule that enhances brightly with gadolinium contrast; T2 may demonstrate vascularity in the form of flow voids and/or an associated cyst or syrinx. Angiographically, a well-circumscribed, hypervascular mass is usually associated with a single feeding artery that arises from one of the posterior spinal arteries, although deep intramedullary lesions may also receive blood from the sulcocommissural branches of the anterior spinal artery. Hemangioblastomas opacify in the arterial phase and drain quickly but can be differentiated from AVMs by the absence of arteriovenous shunting.

Although tumor hemorrhage is rarely a presenting symptom, intraspinal hemangioblastomas often require preoperative embolization due to their robust blood supply and vascularity. Adjunctive embolization has been reported to decrease blood loss, shorten operative time, decrease surgical morbidity, and increase the chances of complete resection.[1] Safe embolization requires occlusion of pathologic vessels, with preservation of the normal vascular supply. In tumors with posterior spinal artery supply, the posterior spinal artery can be catheterized superselectively and embolized, providing that a pedicle does not provide flow to the anterior spinal artery. Liquid embolics, such as n-BCA or Onyx, are the embolic materials of choice when feasible.[2] This allows for penetration into the tumoral capillary bed but does require selective feeding artery catheterization with distal placement. Should distal catheterization prove impossible, particle embolization may be used, but it is imperative that the particles be larger than the diameter of the smallest normal vessel surrounding the tumor to prevent inadvertent embolization of the native blood supply to the spinal cord.

Hemangiomas

Hemangiomas are benign tumors of the vertebral body in which blood vessels replace normal marrow, producing hypertrophic sclerotic bony trabeculations. There is an incidence of 11% in the general population. Most hemangiomas are asymptomatic and are often found in multiple vertebral bodies. In cases of large or giant hemangiomas, vertebral body collapse may occur, resulting in localized back pain or even myelopathy.

Hemangiomas can occur in both the vertebral body and the posterior elements. Due to the presence of bony trabeculations, they usually are characterized as having a "honeycomb" appearance on plain radiographic imaging. On CT, a classic "polka dot" appearance occurs because of the cross-sectional view through the thickened, vertically oriented trabeculae. Most hemangiomas are hyperintense on both T1 and T2 MRI, possibly due to adipose tissue, although large, symptomatic hemangiomas tend to be isointense on T1. The angiographic appearance of hemangiomas has been classified by Djindjian into three groups (**Table 21.2**): Group A consists of patients with extravertebral extension and signs of myelopathy showing dense, heterogeneous opacification of the affected vertebral body without arteriovenous shunting; Group B consists of patients experiencing pain and found to have small lesions, with pooling of contrast material; and Group C consists of asymptomatic patients who did not have any pathologic opacification on angiography.[3]

Hemangiomas are radiosensitive and undergo sclerotic obliteration, which may improve pain, although this takes place over months to years. Embolization may provide rapid relief of pain and can also be used preoperatively for large, symptomatic lesions that will likely be surgically treated.[4] Vertebroplasty may be performed in the angiography suite and is particularly useful for pain control in large hemangiomas with an intact neurological exam and posterior spine elements.[4]

Aneurysmal Bone Cysts

Aneurysmal bone cysts (ABCs) are communicating cystic spaces within bone containing venous blood under pressure. ABCs are most commonly found in children under age 20 and involve the spine in almost 90% of cases. Nonspecific back pain is the most common presenting symptom; however, compression of nerve roots from fractures may result in presenting radiculopathy.

Plain radiographs and CT scans demonstrate a destructive, expansile radiolucent lesion with ballooning of a thin shell of surrounding bone. On T1 and T2 MRI, ABCs are usually hypointense and enhance with gadolinium. Angiography images may vary but usually show a rich vascular network of heterogeneous arterial channels, with occasional arteriovenous shunts and the late disappearance of contrast in the venous phase.[3]

Table 21.2 Djindjian's Angiographic Classification of Spinal Hemangiomas

Group A	Patients with extravertebral extension and signs of myelopathy showing dense, heterogeneous opacification of the affected vertebral body without arteriovenous shunting
Group B	Patients experiencing pain and found to have small lesions, with pooling of contrast material
Group C	Asymptomatic patients who did not have any pathologic opacification on angiography

These highly vascular lesions require treatment only for intractable pain. A percutaneous biopsy should not be performed, as it may result in an extradural hematoma. ABCs are hypothesized to be from impaired venous drainage, which may cause the characteristic bony expansion with pain due to venous blood under pressure.[5] Embolization and/or radiation may result in pain control by occluding the feeding arteries and decreasing intraosseous pressure. Preoperative embolization is often essential in managing intraoperative blood loss when surgical treatment is necessary.

Osteoid Osteoma/Osteoblastoma

Osteoid osteomas are benign primary bone tumors that are differentiated by size (osteoid osteomas <1 cm, osteoblastomas ≥1 cm). They account for 3% of primary bone tumors. These tumors characteristically cause nocturnal back pain that is relieved by aspirin and may be tender to palpation. Neurologic deficits are unusual, presenting in only 22% of osteoid osteomas and 28% of osteoblastomas.

Radiographic and CT imaging demonstrate a radiolucent density with adjacent scleroses, which have a predilection for the posterior elements. Osteoblastomas show more expansion and destruction. On MRI, these lesions are identified on T1 as hypointense lesions, with variable signal seen on T2 and contrast-enhanced images. Angiographically, these tumors are shown to have a hypervascular tumor blush without dilated feeding vessels or arteriovenous shunting. Osteoblastomas are, in general, more vascular than their smaller counterparts.

Osteoid osteomas have a high cure rate with complete excision, while osteoblastomas still have a 10% rate of recurrence and may rarely undergo sarcomatous change. Preoperative embolization is not usually necessary unless the lesion is unusually large.

Giant Cell Tumors

Giant cell tumors are aggressive vascular tumors that can cause significant morbidity, depending on their location and size, and may occasionally lead to death. They are usually found in the long bones, but approximately 4% occur in the sacrum. Patients typically present with radiculopathy from nerve root compression. The affected vertebral body usually displays an expanded, lytic lesion with paravertebral extension on plain radiographs.

T1 MRI usually demonstrates a heterogeneous hypointensity, with cystic areas often seen on T2. Djindjian et al. described the characteristic angiographic pattern of giant cell tumors as dilated arteries branching near the cortex with fine corkscrew vessels running in parallel, prominent arteriovenous shunting, and an absence of pooling blood.[3]

Unfortunately, large giant cell tumors of the spine present a significant challenge, especially given that despite accepted treatment methods, including surgical resection, chemotherapy, and radiation, all are associated with frequent morbid complications and high rates of recurrence. Serial arterial embolization may be a useful primary treatment modality for these tumors. Hosalkar et al. describe 9 patients with large sacral giant cell tumors who underwent repeat embolization every 6 weeks until no new vessels were noted; they found that there was no progression in 7 of the 9 cases at 9 years' follow-up; all patients demonstrated substantial pain relief.[6]

Metastases

Metastases are the most common bony tumor to affect the adult spine. Several types, most commonly renal cell and less often thyroid carcinoma, are highly vascular and benefit from preoperative embolization for safe resection (**Table 21.3**). Epidermoid epithelioma, epithelial carcinoma, and undifferentiated carcinomas may all produce similar angiographic appearances.[3] The clinical course is often marked by pain and rapid neurologic decline, due to bony collapse or extradural tumor extension.

Imaging depends on the type of tumor but in general shows bony destruction and bright enhancement. On angiography, the feeding arteries of vascular metastatic tumors are usually dilated, in contrast to normal vertebral bodies in which no distinct branches are seen. The pathologic blush may extend beyond bony confines and occurs early with vascular lakes. Venous drainage may show arteriovenous shunting, with early filling of the paravertebral plexus.

There are two indications for embolization of vascular spinal metastases: intractable pain and preoperative embolization, which may be performed with coils, particles, and liquid embolics. In matched cohorts, significant reductions in blood loss (1650 cc versus 3880 cc, p = 0.02) and transfusions (3.1 versus 5.8 units, p = 0.05) have been shown, as well as a trend toward reduced operative time.[7] Percutaneous vertebroplasty can also be used to stabilize and treat pain associated with vertebral body collapse, if the posterior elements remain intact.

Evidence-Based Medicine

Currently, no large clinical trials have been performed or are underway with regard to the endovascular management of vascular tumors. Supporting literature does exist, however, and was discussed in the previous tumor-specific sections. The reader is referred to those articles in the Recommended Reading and Reference sections of this chapter for further study.

Table 21.3 Metastatic Tumors of the Spine Thought Amenable to Preoperative Embolization

Renal cell carcinoma
Sarcoma
Neuroendocrine tumor
Thyroid carcinoma
Breast cancer
Liver cancer
Esophageal cancer
Germ cell tumor
Adenocarcinoma of unknown origin

Equipment

Embolization strategies for intracranial tumors are similar to the techniques used for aneurysms, that is, standard microcatheter and microwire techniques are utilized. Embolization of spinal tumors utilizes strategies similar to embolization of spinal vascular malformations. Given that these two technique are different, they will be detailed separately.

Intracranial and Skull Base Tumors

Sheath

A standard short sheath is used, and often a 5 or 6 Fr sheath may be used, depending on the desired guide catheter size. A longer sheath or shuttle sheath is rarely used but may be required in cases of tortuous anatomy.

Guide Catheter

A diagnostic angiogram is performed, using a 5 Fr standard diagnostic catheter.

Microcatheter and Microwire

A standard microcatheter, such as an Echelon or Prowler, is usually able to catheterize selectively the vessels of choice with the use of a standard microwire, such as a Synchro or Transcend. Occasionally, a smaller microcatheter (e.g., Ultraflow or Marathon) and microwire (e.g., Mirage) may be necessary if the vascular supply is very small, as in, for example, distal terminal branches of the external carotid artery. While PVA particle embolization of tumors can be done, it is recommended only if surgical resection is planned within several days. Otherwise, we prefer to achieve intratumoral penetration with a liquid embolic when possible. If Onyx embolization is planned, a DMSO-compatible microcatheter, such as a Marathon (0.013″) or Echelon (0.017″), must also be used.

Technique

Cerebral and cervical angiography are performed using standard biplane fluoroscopy. The level of sedation is dependent on the patient and the interventionist. It is preferred to be able to examine the patient during the embolization of the tumor, but that may be unnecessary due to the preoperative deficits. General anesthesia with neuromonitoring may be necessary for extended cases. Tumor embolization usually requires systemic heparinization to achieve an ACT of at least 200–250 seconds. However, tumor embolization can be painful, and adequate pain medication may not be accomplished with sedation. Therefore, general anesthesia should always be anticipated.

Prior to embolization, a hand-run, super-selective angiogram of the vessel of interest should be performed to confirm that the feeding artery supplies only the lesion and no neural tissue. If there is any question, provocative testing with hand injections of either brevital (10 to 20 mg) and/or lidocaine (10 to 20 mg as well, with similar technique) may be used if the patient is awake, followed by serial neurological examinations to determine the potential effect of embolization. A general principle is the smaller the particle size, the more distal the particles will travel, and thus the greater their potential for affecting vital areas. To minimize the risk of ischemia of vital areas and to facilitate intratumoral penetration, embolization should be performed as close to the lesion as possible. If PVA particles are to be used, occlusion of the feeding artery with the catheter is not recommended, as reflux could occur and, without flow to the tumor, no embolization would occur. Once the embolization is complete, a final angiogram should be performed to assess embolization and to confirm antegrade flow in normal arteries.

Spinal Tumors

Sheath

A short (24 cm) femoral sheath allows the sheath to remain within the iliac artery. This facilitates injection of the iliac arteries, the median sacral artery, and the L4/5 segmental vessels. A 5 or 6 Fr sheath may be used, depending on the desired guide catheter size.

Guide Catheter

A diagnostic angiogram is performed using a 5 Fr Cobra catheter. A Mickelson diagnostic catheter may also be used. The angle of the segmental vessels decreases from the horizontal plane as they descend from the thoracic to the lumbar spine. Therefore, in the lower spine and sacral arteries, switching to a Simmons 2 catheter may be helpful. If segmental injections are to be performed, this may be done through the 5 Fr Cobra catheter. If more distal embolization is desired, a 6 Fr Simmons should be used to allow for contrast injection through the guide catheter.

Glide Wire

A glide wire is not generally needed in spinal angiography; the catheter is puffed into the vessel origin with diluted contrast.

Microcatheter

Intramedullary Spinal Tumors
Distal selective catheterization of feeding arteries is preferable, usually with a 0.014" catheter navigated over a soft, torqueable wire, such as a Synchro, Transcend, or Mirage wire (0.008" diameter) with the Marathon catheter. We prefer to achieve intratumoral penetration with a liquid embolic when possible. If Onyx embolization is planned, a DMSO-compatible microcatheter, such as a Marathon (0.013") or Echelon (0.017"), must also be used.

Extradural Spinal Tumors
Tumors of the vertebrae are often embolized from the segmental vessels. A larger catheter and more robust micro guidewire may be used, but they should still be navigated as distally toward the lesion as possible. If the goal is preoperative devascularization, particle embolization, such as with PVA, may be effective, but embolization for pain control or palliation should be with a permanent liquid embolic agent. We

commonly use a 0.0165″ microcatheter with liquid embolic agents and a slightly larger (0.018″–0.023″) microcatheter for PVA particle injection (250–300 mm).

Microwire

A more robust wire, such as the 0.016″ Fathom (Stryker), may assist in cannulating these vessels. Alternatively, the microcatheter may be puffed into the segmental vessels using a 1 or 3 cc syringe with contrast, which is helpful when using a 5 Fr guide catheter.

Technique

Spinal angiography is performed using AP fluoroscopy, with a radiopaque ruler placed on the table to mark the spinal levels during the procedure. It is important to inject the segmental vessels two levels above and below the lesion to avoid missing feeding arteries. The artery of Adamkiewicz or feeding arteries with concomitant medullary supply must be recognized prior to embolization. The angiogram should be studied for the rapidity of flow to select the appropriate viscosity of the liquid embolic agent.

Tumor embolization usually requires systemic heparinization to achieve an ACT of at least 200–250 seconds. General anesthesia with neurophysiologic monitoring, such as somatosensory or motor-evoked potentials, is frequently found to be helpful. In cooperative patients requiring only proximal segmental vessel injections, conscious sedation is sufficient. However, spinal tumor embolization can be painful, and adequate pain medication may not be accomplished. Therefore, general anesthesia should always be anticipated.

Visualization of the arteries can be enhanced by suspending respiration during image acquisition and by the administration of glucagon to decrease gastrointestinal mobility. If the patients are awake, the injection should be timed so that the patients are holding their breath during the image acquisition.

Prior to embolization, a hand-run, super-selective angiogram of the vessel of interest should be performed to confirm that the feeding artery supplies only the lesion and no neural tissue. To minimize the risk of spinal cord ischemia and to facilitate intratumoral penetration, embolization should be performed as close to the lesion as possible. In addition, provocative testing can be useful if there is a possibility that neural function may be impaired by embolization. This can be done with brevital (10 to 20 mg, given through the microcatheter by hand injection) and/or lidocaine (10 to 20 mg as well with similar technique). Wedging the guide catheter in the segmental artery may be occlusive, which can improve forward flow of the liquid embolic. The exception to this is embolization with PVA, in which embolizing with the microcatheter "wedged" in the distal vessel can result in inadvertent embolization of normal spinal vasculature. During segmental artery injections, it is essential that liquid embolic reflux be kept at a minimum to prevent inadvertent embolization into the aorta. Should the embolic agent reach the guide catheter, that catheter should be discarded, because embolic material may be retained in its lumen. Once the embolization is complete, a final angiogram should be performed to assess embolization and to confirm antegrade flow in normal arteries.

Postprocedure Care

Postprocedural care in these cases is fairly standard postprocedural angiographic care. Regular neurological assessments must be performed, with particular attention to sensory and motor spinal examination. Any deterioration in neurological examination requires further evaluation with a head CT, in the case of intracranial or skull base tumors, or spinal MRI, in the cases of spinal tumors, to rule out spinal cord ischemia, hemorrhage, or tumor swelling. Steroids can reduce inflammation and swelling from embolization.

Technical Pearls and Pitfalls

1. Always hand-inject contrast before embolization to ensure minimal arterial feeding of vital areas.
2. Catheter occlusion of feeding arteries is not recommended when using particles, as this stops flow to the tumor and increases the incidence of reflux of particles into areas of vital tissue.
3. For adequate assessment of spinal cord lesions, the segmental arteries on both sides must be catheterized at least two levels above and below the level of the tumor.
4. For lesions in the cervical region, the vertebral arteries, external carotid arteries, thyrocervical and costocervical trunks, and the supreme intercostal arteries must be angiographed to look for feeding vessels.
5. For lesions of the vertebral body, the right intercostal artery will often supply the anterior vertebral body, while the left supplies the posterior vertebral body.[3]
6. In the lumbosacral area, both iliac arteries and median sacral artery must be injected to look for feeding arteries.
7. Onyx may create sparks when hit by Bovie cautery, which is often used in resection of spine tumors. This should be anticipated if aggressive intratumoral embolization is planned prior to surgery of an extraspinal tumor.

Recommended Reading

Berenstein A, Lasjuanias P, ter Brugge K. Tumors of the spinal column and spinal cord. In: *Surgical Neuroangiography*, vol. 2.2. New York: Springer; 2004:873–909

Choi IS, Tantivatana J. Neuroendovascular management of intracranial and spinal tumors. Neurosurg Clin N Am 2000;11(1):167–185

Cornelius JF, Saint-Maurice JP, Bresson D, George B, Houdart E. Hemorrhage after particle embolization of hemangioblastomas: comparison of outcomes in spinal and cerebellar lesions. J Neurosurg 2007;106(6):994–998

Rodesch G, Gaillard S, Loiseau H, Brotchi J. Embolization of intradural vascular spinal cord tumors: report of five cases and review of the literature. Neuroradiology 2008;50(2):145–151

References

1. Choi IS, Tantivatana J. Neuroendovascular management of intracranial and spinal tumors. Neurosurg Clin N Am 2000;11(1):167–185
2. Rodesch G, Gaillard S, Loiseau H, Brotchi J. Embolization of intradural vascular spinal cord tumors: report of five cases and review of the literature. Neuroradiology 2008; 50(2):145–151
3. Djindjian R, Merland J, Djindjian M, Soteter P. Angiography of spinal column and spinal cord tumors. In: *Neuroradiologic Atlas*. New York: Thieme; 1981
4. Acosta FL Jr, Sanai N, Chi JH, et al. Comprehensive management of symptomatic and aggressive vertebral hemangiomas. Neurosurg Clin N Am 2008;19(1):17–29
5. Berenstein A, Lasjuanias P, ter Brugge K. Tumors of the spinal column and spinal cord. In: *Surgical Neuroangiography*, vol. 2.2. New York: Springer; 2004:873–909
6. Hosalkar HS, Jones KJ, King JJ, Lackman RD. Serial arterial embolization for large sacral giant-cell tumors: mid- to long-term results. Spine (Phila PA 1976) 2007; 32(10):1107–1115
7. Wirbel RJ, Roth R, Schulte M, Kramann B, Mutschler W. Preoperative embolization in spinal and pelvic metastases. J Orthop Sci 2005;10(3):253–257

Appendix A

A1 Conversion Chart/Catheter Sizes

Catheter Sizing Chart								
1 mm = 0.039 in. 1 Fr = 0.333 mm 3 F = 1.0 mm								
●	●	●	●	●	●	●	●	.
French	9	8	7	6	5	4	3	2	1
Gauge	11	12	13	14	16	18	20	22	24
mm	3.0	2.7	2.3	2.0	1.7	1.3	1.0	0.67	0.33
inch	0.118	0.105	0.091	0.078	0.065	0.052	0.039	0.026	0.013

Conversion chart/catheter sizes.

A2 Vascular Anatomy (See Chapters 1–2)

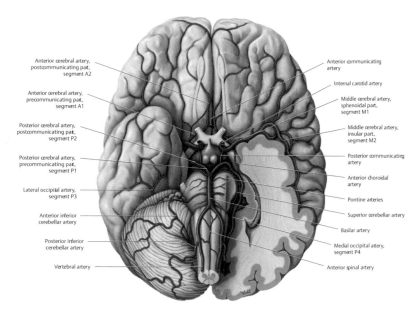

Arteries at the base of the brain. (From THIEME Atlas of Anatomy, Head and Neuro-anatomy, © Thieme 2007, Illustration by Markus Voll.)

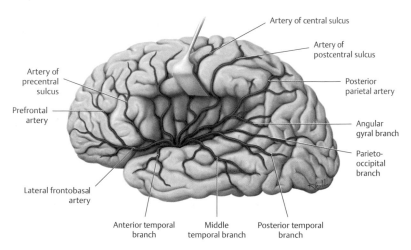

Course of the middle cerebral artery in the interior of the lateral sulcus. Left lateral view. (From THIEME Atlas of Anatomy, Head and Neuroanatomy, © Thieme 2007, Illustration by Markus Voll.)

A2 Vascular Anatomy

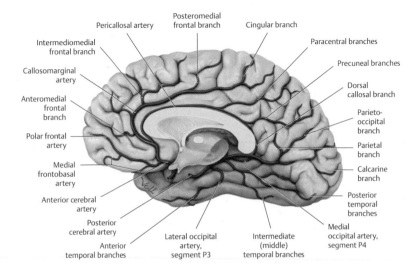

Branches of the anterior and posterior cerebral arteries on the medial surface of the cerebrum. Right cerebral hemisphere viewed from the medial side, with the left cerebral hemisphere and brainstem removed. (From THIEME Atlas of Anatomy, Head and Neuroanatomy, © Thieme 2007, Illustration by Markus Voll.)

A2 Vascular Anatomy

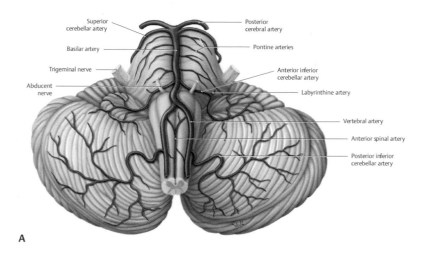

A

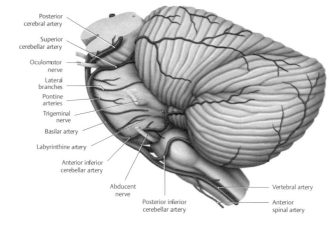

B

Arteries of the brainstem and cerebellum. **(A)** Basal view. **(B)** Lateral view. (From THIEME Atlas of Anatomy, Head and Neuroanatomy, © Thieme 2007, Illustration by Markus Voll.)

A2 Vascular Anatomy

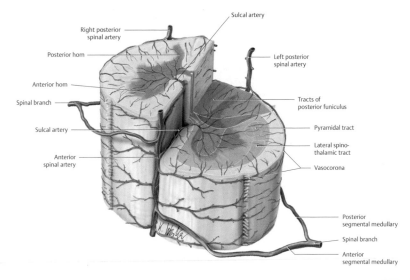

Blood supply to the spinal cord segments. (From THIEME Atlas of Anatomy, Head and Neuroanatomy, © Thieme 2007, Illustration by Karl Wesker.)

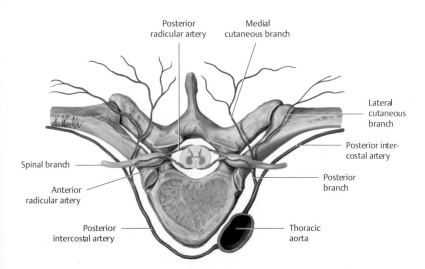

Blood vessels supplying the spinal cord. Thoracic vertebra viewed from above. (From THIEME Atlas of Anatomy, Head and Neuroanatomy, © Thieme 2007, Illustration by Karl Wesker.)

A2 Vascular Anatomy

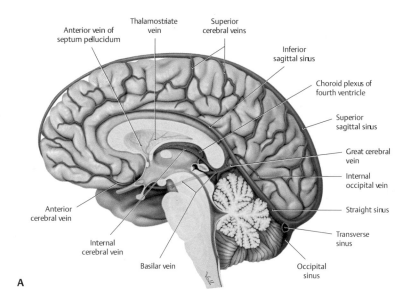

A

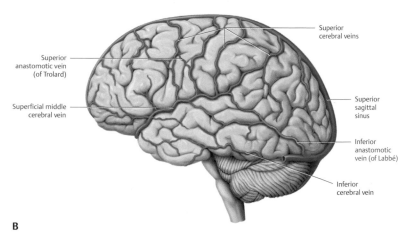

B

Superficial veins of the brain. **(A)** Left lateral view, **(B)** medial view. (From THIEME Atlas of Anatomy, Head and Neuroanatomy, © Thieme 2007, Illustration by Markus Voll.)

A2 Vascular Anatomy

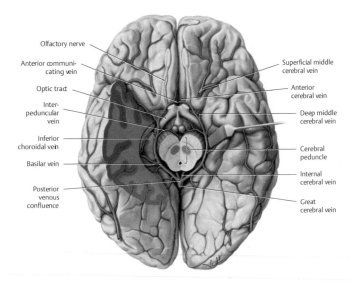

Basal cerebral venous system. (From THIEME Atlas of Anatomy, Head and Neuroanatomy, © Thieme 2007, Illustration by Markus Voll.)

A2 Vascular Anatomy

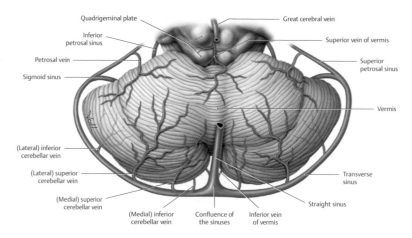

Cerebellar veins, posterior view. (From THIEME Atlas of Anatomy, Head and Neuroanatomy, © Thieme 2007, Illustration by Markus Voll.)

A2 Vascular Anatomy

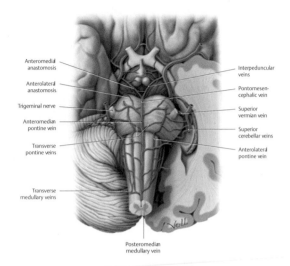

Anteromedial anastomosis
Anterolateral anastomosis
Trigeminal nerve
Anteromedian pontine vein
Transverse pontine veins
Transverse medullary veins

Interpeduncular veins
Pontomesencephalic vein
Superior vermian vein
Superior cerebellar veins
Anterolateral pontine vein

Posteromedian medullary vein

A

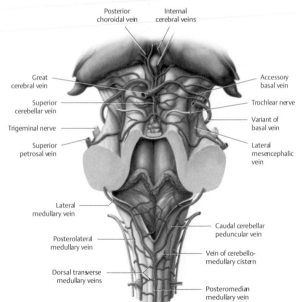

Posterior choroidal vein
Internal cerebral veins

Great cerebral vein
Superior cerebellar vein
Trigeminal nerve
Superior petrosal vein

Accessory basal vein
Trochlear nerve
Variant of basal vein
Lateral mesencephalic vein

Lateral medullary vein
Posterolateral medullary vein
Dorsal transverse medullary veins

Caudal cerebellar peduncular vein
Vein of cerebello-medullary cistern
Posteromedian medullary vein

B

Veins of the brainstem: **(A)** anterior view of the brainstem in situ (the cerebellum and part of the occipital lobe have been removed on the left side) **(B)** posterior view of the isolated brainstem, with the cerebellum removed. (From THIEME Atlas of Anatomy, Head and Neuroanatomy, © Thieme 2007, Illustrations by Markus Voll.)

A3 Angiographic Projections

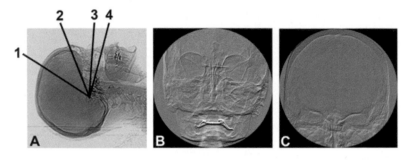

(A) Common angiographic projections (AP): (1) Towne's, (2) carotid angle, (3) transfacial, and (4) transorbital oblique or Stenver's. **(B)** Typical AP view of skull in transfacial projection. **(C)** Typical AP view of skull in carotid angle projection.

Angiographic Projections

Name of projection	Comments
Towne's	The inferior ridge of the petrous bone should be superior to the orbital rim. Maximizes SCA and PCA views, but significantly foreshortens the BA.
Carotid Angle	The superior orbital rim overlies the petrous ridge. Brings carotid terminus, A1, and M1 above the petrous ridge. Also provides good general view of the posterior circulation.
Transfacial	The inferior orbital rim overlies the petrous ridge. Provides good view of the BA and apex. Foreshortens the PCAs, SCAs, and PComAs. Carotid terminus lies within the orbit.
Transorbital Oblique	Centered over the orbit, the optic canal lies in the inferior lateral quadrant of the orbit. Great for visualization of the AComA. Contralateral compression of carotid artery may be necessary.
Stenver's	Centered over the mandibular condyle, the optic canal lies in the inferior lateral quadrant of the orbit. Good visualization of the vertebrobasilar circulation, including PICA.
Haughton's	Using a 45 degree view of the sagital view, this view allows opening up of the carotid siphon and good views of the origins of the PComA and AChorA as well as the MCA candelabra.

A4 Endovascular Medications

Pre-Sedation Checklist

1. Peripheral access lines

   a. Preferably two large-bore access lines, in case rapid fluid resuscitation or drug infusion is necessary.

2. Arterial lines

   a. A direct arterial line is preferred for endovascular interventions rather than transducing through an arterial sheath, due to dampening of the blood pressure readings and the inability to transduce blood pressures once the sheath is removed at the conclusion of the procedure. Accurate blood pressure monitoring is essential in allowing rapid treatment of abrupt periprocedural blood pressure fluctuations.

3. Foley catheter

   a. Preferable in all patients whenever the procedure is likely to be prolonged or the patient will receive high volumes of intravenous fluids.

   b. All patients undergoing intracranial procedures, such as aneurysm coil embolization, AVM embolization, and tumor embolization.

4. Mallampati Score and ASA

5. Co-morbidities:

   a. Diabetes mellitus

   b. Hypertension

   c. Illicit drug ingestion

   d. Pregnancy

   e. Baseline neurological and physical examination

   f. Baseline recent laboratory work, including glucose levels, CBC, basic metabolic profile

   g. Time of last food/liquid intake

   h. Medications: dose and last time taken

   i. Room logistics

      i. Availability of crash cart

      ii. Medication check list, including availability of reversal agents and ease of drug access

      iii. Intubation material check list, including tube extension and status of gas outlets

      iv. Proximity of the anesthesia equipment

   j. Positioning of patient in relation to EVD, lines, etc.

   k. Procedure type and anesthesia considerations, time-out to determine correct patient and procedure

   l. Potential complications and backup mechanisms

   m. Placing the pulse oximetry monitor on the same foot where the arterial sheath will be introduced would provide an early sign of femoral artery obstruction or flow compromise.

   n. Are all lines well secured?

A4 Endovascular Medications

Antiplatelet Agents

Drug	Mechanism of action	Half-life (main compound)	Metabolism	Dosage		Onset of action	Duration of action	Side effects	Contra-indications	Reversal of action	Monitoring	Interruption prior to procedures
Aspirin (Bayer Aspirin, Ecotrin)	Blocks thromboxane A2 (cyclo-oxigenase inhibitor), maximum effect with 160 mg of daily aspirin (range 50–320 mg daily), larger doses don't increase efficacy	20 minutes (plasma) Plasma peak level 30 minutes	Liver	Loading dose	325 mg PO/per rectum	20–30 minutes	4–6 hours	Gastric irritation, nausea, abdominal irritation, ringing in ears	Active gastrointestinal bleeding, hypersensitivity to aspirin, and patients younger than 13 years old.	Drug interruption and platelet transfusion	N/A	N/A
				Maintenance	325 mg PO daily							
Clopi-dogrel (Plavix)	Blocks platelet ADP-binding site. Inhibits ADP-mediated activation of GP IIb/IIIa complex	8 hours for the main compound. 2% of platelets are covalently bound to clopidogrel by day 11		Loading dose	300–600 mg PO/per rectum	2 hours. Steady state platelet inhibition 3–7 days after utilization	5–11 days once steady state reached (40–60% platelet function inhibition)	Bleeding, allergic reactions, ecchymoses	Acute bleeding, hypersensitivity to the drug			5–7 days
				Maintenance	75–150 mg PO daily							

| Ticlopidine (Ticlid) | Persistently inhibits ADP-mediated paltelet-fibrinogen binding and subsequent platelet-platelet interactions | 2 hours to 5 days (elderly patients) | Liver | Mainte-nance | 250 mg PO BID | 2 hours. Steady state within 5 days | 14–21 days (platelet inhibition rises to 60–70%) | GI bleeding, diarrhea, rash, nausea, and severe neutropenia, agranulocytosis (FDA Boxed warnings), leukemia, pancytopenia, and thrombocytosis | GI bleeding, liver and kidney failure | Methylprednisolone 20 mg IV (prolonged bleeding time normalized after 2 hours) | CBC prior to starting treatment and every 2 weeks for 3 months | 10–14 days |

A4 Endovascular Medications

Thrombolytic Agents

Drug	Mechanism of action	Half-life (main compound)	Metabolism	Dosage			Onset of action	Duration of action	Side effects	Contra-indications	Reversal of action	Monitoring	Interruption prior to procedures
Alteplase	Binds to fibrin in a thrombus and converts entrapped plasminogen to plasmin. This will initiate fibrinolysis with limited systemic proteolysis.	Less than 5 minutes	Liver	Acute stroke (NINDS trial)	Bolus	0.1 mg/kg	5–10 minutes (80% of alteplase unbound after 10 minutes)	1 hour	Bleeding, allergic reactions, ecchymoses	Active internal bleeding, history of stroke, recent intracranial or intraspinal surgery (3 months), intracranial neoplasms, severe uncontrolled hypertension	Stop medication immediately and transfuse fresh frozen plasma + packed red cells or whole blood.	N/A	N/A
					Infusion	0.8 mg/kg over 1 hour							
				Acute stroke (IMS trial)	Bolus	0.1 mg/kg							
					Infusion	0.6 mg/kg IV, 0.3 mg/kg IA							
				Intervention		6–22 mg at clot level							

A4 Endovascular Medications

Anticoagulant Agents

Drug	Mechanism of action	Half-life (main compound)	Metabolism	Dosage		Onset of action	Duration of action	Side effects	Contra-indications	Reversal of action	Monitoring	Interruption prior to procedures
Heparin	Inactivation of factor X, inhibiting conversion of prothrombin to thrombin. After thrombosis development, larger amounts of heparin prevent conversion of fibrinogen to fibrin.	90 minutes	Liver	Intraprocedural	50–100 units/kg bolus at positioning of guide-catheter, followed by 1,000 units every hour till the end of procedure, to achieve ACTs between 200–300. Higher doses generally considered for higher-risk procedures.	Immediate after IV injection, delayed after SC injections	2–4 hours	Thrombocytopenia	Hemophilia, recent surgery, clotting disorders	Protamine sulfate 10 mg for every 1,000 units of heparin given. However, dose should be calculated based upon the time of last heparin infusion. Between 30–60 minutes of infusion, half a dose of protamine should be sufficient to reverse heparin effects.	N/A	N/A
				Maintenance	12–18 units per kilogram to achieve PTT between 70 and 90							

A4 Endovascular Medications

IIb/IIIa Inhibitor Agents

Drug	Mechanism of action	Half-life (main compound)	Metabolism	Dosage		Onset of Action	Duration of action	Side effects	Contra-indications	Reversal of action	Monitoring	Interruption prior to procedures
Eptifi-batide (Integril-lin)	Reversibly in-hibits platelet aggregation and prevents fibrinogen, von Wil-lebrand factor, and other adhesive ligand binding to GP IIb/IIIa. Dissociation between ep-tifibatide and platelet results in cessation of effects.	2.5 hours	Liver	Loading dose	180 mcg/kg bolus for normal creatinine clearance if ClCr <50 ml/min, give 180 mcg/kg prior to the procedure, followed by a second bolus of 180 mcg/kg 10 minutes after the first.	15 minutes after bolus, there is 84% of platelet inhibition utilizing the standard doses	4–6 hours (elimination half-life 2.5 hours)	Hemorrhage, allergic reactions, ecchymoses, intracranial hemorrhages	History of bleeding diathesis, hypertension, major surgery within the past 6 weeks, history of stroke within the past 30 days, patients on renal dialysis, known hypersensitivity to the product	Drug interruption and platelet transfusion	N/A	N/A
				Maintenance	2 mcg/kg/min for normal ClCr: 1 mcg/kg/min for ClCr <50 ml/min.							

Abciximab (Reopro)	Binds to IIb/IIIa platelet receptors and inhibits platelet aggregation	Several minutes to 30 minutes	Liver	Intravenous Intraarterial	0.25 mg/kg bolus, followed by 0.125 mcg/kg/minute infusion Range 2–30 mg intraprocedural for thromboembolic complications	10 minutes	After IV infusion, effects decrease substantially after 10 minutes; platelet function generally recovers within 48 hours of administration, although the drug may remain in the circulation for up to 15 days.	Bleeding (10–25%), thrombocytopenia, allergic reactions, hypotension, bradycardia, anxiety, vertigo	Active internal bleeding, recent (within 6 weeks) GI or GU bleeding, bleeding diathesis, oral anticoagulants within seven days, thrombocytopenia, recent surgery or trauma, intracranial neoplasm, uncontrolled hypertension, h/o vasculitis	N/A	N/A	N/A	N/A
Tirofiban (Aggrastat)	Reversible inhibition of GP IIb/IIIa receptor in a dose-dependent manner. Over 90% platelet inhibition obtained in a concentration-dependent manner	2 hours	Limited, urinary excretion	Intravenous (not FDA approved for stroke management)	0.4 mcg/kg/min for 30 minutes then continued infusion to 0.1 mcg/kg/min. Renal patients should receive half the dose	Immediate	4–8 hours after drug is interrupted	Hemorrhage, which may be severe, requiring massive platelet transfusions.	Known hypersensitivity to any component of the product, active internal bleeding, intracranial hemorrhage, intracranial neoplasms, aneurysm, major surgical procedures, aortic dissection, severe hypertension, another concomitant IIb/IIIa inhibitor.	Platelet transfusion and drug interruption	N/A

A4 Endovascular Medications

Contrast Agents

Drug	Class	Trade name	Iodine content	Osmolality	Relative osmolality	Comfort during angiography
Sodium and/or methylglucamine diatrizoate	High osmolality -ionic	Hypaque	141	633	High osmolar	→
			282	1415		
			370	2016		
Iopamidol	Non-ionic monomer	Isovue 370	370	796	Low osmolar	↑
Iohexol	Non-ionic	Omnipaque 350	350	884	Low osmolar	↑
Iodixanol	Non-ionic dimer	Visipaque 320	320	290	Iso-osmolar	↑↑

A5 Endovascular Equipment (See Chapter 7)

Traditional and Intermediate Guide Catheters

Name	Outer diameter	Inner diameter	Length (cm)	Special features
Envoy	5.0 Fr/6.0 Fr	5.3 Fr (0.070")	90, 100	Multiple shapes, more stiff.
DAC 038	3.9 Fr (0.050")	2.9 Fr (0.038")	125, 136	Smallest intermediate guide catheter.
DAC 044	4.3 Fr (0.056")	3.3 Fr (0.044")	115, 130, 136	Compatible with Merci microcatheters.
DAC 057	5.2 Fr (0.068")	4.3 Fr (0.057")	115, 125	Long working length available.
Neuron 6 F 070	6.0 Fr/6.0 Fr	(0.070")	95, 105	Straight or angled tip available.
Neuron 6 F 053	6.0 Fr/5.0 Fr	(0.053")	105, 115	Straight or angled tip available. Distal flexible zone choice on each catheter 6 cm or 12 cm.

Flow-Guided Microcatheters

Catheter	Prox. OD	OD at tip	Length (cm)	Wire diameter	DMSO compatible?	Tip properties
Magic (Balt)	2.7 Fr	1.2 Fr*	165 or 180	.008	No	non-braided
Baltacci (Balt)	2.7 Fr	1.2 Fr*	165 or 180	.008	Yes	non-braided
Sonic (Balt)	2.7 Fr	1.2 Fr	165 or 180	.008	Yes	braided with non-braided detachable tip
Ultraflow (ev3)	3.0 Fr	1.5 Fr	165	.010	Yes	non-braided
Marathon (ev3)	3.0 Fr	1.3 Fr	165	.010	No	nitinol braid

*Olive tip available

A5 Endovascular Equipment

Medium-Length Microcatheters

Catheter	Company	ID	Prox OD	Dist OD	Length	Min. guide ID	Max wire	Construction	Shapes
Rebar 10	ev3	0.015"	2.3 Fr	1.7 Fr	153 cm	0.035"	0.012"	stainless steel coil	0
Prowler 10	Cordis	0.015"	2.3 Fr	1.7 Fr	150/170 cm	0.035"	0.012"	stainless steel braid, distal platinum coil	0,45,90,J
Prowler 14	Cordis	0.0165"	2.3 Fr	1.9 Fr	150/170 cm	0.035"	0.014"	stainless steel braid, distal platinum coil	0,45,90,J
Prowler Select	Cordis	0.0165"	2.3 Fr	1.9 Fr	150 cm	0.035"	0.014"	stainless steel braid, distal platinum coil	0,45,90,J
Excelsior SL-10	Boston Sci	0.0165"	2.4 Fr	1.7 Fr	150 cm	0.038"	0.014"	stainless steel braid, distal coil	0,45,90,J,S,C
Tracker Excel-14	Boston Sci	0.017"	2.4 Fr	1.9 Fr	150 cm	0.038"	0.014"	stainless steel braid	0
Echelon 10	ev3	0.017"	2.1 Fr	1.7 Fr	150 cm	0.035"	0.014"	nitinol braid	0,45,90
Echelon 14	ev3	0.017"	2.4 Fr	1.9 Fr	150 cm	0.050"	0.014"	nitinol braid	0,45,90
Rebar 14	ev3	0.017"	2.4 Fr	1.9 Fr	153 cm	0.035"	0.014"	stainless steel coil	0
Courier 170	Micrus	0.017"	2.3 Fr	1.8 Fr	150 cm	0.035"	0.014"	stainless steel braid	0,45,90
Concourse 14	Micrus	0.0165"	2.3 Fr	1.9 Fr	150 cm	0.035"	0.014"	stainless steel braid	0

A5 Endovascular Equipment

Large Microcatheters

Catheter	Company	ID	Prox OD	Dist OD	Length	Min. guide ID	Max wire	Construction	Shapes
Courier 190	Micrus	0.019"	2.4 Fr	1.9 Fr	150 cm	0.042"	0.014"	stainless steel braid	0,45,90
Excelsior 1018	Boston Sci	0.019"	2.6 Fr	2.0 Fr	150 cm	0.038"	0.016"	stainless steel braid with distal coil reinforcement	0,45,90,J,S,C
Nautica 14XL	ev3	0.018"	2.8 Fr	2.2 Fr	150 cm	0.050"	0.016"	nitinol braid	0
Prowler Plus	Cordis	0.021"	2.8 Fr	2.3 Fr	135, 150 cm	0.042"	0.018"	stainless steel braid and distal platinum coil	0,45,90,J
Prowler Select Plus	Cordis	0.021"	2.8 Fr	2.3 Fr	150, 170 cm	0.042"	0.018"	stainless steel braid and distal platinum coil	0,45,90,J
Rapid Transit	Cordis	0.021"	2.8 Fr	2.3 Fr	150, 170 cm	0.042"	0.018"	stainless steel braid with distal platinum coil	0
Rebar-18	ev3	0.021"	2.8 Fr	2.3 Fr	130, 153 cm	0.035"	0.018"	stainless steel coil	0
Renegade 18	Boston Sci	0.021"	3.0 Fr	2.5 Fr	150 cm	0.042"	0.018"	fiber braid	0

A5 Endovascular Equipment

Standard Microwires (0.014" to 0.016")

Wire	Vendor	Diameter	Length (cm)	Material	Options
Glidewire Gold 0.016	MV	0.016"	180	nitinol/tungsten	45/70 pre-shaped
Headliner 0.016	MV	0.016"	200	nitinol/tungsten	floppy,0,45,90,90/60/J
Traxcess	MV	0.014"	200	nitinol/SS	EX (Stiff)
Synchro-14	BS	0.014"	200/300	nitinol HT/SS	none
Synchro²	BS	0.014"	200	nitinol HT/SS	soft, pre-shaped
Synchro² 300	BS	0.014"	300	nitinol HT/SS	soft, pre-shaped
Transend EX	BS	0.014"	182	scitanium	soft, floppy, plat
Transend 300	BS	0.014"	300	scitanium	ES, floppy
Glidewire Gold 0.014	Ter	0.014"	180	nitinol/tungsten	45/70 pre-shaped
Agility	Cor	0.014"	205/350	SS/plat/tungsten	soft
Silverspeed 14	EV3	0.014"	175/200	SS/plat	none
X-Pedion 14	EV3	0.014"	175/200	SS/plat	none
X-Celerator	EV3	0.014"	300	SS/plat	none
Watusi	Mic	0.014"	205	SS/plat	none
Steel	Balt	0.014"	200	SS	
Sorcerer	Balt	0.014"	200	nitinol	n/a

Abbreviations: BS, Boston Scientific; MV, Microvention; Cor, Cordis; Mic, Micrus; SS, stainless steel; HT, hypotube; plat, platinum; ES, extra support.

A5 Endovascular Equipment
Small Microwires (0.007" to 0.012")

Wires	Vendor	Diameter	Length (cm)	Material	Options
Headliner 0.012	MV	0.012"	200	nitinol/tungsten	0,45,90,90/60
Sorcerer	Balt	0.012"	200	nitinol	n/a
Steel	Balt	0.012"	200	SS	n/a
Glidewire 0.011	MV	0.011"	180	nitinol/tungsten	0,45,70
Syncho 10	BS	0.010"	200/300	nitinol HT/SS	n/a
Transend 0.010	BS	0.010"	205	scitanium	n/a
Agility 10	Cor	0.010"	195	SS/plat/tungsten	Soft
Silverspeed 10	ev3	0.010"	200	SS/plat	n/a
X-Pedion 10	ev3	0.010"	200	SS/plat	n/a
X-Celerator 10	ev3	0.010"	300	SS/plat	n/a
Sorcerer	Balt	0.009"	200	nitinol	n/a
Steel	Balt	0.009"	200	SS	n/a
Mirage 0.008	ev3	0.008"	200	SS/plat	n/a
Steel	Balt	0.008"	200	SS	n/a
Steel	Balt	0.007"	200	SS	n/a
Sorcerer	Balt	0.007"	200	nitinol	n/a

Abbreviations: BS, Boston Scientific; MV, Microvention; Cor, Cordis; Mic, Micrus; SS, stainless steel; HT, hypotube; plat, platinum; ES, extra support.

A5 Endovascular Equipment
Comparison of Commonly Used Carotid Stents

Stent	Vendor	Cell design	Sheath req.	Material	Protection device	Special features
Protégé Rx	ev3	Open	6.0 Fr	nitinol	Spyder	No foreshortening. Can cross lesion with wire of choice in combination with Spyder EPD.
Precise	Cordis	Open	5.5/6.0 Fr	nitinol	Angioguard	Up to 0.018" guide ok
Precise Pro RX	Cordis	Open	5.0/6.0 Fr	nitinol	Angioguard	High radial stiffness
Acculink	Abbott	Open	6.0 Fr	nitinol	Accunet	Highest cell area
Xact	Abbott	Closed	5.7 Fr	nitinol	EmboShield	Can cross lesion with wire of choice in combination with EmboShield EPD.
Nexstent	Boston Sci	Closed	5.0 Fr	nitinol	Filterwire EZ	Self-sizing
Wallstent	Boston Sci	Closed	5.0/6.0 Fr	Elgiloy	Filterwire EZ	Reconstrainable if less than 90% deployed
Cristallo	Invatec	Both	5.0 Fr	nitinol	Fibernet	Dual cell design

A5 Endovascular Equipment

Most Commonly Used Endovascular Coils in the US Market (Not All Internationally Available Coils Listed)

OD primary coil (in)	Delivery wire	Company	Specific coils	Available lengths (cm)	Available diameters (mm)	Length	Detachment mechanism
0.012	0.012	Codman/Cordis	TRUFILL DCS Orbit Complex Fill TDL	7–30	4–12	175	Hydraulic
0.012	0.012	Codman/Cordis	TRUFILL DCS Orbit Complex Std TDL	15–30	6–20	175	Hydraulic
0.012	0.012	Codman/Cordis	TRUFILL DCS Orbit Helical Fill	2–30	2–12	175	Hydraulic
0.012	0.012	Codman/Cordis	TRUFILL DCS Orbit Complex Std	15–30	6–20	175	Hydraulic
0.012	0.012	Codman/Cordis	TRUFILL DCS Orbit Mini Complex Fill	1.5–10	2–4	175	Hydraulic
0.012	0.012	Codman/Cordis	TRUFILL DCS Orbit Mini Complex Fill TDL	7–10	4	175	Hydraulic
0.012	0.012	Codman/Cordis	Galaxy XTRASOFT Complex	1.5–10	2–4	175	Hydraulic
0.012	0.012	Codman/Cordis	Galaxy XTRASOFT Helical	1.5–10	2–4	175	Hydraulic
0.014	0.014	Codman/Cordis	Galaxy Frame Coil	20–30	6–20	175	Hydraulic
0.012	0.012	Codman/Cordis	Galaxy Fill Coil	1.5–30	2–12	175	Hydraulic
0.0145	0.014	ev3	Axium SR >11	30–50	12–20	180	Mechanical
0.0125	0.013	ev3	Axium SR 4–6	8–20	4–6	180	Mechanical
0.0135	0.013	ev3	Axium SR 7–10	30	7–10	180	Mechanical
0.0115	0.012	ev3	Axium SR	1–8	1.5–4	180	Mechanical
0.0115	0.012	ev3	Nexus Tetris 3D CSR Small	4–15	3–7	180	Mechanical
0.0125	0.013	ev3	Nexus Tetris 3D CSR Medium	16–20	8–10	180	Mechanical
0.0145	0.014	ev3	Nexus Tetris 3D CSR Large	23–29	12–18	180	Mechanical

(Continued on page 424)

A5 Endovascular Equipment

(Continued) Most Commonly Used Endovascular Coils in the US Market (Not All Internationally Available Coils Listed)

OD primary coil (in)	Delivery wire	Company	Specific coils	Available lengths (cm)	Available diameters (mm)	Length	Detachment mechanism
0.0115–0.0135	0.01–0.013	ev3	Nexus Multidiameter CSR	10–30	4–10	180	Mechanical
0.0115–0.0135	0.01–0.13	ev3	Nexus Helix Supersoft CSR	1–30	2–10	180	Mechanical
0.0145	0.014	ev3	Axium 3D SR >11	40–50	12–25	180	Mechanical
0.0125	0.013	ev3	Axium 3D SR 4–6	8–20	4–6	180	Mechanical
0.0135	0.013	ev3	Axium 3D SR 7–10	20–30	7–10	180	Mechanical
0.0115	0.012	ev3	Axium 3D SR	2–8	2–4	180	Mechanical
0.0115	0.012	ev3	Axium MicroFX 3D PGLA 2–3	2–8	2–3	180	Mechanical
0.0125	0.013	ev3	Axium MicroFX 3D PGLA 4–6	8–20	4–6	180	Mechanical
0.0145	0.014	ev3	Axium MicroFX 3D PGLA 7–10	20–30	7–10	180	Mechanical
0.0125	0.013	ev3	Axium MicroFX Helix PGLA SR 7–10	30	7–10	180	Mechanical
0.0135	0.013	ev3	Axium MicroFX Helix PGLA SR 4–6	8–20	4–6	180	Mechanical
0.0115	0.012	ev3	Axium MicroFX Helix PGLA SR 2–3	1–8	2–3	180	Mechanical
0.0125	0.013	ev3	Axium MicroFX Helix Nylon SR 4	8–10	4	180	Mechanical
0.0115	0.012	ev3	Axium MicroFX Helix Nylon SR 2–3	1–8	2–3	180	Mechanical
.01–0.012	0.0145	Microvention	Microplex - Cosmos 10-SR	6–31	3–7	175	Electrothermal
0.0145–0.015	0.0145	Microvention	Microplex - Cosmos 18	23–68	7–24	175	Electrothermal
0.0095–0.01	0.0145	Microvention	Microplex - 10 Complex 3D	4–26	2–10	175	Electrothermal

OD primary coil (in)	Delivery wire	Company	Specific coils	Available lengths (cm)	Available diameters (mm)	Length	Detachment mechanism
0.0135–0.015	0.0145	Microvention	Microplex - 18 Complex 3D	10–50	4–20	175	Electrothermal
0.0095–0.01	0.0145	Microvention	Microplex - 10 Complex Compass	3–30	2–10	175	Electrothermal
0.0135–0.015	0.0145	Microvention	Microplex - 18 Complex Compass	9–60	4–20	175	Electrothermal
0.010–0.011	0.0145	Microvention	Microplex - 10 Hypersoft	1–8	1.5–6	175	Electrothermal
0.0095	0.0145	Microvention	Microplex - 10 Helical SR Soft	2–10	2–4	175	Electrothermal
0.01	0.0145	Microvention	Microplex - 10 Helical SR Regular	15–30	5–10	175	Electrothermal
0.0135	0.0145	Microvention	Microplex - 18 Helical Soft	4–15	2–6	175	Electrothermal
0.014	0.0145	Microvention	Microplex - 18 Helical Regular	20–30	5–20	175	Electrothermal
0.013 (0.022)	0.0145	Microvention	Hydrocoil 10 Helical Regular	2–10	2–6	175	Electrothermal
0.014 (0.027)	0.0145	Microvention	Hydrocoil 14 Helical Regular	3–20	2–10	175	Electrothermal
0.018 (0.034)	0.0145	Microvention	Hydrocoil 18 Helical Regular	10–20	6–20	175	Electrothermal
0.012–0.0125	0.0145	Microvention	Hydroframe 10 Framing Coil	6–36	3–10	175	Electrothermal
0.014–0.015	0.0145	Microvention	Hydroframe 18 Framing Coil	19–48	6–20	175	Electrothermal
0.013	0.0145	Microvention	Hydrosoft Helical Coil	1–8	2–6	175	Electrothermal
0.01–0.011	0.0145	Microvention	HyperSoft 10	1–8	2–6	175	Electrothermal
0.0135	0.014	Micrus	Cashmere-14	2.5–30	2–12	190	Electrothermal
0.01	0.01	Micrus	DeltaPlush-10 (Cerecyte)	1–8	1.5–4	190	Electrothermal
0.01	0.01	Micrus	DeltaPlush SR-10	1–8	1.5–4	190	Electrothermal
0.01	0.01	Micrus	Micrusphere 10 (Cerecyte)	2.5–20.3	2–10	190	Electrothermal

(Continued on page 426)

A5 Endovascular Equipment

(Continued) Most Commonly Used Endovascular Coils in the US Market (Not All Internationally Available Coils Listed)

OD primary coil (in)	Delivery wire	Company	Specific coils	Available lengths (cm)	Available diameters (mm)	Length	Detachment mechanism
0.015	0.01	Micrus	Micrusphere 18 (Cerecyte)	2.7–30	2–18	190	Electrothermal
0.01	0.01	Micrus	Micrusphere 10	2.5–30	2–10	190	Electrothermal
0.015	0.01	Micrus	Micrusphere 18	2.7–30	2–18	190	Electrothermal
0.01	0.01	Micrus	UltiPaq-10	1–8	2–4	190	Electrothermal
0.01	0.01	Micrus	UltiPaq-10 (Cerecyte)	1–8	2–4	190	Electrothermal
0.0105	0.012	Micrus	Presidio-10 (Cerecyte)	11.5–29	4–8	190	Electrothermal
0.015	0.012	Micrus	Presidio-18 (Cerecyte)	30–50	8–20	190	Electrothermal
0.0105	0.012	Micrus	DeltaPaq (Cerecyte)	2–25	1.5–10	190	Electrothermal
0.0105	0.012	Micrus	DeltaPaq SR	2–25	1.5–10	190	Electrothermal
0.01	0.012	Micrus	HeliPaq 10 (Cerecyte)	1–30	2–10	190	Electrothermal
0.01	0.012	Micrus	Helipaq SR 10	1–30	2–10	190	Electrothermal
0.014	0.012	Micrus	HeliPaq SR 18 (Cerecyte)	4–30	2–20	190	Electrothermal
0.01	0.012	Micrus	InterPaq 10	10–30	4–6	190	Electrothermal
0.014	0.015	Micrus	HeliPaq 18	4–30	2–20	190	Electrothermal
0.02	0.02	Penumbra	Penumbra Complex Standard	1–60	2–24	175	Mechanical
0.02	0.02	Penumbra	Penumbra Complex Soft	1–60	2–24	175	Mechanical
0.02	0.02	Penumbra	Penumbra J Soft	1–60	2–24	175	Mechanical

OD primary coil (in)	Delivery wire	Company	Specific coils	Available lengths (cm)	Available diameters (mm)	Length	Detachment mechanism
0.02	0.02	Penumbra	Penumbra Curve Extra Soft	1–60	2–24	175	Mechanical
0.01–0.012	0.01	Stryker	Target 360 Standard (SFL)	6–40	3–15	185	Electrolytic
.0095–.010	0.01	Stryker	Target 360 Soft (SFL)	4–30	2–14	185	Electrolytic
0.01	0.01	Stryker	Target 360 Ultra (SFL)	3–10	2–5	185	Electrolytic
0.01	0.01	Stryker	Target Helical Ultra	1–8	2–4	185	Electrolytic
0.015	0.01	Stryker	GDC-18 360 (SFL)	15–40	6–24	185	Electrolytic
0.01–0.012	0.01	Stryker	GDC-10 360 SR (SFL)	5–40	3–15	185	Electrolytic
0.0095–0.01	0.01	Stryker	GDC-10 360 Soft SR (SFL)	4–23	2–14	185	Electrolytic
0.014–0.015	0.01	Stryker	GDC-18 3D	15–30	6–20	185	Electrolytic
0.01	0.01	Stryker	GDC-10 3D	4–30	3–10	185	Electrolytic
0.015	0.01	Stryker	GDC-18 2D (SFL)	20–30	5–20	185	Electrolytic
0.01	0.01	Stryker	GDC-10 2D (SFL)	8–30	3–10	185	Electrolytic
0.0095	0.01	Stryker	GDC-10 Soft 2D SR (SFL)	2–15	3–7	185	Electrolytic
0.0135	0.01	Stryker	GDC-18 Spft	4–15	2–6	185	Electrolytic
0.0095	0.01	Stryker	GDC-10 Soft	2–10	2–4	185	Electrolytic
0.0095	0.01	Stryker	GDC-10 Soft SR	1–8	2	185	Electrolytic
0.01	0.01	Stryker	GDC-10 Ultrasoft	1–8	2–4	175	Electrolytic
0.011	0.01	Stryker	Matrix2 Ultrasoft SR 360	4–15	2–6	185	Electrolytic
0.011	0.01	Stryker	Matrix2 Ultrasoft SR Helical	2–20	2–6	185	Electrolytic

(Continued on page 428)

A5 Endovascular Equipment

(*Continued*) Most Commonly Used Endovascular Coils in the US Market (Not All Internationally Available Coils Listed)

OD primary coil (in)	Delivery wire	Company	Specific coils	Available lengths (cm)	Available diameters (mm)	Length	Detachment mechanism
0.0115	0.01	Stryker	Matrix2 Helical Soft SR	4–8	2	185	Electrolytic
0.0115	0.01	Stryker	Matrix2 Soft SR	4–30	3–8	185	Electrolytic
0.0115	0.01	Stryker	Matrix2 360 Soft SR	4–30	3–8	185	Electrolytic
0.012	0.01	Stryker	Matrix2 Standard 2D SR	8–30	3–10	185	Electrolytic
0.012	0.01	Stryker	Matrix2 Standard 3D Omega	4–30	3–10	185	Electrolytic
0.012	0.01	Stryker	Matrix2 Standard 360 SR	8–30	3–12	185	Electrolytic
0.012	0.01	Stryker	Matrix2 360 Firm (5–14mm)	15–30	5–12	185	Electrolytic
0.0118	0.01	Stryker	Matrix2 360 Firm (16–24mm)	30–40	14–24	185	Electrolytic

A6 Test Balloon Occlusion (TBO)

Hemodynamic requirement	TBO and perfusion results
Parent artery sacrifice without bypass	No clinical exam failure during occlusion; no cerebral perfusion abnormalities
Low-flow bypass	Minimal clinical changes at end of exam; EEG or failure of hypotensive challenge; no cerebral perfusion abnormalities
High-flow bypass	Failure of all clinical exams; cerebral perfusion abnormalities

Abbreviations: TBO, trial balloon occlusion; EEG, electroencephalogram.

A7 National Institutes of Health Stroke Scale

**N I H
STROKE
SCALE**

Patient Identification. ___ ___-___ ___ ___-___ ___ ___

Pt. Date of Birth ___ ___/___ ___/___ ___

Hospital _____ (___ ___.___ ___)

Date of Exam ___ ___/___ ___/___ ___

Interval: [ ] Baseline [ ] 2 hours post treatment [ ] 24 hours post onset of symptoms ±20 minutes [ ] 7-10 days
[ ] 3 months [ ] Other _____ (___ ___)

Time: ___ ___:___ ___ [ ] am [ ] pm

Person Administering Scale _____

Administer stroke scale items in the order listed. Record performance in each category after each subscale exam. Do not go back and change scores. Follow directions provided for each exam technique. Scores should reflect what the patient does, not what the clinician thinks the patient can do. The clinician should record answers while administering the exam and work quickly. Except where indicated, the patient should not be coached (i.e., repeated requests to patient to make a special effort).

Instructions	Scale Definition	Score
1a. Level of Consciousness: The investigator must choose a response if a full evaluation is prevented by such obstacles as an endotracheal tube, language barrier, orotracheal trauma/bandages. A 3 is scored only if the patient makes no movement (other than reflexive posturing) in response to noxious stimulation.	0 = **Alert;** keenly responsive. 1 = **Not alert,** but arousable by minor stimulation to obey, answer, or respond. 2 = **Not alert;** requires repeated stimulation to attend, or is obtunded and requires strong or painful stimulation to make movements (not stereotyped). 3 = Responds only with reflex motor or autonomic effects or totally unresponsive, flaccid, and areflexic.	_____
1b. LOC Questions: The patient is asked the month and his/her age. The answer must be correct - there is no partial credit for being close. Aphasic and stuporous patients who do not comprehend the questions will score 2. Patients unable to speak because of endotracheal intubation, orotracheal trauma, severe dysarthria from any cause, language barrier, or any other problem not secondary to aphasia are given a 1. It is important that only the initial answer be graded and that the examiner not "help" the patient with verbal or non-verbal cues.	0 = **Answers** both questions correctly. 1 = **Answers** one question correctly. 2 = **Answers** neither question correctly.	_____
1c. LOC Commands: The patient is asked to open and close the eyes and then to grip and release the non-paretic hand. Substitute another one step command if the hands cannot be used. Credit is given if an unequivocal attempt is made but not completed due to weakness. If the patient does not respond to command, the task should be demonstrated to him or her (pantomime), and the result scored (i.e., follows none, one or two commands). Patients with trauma, amputation, or other physical impediments should be given suitable one-step commands. Only the first attempt is scored.	0 = **Performs** both tasks correctly. 1 = **Performs** one task correctly. 2 = **Performs** neither task correctly.	_____
2. Best Gaze: Only horizontal eye movements will be tested. Voluntary or reflexive (oculocephalic) eye movements will be scored, but caloric testing is not done. If the patient has a conjugate deviation of the eyes that can be overcome by voluntary or reflexive activity, the score will be 1. If a patient has an isolated peripheral nerve paresis (CN III, IV or VI), score a 1. Gaze is testable in all aphasic patients. Patients with ocular trauma, bandages, pre-existing blindness, or other disorder of visual acuity or fields should be tested with reflexive movements, and a choice made by the investigator. Establishing eye contact and then moving about the patient from side to side will occasionally clarify the presence of a partial gaze palsy.	0 = **Normal.** 1 = **Partial gaze palsy;** gaze is abnormal in one or both eyes, but forced deviation or total gaze paresis is not present. 2 = **Forced deviation,** or total gaze paresis not overcome by the oculocephalic maneuver.	_____

Rev 10/1/2003

National Institutes of Health Stroke Scale.

A7 National Institutes of Health Stroke Scale

N I H
STROKE
SCALE

Patient Identification. ___ ___·___ ___ ___·___ ___ ___

Pt. Date of Birth ___ ___/___ ___/___ ___

Hospital _____ (___ ___·___ ___)

Date of Exam ___ ___/___ ___/___ ___

Interval: [ ] Baseline   [ ] 2 hours post treatment   [ ] 24 hours post onset of symptoms ±20 minutes   [ ] 7-10 days   [ ] 3 months [ ] Other _____ (___ ___)

3. Visual: Visual fields (upper and lower quadrants) are tested by confrontation, using finger counting or visual threat, as appropriate. Patients may be encouraged, but if they look at the side of the moving fingers appropriately, this can be scored as normal. If there is unilateral blindness or enucleation, visual fields in the remaining eye are scored. Score 1 only if a clear-cut asymmetry, including quadrantanopia, is found. If patient is blind from any cause, score 3. Double simultaneous stimulation is performed at this point. If there is extinction, patient receives a 1, and the results are used to respond to item 11.	0 = **No visual loss.** 1 = **Partial hemianopia.** 2 = **Complete hemianopia.** 3 = **Bilateral hemianopia** (blind including cortical blindness).	____
4. Facial Palsy: Ask — or use pantomime to encourage — the patient to show teeth or raise eyebrows and close eyes. Score symmetry of grimace in response to noxious stimuli in the poorly responsive or non-comprehending patient. If facial trauma/bandages, orotracheal tube, tape or other physical barriers obscure the face, these should be removed to the extent possible.	0 = **Normal** symmetrical movements. 1 = **Minor paralysis** (flattened nasolabial fold, asymmetry on smiling). 2 = **Partial paralysis** (total or near-total paralysis of lower face). 3 = **Complete paralysis** of one or both sides (absence of facial movement in the upper and lower face).	____
5. Motor Arm: The limb is placed in the appropriate position: extend the arms (palms down) 90 degrees (if sitting) or 45 degrees (if supine). Drift is scored if the arm falls before 10 seconds. The aphasic patient is encouraged using urgency in the voice and pantomime, but not noxious stimulation. Each limb is tested in turn, beginning with the non-paretic arm. Only in the case of amputation or joint fusion at the shoulder, the examiner should record the score as untestable (UN), and clearly write the explanation for this choice.	0 = **No drift;** limb holds 90 (or 45) degrees for full 10 seconds. 1 = **Drift;** limb holds 90 (or 45) degrees, but drifts down before full 10 seconds; does not hit bed or other support. 2 = **Some effort against gravity;** limb cannot get to or maintain (if cued) 90 (or 45) degrees, drifts down to bed, but has some effort against gravity. 3 = **No effort against gravity;** limb falls. 4 = **No movement.** UN = **Amputation** or joint fusion, explain: _____ **5a. Left Arm** **5b. Right Arm**	____ ____
6. Motor Leg: The limb is placed in the appropriate position: hold the leg at 30 degrees (always tested supine). Drift is scored if the leg falls before 5 seconds. The aphasic patient is encouraged using urgency in the voice and pantomime, but not noxious stimulation. Each limb is tested in turn, beginning with the non-paretic leg. Only in the case of amputation or joint fusion at the hip, the examiner should record the score as untestable (UN), and clearly write the explanation for this choice.	0 = **No drift;** leg holds 30-degree position for full 5 seconds. 1 = **Drift;** leg falls by the end of the 5-second period but does not hit bed. 2 = **Some effort against gravity;** leg falls to bed by 5 seconds, but has some effort against gravity. 3 = **No effort against gravity;** leg falls to bed immediately. 4 = **No movement.** UN = **Amputation** or joint fusion, explain: _____ **6a. Left Leg** **6b. Right Leg**	____

Rev 10/1/2003

(Continued on page 432)

A7 National Institutes of Health Stroke Scale

(Continued from page 431)

Patient Identification. ___ ___-___ ___ ___-___ ___ ___

Pt. Date of Birth ___ ___/___ ___/___ ___

Hospital _____ (___ ___-___ ___)

Date of Exam ___ ___/___ ___/___ ___

Interval: [ ] Baseline   [ ] 2 hours post treatment   [ ] 24 hours post onset of symptoms ±20 minutes   [ ] 7-10 days   [ ] 3 months   [ ] Other _____ (___ ___ ___)

7. Limb Ataxia: This item is aimed at finding evidence of a unilateral cerebellar lesion. Test with eyes open. In case of visual defect, ensure testing is done in intact visual field. The finger-nose-finger and heel-shin tests are performed on both sides, and ataxia is scored only if present out of proportion to weakness. Ataxia is absent in the patient who cannot understand or is paralyzed. Only in the case of amputation or joint fusion, the examiner should record the score as untestable (UN), and clearly write the explanation for this choice. In case of blindness, test by having the patient touch nose from extended arm position.	0 = **Absent.** 1 = **Present in one limb.** 2 = **Present in two limbs.** UN = **Amputation** or joint fusion, explain: _____	___
8. Sensory: Sensation or grimace to pinprick when tested, or withdrawal from noxious stimulus in the obtunded or aphasic patient. Only sensory loss attributed to stroke is scored as abnormal and the examiner should test as many body areas (arms [not hands], legs, trunk, face) as needed to accurately check for hemisensory loss. A score of 2, "severe or total sensory loss," should only be given when a severe or total loss of sensation can be clearly demonstrated. Stuporous and aphasic patients will, therefore, probably score 1 or 0. The patient with brainstem stroke who has bilateral loss of sensation is scored 2. If the patient does not respond and is quadriplegic, score 2. Patients in a coma (item 1a=3) are automatically given a 2 on this item.	0 = **Normal;** no sensory loss. 1 = **Mild-to-moderate sensory loss;** patient feels pinprick is less sharp or is dull on the affected side; or there is a loss of superficial pain with pinprick, but patient is aware of being touched. 2 = **Severe to total sensory loss;** patient is not aware of being touched in the face, arm, and leg.	___
9. Best Language: A great deal of information about comprehension will be obtained during the preceding sections of the examination. For this scale item, the patient is asked to describe what is happening in the attached picture, to name the items on the attached naming sheet and to read from the attached list of sentences. Comprehension is judged from responses here, as well as to all of the commands in the preceding general neurological exam. If visual loss interferes with the tests, ask the patient to identify objects placed in the hand, repeat, and produce speech. The intubated patient should be asked to write. The patient in a coma (item 1a=3) will automatically score 3 on this item. The examiner must choose a score for the patient with stupor or limited cooperation, but a score of 3 should be used only if the patient is mute and follows no one-step commands.	0 = **No aphasia;** normal. 1 = **Mild-to-moderate aphasia;** some obvious loss of fluency or facility of comprehension, without significant limitation on ideas expressed or form of expression. Reduction of speech and/or comprehension, however, makes conversation about provided materials difficult or impossible. For example, in conversation about provided materials, examiner can identify picture or naming card content from patient's response. 2 = **Severe aphasia;** all communication is through fragmentary expression; great need for inference, questioning, and guessing by the listener. Range of information that can be exchanged is limited; listener carries burden of communication. Examiner cannot identify materials provided from patient response. 3 = **Mute, global aphasia;** no usable speech or auditory comprehension.	___
10. Dysarthria: If patient is thought to be normal, an adequate sample of speech must be obtained by asking patient to read or repeat words from the attached list. If the patient has severe aphasia, the clarity of articulation of spontaneous speech can be rated. Only if the patient is intubated or has other physical barriers to producing speech, the examiner should record the score as untestable (UN), and clearly write an explanation for this choice. Do not tell the patient why he or she is being tested.	0 = **Normal.** 1 = **Mild-to-moderate dysarthria;** patient slurs at least some words and, at worst, can be understood with some difficulty. 2 = **Severe dysarthria;** patient's speech is so slurred as to be unintelligible in the absence of or out of proportion to any dysphasia, or is mute/anarthric. UN = **Intubated** or other physical barrier, explain: _____	___

Rev 10/1/2003

N I H
STROKE
SCALE

Patient Identification. ___ ___-___ ___ ___-___ ___ ___

Pt. Date of Birth ___ ___/___ ___/___ ___

Hospital _____ (___ ___-___ ___)

Date of Exam ___ ___/___ ___/___ ___

Interval: [ ] Baseline   [ ] 2 hours post treatment   [ ] 24 hours post onset of symptoms ±20 minutes   [ ] 7-10 days   [ ] 3 months   [ ] Other _____ (___ ___ ___)

11. Extinction and Inattention (formerly Neglect): Sufficient information to identify neglect may be obtained during the prior testing. If the patient has a severe visual loss preventing visual double simultaneous stimulation, and the cutaneous stimuli are normal, the score is normal. If the patient has aphasia but does appear to attend to both sides, the score is normal. The presence of visual spatial neglect or anosognosia may also be taken as evidence of abnormality. Since the abnormality is scored only if present, the item is never untestable.	0 = **No abnormality.** 1 = **Visual, tactile, auditory, spatial, or personal inattention** or extinction to bilateral simultaneous stimulation in one of the sensory modalities. 2 = **Profound hemi-inattention or extinction to more than one modality;** does not recognize own hand or orients to only one side of space.	

A7 National Institutes of Health Stroke Scale

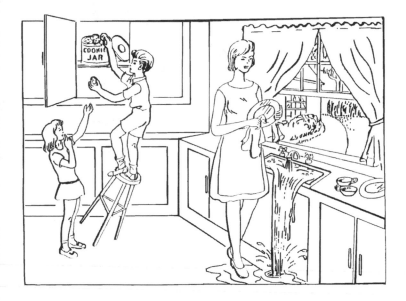

You know how.

Down to earth.

I got home from work.

Near the table in the dining
room.

They heard him speak on the
radio last night.

(Continued on page 434)

A7 National Institutes of Health Stroke Scale

(Continued from page 433)

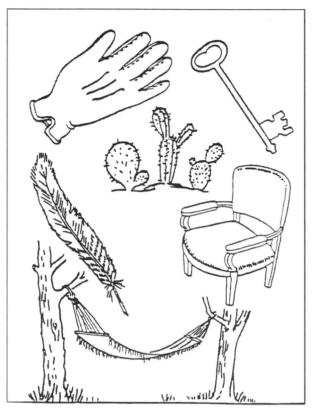

MAMA

TIP – TOP

FIFTY – FIFTY

THANKS

HUCKLEBERRY

BASEBALL PLAYER

A8 Aneurysm/AVM/dAVF Classifications

ISUIA-1: Relative Risk of Aneurysm Rupture, Based on Location (See Chapter 13)

	Annual rupture risk	
Location	**Group 1**	**Group 2**
Basilar tip	13.8	5.1
Vertebrobasilar artery	13.6	—
Posterior communicating artery	8	—

ABCVs of SAH: Recommendations for Preprocedural Preparation (See Chapter 13)

Assessment	Result	Action
Airway	Unable to protect airway, GCS£8	Intubation
Breathing	Required intubation	Mechanical ventilation (pCO_2 35–45)
Circulation	Hypertension, cardiac ischemia, arrhythmia	Normotensive (SBP 90–130), cardiac enzymes
Ventricles	Hydrocephalus	EVD at 15 cm, ICP <20 cm H_2O

Spetzler-Martin Grading Scale (See Chapter 14)

Graded feature	Points assigned
Size	
Small (<3 cm)	1
Medium (3–6 cm)	2
Large (>6 cm)	3
Eloquence of adjacent brain	
Non-eloquent	0
Eloquent	1
Pattern of venous drainage	
Superficial	0
Deep	1

A8 Aneurysm/AVM/dAVF Classification

Benefits of AVM Embolization before Microsurgery and Radiosurgery (See Chapter 14)

Microsurgery	Radiosurgery
Occludes the deep and surgically inaccessible feeding pedicles.	Decreases the size of large AVM (>3 cm) so radiosurgery can be performed.
Decreases blood flow and nidal size, resulting in less blood loss during the surgery.	Treat AVM-associated aneurysms prior to radiosurgery (radiosurgery may not be effective for the aneurysms).
Onyx or n-BCA in the feeding arteries or nidus provides a good road map during resection.	Smaller residual AVMs have higher radiosurgical cure rate.
Treat AVM-associated aneurysms prior to the surgical resection.	

Barrow Classification of Carotid-Cavernous Fistulae (See Chapter 15)

Type	Fistulous vessels	Comments
A	Carotid artery to cavernous sinus (CS)	Direct, high flow, most common
B	Dural ICA branches to CS: Meningohypophyseal trunk (66%), inferolateral trunk (30%)	Indirect, low flow
C	ECA branches to CS: internal max (67%), middle mening (59%), accessory mening (31%), ascending pharyn (24%)	Indirect, low flow
D	Both ICA and ECA branches	Indirect, most common low flow

A8 Aneurysm/AVM/dAVF Classification

Cognard DAVF Classification (See Chapter 15)

Type I: Anterograde drainage into a venous sinus
Type IIa: Retrograde drainage into a venous sinus
Type IIb: Anterograde drainage into a venous sinus and cortical veins
Type III: Drainage into cortical veins only
Type IV: Drainage into cortical veins only with venous ectasias

Cognard C, Gobin Y, Pierot L, et al. Cerebral dural arteriovenous fistulas: clinical and angiographic correlation with a revised classification of venous drainage. Radiology 1995;194:671–680

Borden DAVF Classification (See Chapter 15)

Type I: Antegrade flow into a venous sinus
Type II: Retrograde flow into a venous sinus
Type III: Retrograde into cortical veins

Borden JA, Wu JK, Shucart WA. A proposed classification for spinal and cranial dural arteriovenous fistulous malformations and implications for treatment. J Neurosurg 1995;82:166–179

A9 Clinical Stenosis Trials

Stroke Risks (See Chapter 16)

Symptomatology	Stenosis severity	Stroke risk
Asymptomatic	>60%	2% annual
Symptomatic*	50–69%	4% annual
Symptomatic*	>70%	13% in the first year after first stroke/TIA

*Symptomatic usually involves neurological changes or transient ischemic attacks (TIAs).

Recanalization and Revascularization Scores (See Chapter 16)

Score	AOL recanalization	Score	TIMI reperfusion
0	No recanalization of the primary occlusive lesion	0	No perfusion
I	Incomplete or partial recanalization of the primary occlusive lesion with no distal flow	1	Perfusion past the initial occlusion but no distal branch filling
II	Incomplete or partial recanalization of the primary occlusive lesion with any distal flow	2	Perfusion with incomplete or slow distal branch filling
III	Complete recanalization of the primary occlusive lesion with any distal flow	3	Full perfusion with filling of all distal branches, including M 3, 4

Abbreviations: AOL, arterial occlusive lesion; TIMI, thrombolysis in myocardial infarction.

A9 Clinical Stenosis Trials

TICI Reperfusion Score Terminology and Definition of TICI Reperfusion (I) and AOL Recanalization Scores (II)* (See Chapter 16)

I. Posttreatment TICI reperfusion grade
0 = No perfusion
1 = Perfusion past the initial obstruction but limited distal branch filling with little or slow distal perfusion
2A = Perfusion of less than half of the vascular distribution of the occluded artery (e.g., filling and perfusion through 1 M2 division)
2B = Perfusion of half or greater of the vascular distribution of the occluded artery (e.g., filling and perfusion through 2 M2 divisions)
3 = Full perfusion with filling of all distal branches
II. Posttreatment AOL recanalization grade
0 = No recanalization of the occlusion
1 = Incomplete or partial recanalization of the occlusion, with no distal flow
2 = Incomplete or partial recanalization of the occlusion, with any distal flow
3 = Complete recanalization of the occlusion with any distal flow

*The modified TICI reperfusion score was essentially equivalent to TIMI score applied in IMS I, with grade 2 further divided into A and B for post hoc analysis
Abbreviations: AOL, arterial occlusive lesion; TICI score, thrombolysis in cerebral infarction score.

A9 Clinical Stenosis Trials

Summary of Major Trials Comparing CEA and Medical Therapy for Carotid Stenosis (See Chapter 17)

	Purpose	Eligibility	Results	Criticism
Asymptomatic Carotid Atherosclerosis Study (ACAS)	Randomized prospective 5-year multicenter study comparing medical management to CEA for asymptomatic patients with carotid stenosis (via ultrasound and arteriogram) in 1662 patients.	Patients had at least 60% asymptomatic carotid stenosis and were randomized to aspirin only (325 mg daily) or aspirin plus CEA. Barred further participation of some surgeons who had adverse outcomes during the trial.	For the CEA group, the risk of death, any perioperative stroke or ipsilateral stroke over 5 years was half that of the aspirin-only group (5.1% in the surgery group versus 11% in the non-surgical group). There was no significant benefit of CEA in women.	(1) Absolute risk reduction with CEA was only ~1% per year. (2) The low operative risk may not be matched in "real world" practice. (3) Non-significant absolute risk reduction of disabling or fatal stroke with surgery (2.7%). (4) The trial had insufficient power for subgroup analysis compared with ACST.
Asymptomatic Carotid Surgery Trial (ACST)	A 5-year prospective, randomized trial that included 126 hospitals and randomized 3120 asymptomatic patients with carotid stenosis (by ultrasound) to either receive immediate CEA or deferral of CEA until treatment was indicated.	At least 60% unilateral or bilateral carotid stenosis without any TIA or stroke within 6 months prior to the study. Very few exclusion criteria.	Similar results to ACAS. Absolute reduction in 5 year stroke risk was 6.4% in the CEA group versus 11.8% in the deferral group. Unlike ACAS, there was a significant absolute reduction with CEA in risk of disabling or fatal stroke. Because of larger enrollment, the study had sufficient power for subgroup analysis.	(1) Medical management in the deferral group was variable. (2) The study excluded patients who had neurological symptoms or stroke for up to 6 months prior to the study; however, around 300 patients were admitted into the study who had neurological symptoms more than 6 months prior to the study onset.

Trial	Description	Patient Population	Results	Comments
North American Symptomatic Carotid Endarterectomy Trial (NASCET)	One of the original multicenter, randomized, controlled prospective trials designed to compare CEA to medical therapy for secondary stroke prevention in patients with symptomatic carotid stenosis. The trial studied 2885 patients at 106 centers. Primary outcome was fatal or nonfatal stroke ipsilateral to the stenosis for which patient was treated. Secondary outcome was all strokes and deaths.	Hemispheric or retinal TIA or nondisabling stroke within 120 days prior to enrollment. Patients were divided into two categories based on severity of carotid stenosis: 30–69% and 70–99%. 659 patients were randomized in the high-grade category, and 858 patients were in the 50–69% category. The remainder were in the <50% stenosis group.	The 2-year ipsilateral stroke risk was significantly lower in the CEA group compared with medical group (9% in the surgery group versus 26% in the medical group, p < 0.001). The moderate stenosis group achieved a statistically significant 5-year stroke risk reduction with CEA (15.7% versus 22.2% in medical group). CEA was clearly beneficial for symptomatic high-grade (≥70%) stenosis. CEA was beneficial in carefully selected patients with symptomatic moderate stenosis. There was no benefit with CEA for stenosis <50%.	(1) There were no standardized guidelines for the medical management group. (2) Patients ≥80 years and medical comorbidities were excluded; study population not reflective of entire population at risk of stroke from carotid stenosis. (3) The low surgical complication rates in the trial are not reflective of "real world" practice. (4) Medical management has improved since this trial and the results in the medical arm may no longer be applicable.
European Carotid Surgery Trial (ECST)	ECST was a randomized, multicenter, prospective trial that compared CEA to medical management in 3024 patients with symptomatic carotid stenosis. The trial was conducted at 100 centers in 14 countries.	Similar to NASCET. Patients with any degree of carotid stenosis were eligible for ECST. 501 patients had stenosis ≥70% and 684 patients were in the moderate stenosis category. Method of measurement of stenosis was different than in NASCET. The ECST method resulted in higher degrees of stenosis compared with NASCET. Very few exclusion criteria.	Results were similar to NASCET with regard to high-grade (≥70%) stenosis. Two-year risk of ipsilateral stroke was 7% for CEA compared with 19.9% for medical therapy. ECST showed negative benefit with CEA in patients with moderate stenosis (50–69%). There was no benefit with CEA for stenosis <50%.	(1) When stenosis was remeasured using NASCET criteria, CEA reduced 5-year stroke and death risk by 5.7%, a modest reduction similar to the results seen in NASCET. (2) ECST defined follow-up stroke as a deficit persisting more than 7 days and did not include retinal TIAs. (3) Medical management has improved since this trial was conducted.

Abbreviations: CEA, carotid endarterectomy; TIA, transient ischemic attack.

A9 Clinical Stenosis Trials

Major CAS Trials (See Chapter 17)

	Purpose	Eligibility	Results	Criticism
Stent-Protected Angioplasty versus Carotid Endarterectomy Trial (SPACE)	Prospective, randomized trial, designed to establish non-inferiority of CAS compared with CEA for symptomatic extracranial carotid stenosis in low surgical risk patients.	Inclusion criteria—patients from 35 different centers throughout Europe with symptomatic severe carotid stenosis (≥70% on duplex ultrasound, ≥50% by NASCET criteria, ≥70% by ECST criteria). 1183 patients were randomized within 6 months of a TIA or stroke to receive either CAS or CEA. High-risk surgical candidates were excluded from the study. Primary endpoint was stroke or death, with follow-up at 30 days and at 2 years following treatment.	The 30-day post-treatment results failed to support non-inferiority of CAS compared with CEA. The rate of ipsilateral stroke or death was 6.34% in the CEA group and 6.84% in the CAS group, which was not statistically significant. The 2-year post-treatment results showed that the rates of ipsilateral stroke between the two modalities are similar (8.8% in the CEA group and 9.5% in the CAS group, p = 0.62).	(1) Enrollment was halted well short of intended enrollment of 1900 patients. Interim analysis suggested that 2500 patients would be needed to demonstrate significance. The trial did not have funds to meet this goal and was terminated early. (2) Use of embolic protection devices was not required and was used in 27% of the CAS cases.

Trial	Design	Patients	Results	Comments
Endarterectomy versus Angioplasty in Patients with Symptomatic Severe Carotid Stenosis (EVA-3S)	Prospective, randomized, assessor-blinded trial designed to compare CEA versus CAS in patients with symptomatic extracranial carotid stenosis.	527 patients with symptomatic severe carotid artery stenosis ($\geq$60% on angiography or duplex ultrasound and MRA) from 30 different centers in France were randomized within 4 months of stroke. Primary endpoint was stroke or death within 30 days following treatment. The trial was stopped prematurely after it was estimated that at least 4000 patients would have to be enrolled to test the non-inferiority of carotid stenting. As in the SPACE trial, high-risk surgical candidates were excluded from this trial.	30-day rate of death or any stroke was 3.9% in the CEA group versus 9.6% in the CAS group (significant). 6-month rate of death or stroke was 6.1% for CEA and 11.7% for CAS. 30-day rate of disabling stroke was 1.3% for CEA and 3.4% for CAS (not significant).	(1) The inexperience of the operators performing CAS in this trial has been cited as one factor for the high complication rate for CAS. The complication rate for CAS was much higher than described in previously published papers. (2) Embolic protection devices were recommended after half the trial duration was completed. (3) Dual antiplatelet therapy was used in fewer than 50% of the CAS patients. (4) Rates of MI were not assessed.
Stenting and Angioplasty with Protection in Patients at High Risk for Endarterectomy (SAPPHIRE)	A prospective observational randomized trial that included North American that included 29 centers throughout North America. This study compared high-risk surgical patients who were symptomatic with $\geq$50% carotid stenosis (with duplex ultrasound or angiography) to high-risk surgical patients who were asymptomatic with $\geq$80% stenosis. Primary endpoints were major adverse events that included stroke, death, and MI (unlike EVA-3S and SPACE).	Only high-risk surgical candidates were included in the study. They defined high-risk as having one or more of the co-morbidities listed in Table 15.3.	This trial demonstrated that CAS was not inferior to CEA in high-risk patients. The 30-day rates of death, stroke, or MI were 5.8% for CAS and 12.6% for CEA. At 6 months, combined major adverse events rate was 12.2% with CAS and 20.1% in the CEA group. There was a significant decrease in cranial nerve injuries with CAS.	(1) Almost 29% of patients in both treatment groups had recurrent arterial, which favors carotid stenting. This is because repeat surgery is associated with a higher complication rate. (2) Many patients were lost to follow-up at 3 years. (3) The inclusion of MI as an endpoint was not part of the NASCET or ECST trials.

(Continued on page 444)

A9 Clinical Stenosis Trials

(Continued) Major CAS Trials

	Purpose	Eligibility	Results	Criticism
Carotid Revascularization Endarterectomy versus Stenting Trial (CREST) (REF)	CREST was a randomized, multicenter, prospective trial that compared CEA to CAS in 2502 patients with symptomatic and asymptomatic carotid stenosis. The trial was conducted at 117 centers in the US and Canada.	Symptomatic: transient ischemic attack (TIA), amaurosis fugax (AF), or non-disabling stroke within the past 180 days, and who have an ipsilateral carotid stenosis ≥50% by angiography or ≥70% by ultrasound or ≥70% by CTA or MRA. Asymptomatic subjects: Patients who have carotid stenosis ≥60% by angiography or ≥70% by ultrasound or ≥80% by CTA or MRA are eligible for this study. (Subjects with symptoms beyond 180 days are considered asymptomatic.) Outcome: Mortality, stroke, or myocardial infarction at 30 days postoperatively; ipsilateral stroke at 30 days postoperatively.	For 2502 patients (median follow-up 2.5 years), there was no significant difference in the estimated 4-year rates of the primary endpoint between the CAS group and the CEA group (7.2% and 6.8%, respectively; hazard ratio with CAS, 1.11; 95% confidence interval, 0.81 to 1.51; $p = 0.51$). There was no differential treatment effect with regard to the primary endpoint according to symptomatic status ($p = 0.84$) or sex ($p = 0.34$). The 4-year rate of stroke or death was 6.4% with CAS and 4.7% with CEA (hazard ratio, 1.50; $p = 0.03$); the rates among symptomatic patients were 8.0 and 6.4% (hazard ratio, 1.37; $p = 0.14$), and the rates among asymptomatic patients were 4.5% and 2.7% (hazard ratio, 1.86; $p = 0.07$), respectively. Periprocedural rates of individual components of the endpoints differed between the CAS group and the CEA group: for death (0.7% versus 0.3%, $p = 0.18$), for stroke (4.1% versus 2.3%, $p = 0.01$), and for myocardial infarction (1.1% versus 2.3%, $p = 0.03$). After this period, the incidences of ipsilateral stroke with CAS and with CEA were similarly low (2.0% and 2.4%, respectively; $p = 0.85$).	N/A

A9 Clinical Stenosis Trials

Stent Selection in Carotid Artery Disease (See Chapter 17)

Stent design	Pro	Con
Closed cell	Can completely cover and stabilize plaque decreasing distal embolization risk	Cannot cross into the CCA if plaque extends into CCA; cannot be used in the ECA; difficulty with navigation in tortuous anatomy
Open small cell	Improved navigation in tortuous anatomy; can be used in CCA-ICA plaques	Should not be used in CCA-ECA due to small perforating vessels off ECA; some reports of "watermelon seeding"; can erode into plaque, causing distal embolization
Open large cell	Improved navigation in tortuous anatomy; can be used in CCA-ICA and CCA-ECA plaques	Erosion into plaque can cause distal embolization

Abbreviations: CCA, common carotid artery; ECA, external carotid artery; ICA, internal carotid artery.

Appendix B

B1 Vascular Access

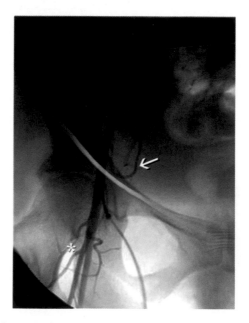

Anatomy of the femoral artery. Common femoral artery angiogram, showing the bifurcation (*asterisk*) into the profundus and superficialis branches distal to the femoral head and cannulation over the upper, inner quadrant of the femoral head to prevent vascular complications. Note the location of the inferior epigastric artery (*arrow*) just above the inguinal ligament. (See Chapter 6, Vascular Access and Arteriotomy Closures.)

B2 Basic Catheterization (See Chapter 8, Endovascular Techniques)

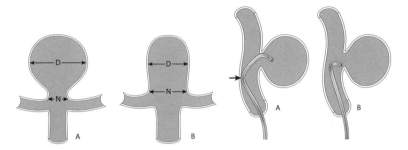

Aspect Ratio. The length of the dome (D) divided by the length of the neck (N) is the dome:neck ratio. **(A)** A favorable dome:neck ratio is 2 or greater. **(B)** A smaller dome:neck ratio may require adjunctive techniques like balloon or stent assistance for best results.

Aneurysm catheterization. The double-bend "headhunter" shape **(A)** will allow the body of the catheter to lean against the back wall of the parent (*arrow*) providing more support than a simple curve **(B)**.

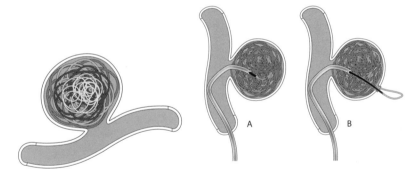

Framing coils. Framing coils can be used to fill an aneurysm. The first coil (lightest gray) should be the same size as the dome of the aneurysm. Progressively smaller framing coils can then be deployed inside it until the aneurysm is filled. This has been referred to as the "Russian doll" technique.

Detaching coils. **(A)** Ideally the pusher should extend just past the tip of the catheter during detachment. This is particularly important on the last coil as deploying the coil inside the microcatheter will often leave a "tail" of coil in the parent vessel when the microcatheter is removed. **(B)** If the stiff detachment zone of the coil is deployed too far into the aneurysm, however, it may perforate the aneurysm.

B3 Coil Embolization

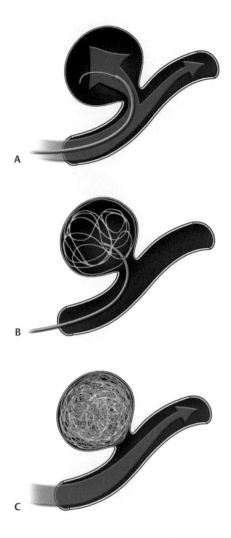

Steps in coil embolization of an intracranial aneurysm. **(A)** Catheterization of aneurysm sac. **(B)** Deployment of the coil into the aneurysm sac. **(C)** Complete coil embolization and removal of microcatheter. (See Chapters 8, 13.)

B4 Stent Placement

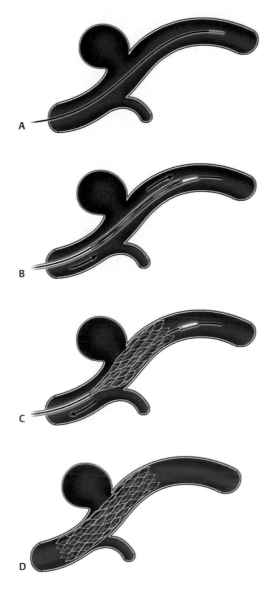

Steps in placement of vascular reconstruction device (stent). **(A)** Placement of microwire beyond lesion. **(B)** Navigate stent across lesion. **(C)** Slowly unsheath/deploy stent. **(D)** Complete deployment and remove microwire or delivery system. (See Chapter 8.)

B5 Stent-Coil Aneurysm Embolization

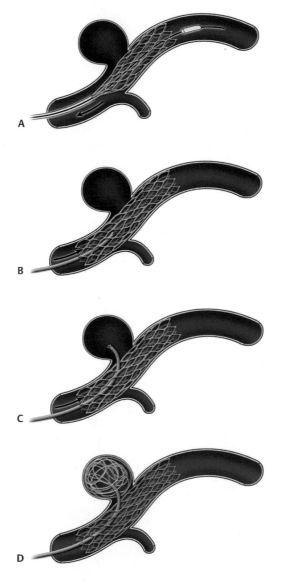

Steps in placement of vascular reconstruction device (stent) and coil embolization of intracranial aneurysm. **(A)** Stent deployment. **(B)** Navigation of microcatheter inside stent. **(C)** Catheterization of aneurysm through stent tines. **(D)** Deployment of coils into aneurysm through stent. (See Chapters 8, 13.)

B6 Liquid/Particle Embolization of AVM

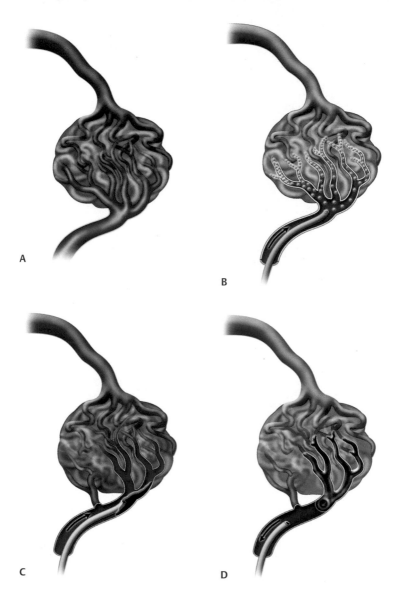

AVMs **(A)** can be embolized with both particles, e.g., PVA **(B)** and liquid embolics, e.g., Onyx **(C,D)**. Onyx requires that a plug **(C)** be slowly built up. Once the vessel is occluded, the microcatheter should be carefully removed **(D)**. (See Chapter 14.)

B7 Balloon Angioplasty

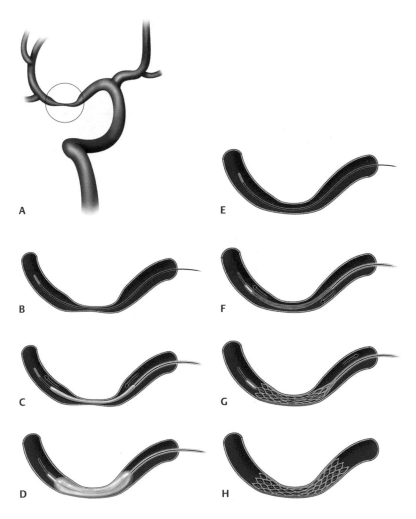

A

B

C

D

E

F

G

H

Balloon angioplasty and stent placement. **(A–D)** Navigation of angioplasty balloon across stenotic lesion and inflation of balloon. **(E–H)** Placement of stent across stenotic lesion. (See Chapter 18.)

B8 Mechanical Thrombolysis

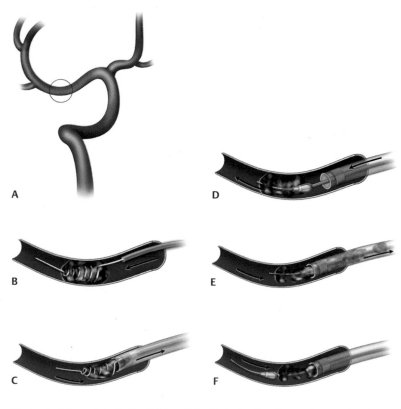

Mechanical thrombolysis. **(A–C)** Use of MERCI device. **(D–F)** Use of Penumbra device. (See Chapter 16.)

Index

A treasure trove of patient education pictorials from *Handbook of Neuroendovascular Surgery* online at MediaCenter.thieme.com!

Appendix B available online: Ready for downloading to your multimedia device, this collection of beautiful, full-color pictorials covering Vascular Access, Basic Catheterization, and Coil Embolization, to name a few, can be used for teaching and patient education. These professional diagrams will come in handy time and time again not only in working with trainees but also in clinic appointments and hospital visits with your patients.

System requirements:

	WINDOWS	MAC	TABLET
Recommended Browser(s)**	Microsoft Internet Explorer 8.0 or later, Firefox 3.x	Firefox 3.x, Safari 4.x	HTML5 mobile browser. iPad — Safari. Opera Mobile — Tablet PCs preferred.
	** all browsers should have JavaScript enabled		
Flash Player Plug-in	Flash Player 9 or Higher* *Mac users: ATI Rage 128 GPU does not support full-screen mode with hardware scaling		Tablet PCs with Android OS support Flash 10.1
Minimum Hardware Configurations	Intel® Pentium® II 450 MHz, AMD Athlon™ 600 MHz or faster processor (or equivalent) 512 MB of RAM	PowerPC® G3 500 MHz or faster processor Intel Core™ Duo 1.33 GHz or faster processor 512MB of RAM	Minimum CPU powered at 800MHz 256MB DDR2 of RAM
Recommended for optimal usage experience	Monitor resolutions: • Normal (4:3) 1024×768 or Higher • Widescreen (16:9) 1280×720 or Higher • Widescreen (16:10) 1440×900 or Higher DSL/Cable internet connection at a minimum speed of 384.0 Kbps or faster WiFi 802.11 b/g preferred.		7-inch and 10-inch tablets on maximum resolution. WiFi connection is required.